# Radiation Therapy Treatment Effects

An Evidence-Based Guide to Managing Toxicity

Editor

**Bridget F. Koontz, MD**
*Associate Professor of Radiation Oncology*
*Duke University School of Medicine*
*Durham, North Carolina*

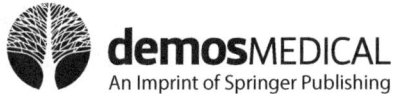

Visit our website at www.demosmedical.com

*ISBN:* 9780826181138
*ebook ISBN:* 9780826181145

*Acquisitions Editor:* David D'Addona
*Compositor:* Exeter Premedia Services Private Ltd.

Copyright © 2018 Springer Publishing Company.
Demos Medical Publishing is an imprint of Springer Publishing Company, LLC.

All rights reserved. This book is protected by copyright. No part of it may be reproduced, stored in a retrieval system, or transmitted in any form or by any means, electronic, mechanical, photocopying, recording, or otherwise, without the prior written permission of the publisher.

Medicine is an ever-changing science. Research and clinical experience are continually expanding our knowledge, in particular our understanding of proper treatment and drug therapy. The authors, editors, and publisher have made every effort to ensure that all information in this book is in accordance with the state of knowledge at the time of production of the book. Nevertheless, the authors, editors, and publisher are not responsible for errors or omissions or for any consequences from application of the information in this book and make no warranty, expressed or implied, with respect to the contents of the publication. Every reader should examine carefully the package inserts accompanying each drug and should carefully check whether the dosage schedules mentioned therein or the contraindications stated by the manufacturer differ from the statements made in this book. Such examination is particularly important with drugs that are either rarely used or have been newly released on the market.

**Library of Congress Cataloging-in-Publication Data**

Names: Koontz, Bridget F., editor.
Title: Radiation therapy treatment effects: an evidence-based guide to managing toxicity / editor, Bridget F. Koontz.
Description: New York: Demos, [2018] | Includes bibliographical references and index.
Identifiers: LCCN 2017017568 | ISBN 9780826181138 | ISBN 9780826181145 (e-book)
Subjects: | MESH: Neoplasms—radiotherapy | Radiation Effects | Radiation Protection—methods | Radiation Injuries—prevention & control | Evidence-Based Medicine
Classification: LCC RC271.R3 | NLM QZ 269 | DDC 616.99/40642—dc23
LC record available at https://lccn.loc.gov/2017017568

---

Contact us to receive discount rates on bulk purchases.
We can also customize our books to meet your needs.
For more information please contact: sales@springerpub.com

---

Printed in the United States of America by McNaughton & Gunn.
19 20 21 22 23 / 7 6 5 4 3

*For my colleagues, my patients, and my children—from whom
I learn every day.*

# Contents

*Contributors  ix*
*Preface  xiii*

1. Radiation Therapy Effects on the Central Nervous System  1
   *Christina K. Cramer, Michael D. Chan, and John P. Kirkpatrick*

2. Radiation Therapy Effects in Head and Neck Cancer  19
   *Thomas J. Galloway and Sue S. Yom*

3. Radiation Therapy Effects on the Thorax  59
   *Orit Kaidar-Person, Timothy M. Zagar, and Lawrence B. Marks*

4. Radiation Therapy Effects in Breast Cancer  79
   *D. Hunter Boggs and Jennifer De Los Santos*

5. Radiation Therapy Effects on the Abdomen  101
   *John Cuaron and Abraham Wu*

6. Radiation Therapy Effects on the Pelvis  117
   *Elizabeth B. Jeans and Peter J. Rossi*

7. Radiation Therapy Effects on Skin and Extremities  167
   *Adam A. Garsa and Alexander R. Gottschalk*

8. Radiation Toxicity Management in Children  173
   *Clayton B. Hess and Torunn I. Yock*

9. Systemic Effects of Radiation Therapy  197
   *Monica Krishnan and Ron Shiloh*

10. Radioprotection for Radiation Therapy  211
    *Noah S. Kalman, Sherry Zhao, Mitchell S. Anscher, and Alfredo I. Urdaneta*

11. Risk and Prevention of Radiation-Induced Cancers  277
    *Sophia C. Kamran and Akila N. Viswanathan*

12. Cancer Survivorship: Approaches and Challenges  295
    *Sophia K. Smith*

13. Maximizing the Health and Wellness of Cancer Survivors Through Healthy Lifestyle Behaviors     305
    Denise Spector

*Index     317*

# Contributors

**Mitchell S. Anscher, MD**   Professor Emeritus, Department of Radiation Oncology, Virginia Commonwealth University Medical Center, Richmond, Virginia; Professor, Department of Radiation Oncology, University of Texas MD Anderson Cancer Center, Houston, Texas

**D. Hunter Boggs, MD**   Assistant Professor, Department of Radiation Oncology, University of Alabama at Birmingham, Birmingham, Alabama

**Michael D. Chan, MD**   Associate Professor, Department of Radiation Oncology, Wake Forest Baptist Medical Center, Winston-Salem, North Carolina

**Christina K. Cramer, MD**   Assistant Professor, Department of Radiation Oncology, Wake Forest Baptist Medical Center, Winston-Salem, North Carolina

**John Cuaron, MD**   Radiation Oncologist, Memorial Sloan Kettering Cancer Center, New York, New York

**Jennifer De Los Santos, MD**   Professor, Department of Radiation Oncology, University of Alabama at Birmingham, Birmingham, Alabama

**Thomas J. Galloway, MD**   Assistant Professor, Department of Radiation Oncology, Chief, Division of Head and Neck Radiation Oncology, Medical Director, Clinical Research, Fox Chase Cancer Center, Temple University Health System, Philadelphia, Pennsylvania

**Adam A. Garsa, MD**   Assistant Professor, Department of Radiation Oncology, University of Southern California, Los Angeles, California

**Alexander R. Gottschalk, MD, PhD**   Professor, Department of Radiation Oncology, University of California, San Francisco, California

**Clayton B. Hess, MD**   Pediatric Proton Therapy Clinical and Research Fellow, Pediatric Radiation Oncology, Department of Radiation Oncology, Massachusetts General Hospital, Francis H. Burr Proton Therapy Center, Harvard University, Boston, Massachusetts

**Elizabeth B. Jeans, MD**   Resident Physician, Department of Radiation Oncology, Mayo Clinic, Rochester, Minnesota

**Orit Kaidar-Person, MD**   Clinical Fellow, Department of Radiation Oncology, University of North Carolina, Chapel Hill, North Carolina

**Noah S. Kalman, MD, MBA**   Resident Physician, Department of Radiation Oncology, Virginia Commonwealth University Medical Center, Richmond, Virginia

**Sophia C. Kamran, MD**   Resident Physician, Department of Radiation Oncology, Harvard Radiation Oncology Program, Boston, Massachusetts

**John P. Kirkpatrick, MD, PhD**   Associate Professor and Clinical Director, Departments of Radiation Oncology and Neurosurgery, Duke University Medical Center, Durham, North Carolina

**Monica Krishnan, MD**   Clinical Assistant Professor, Department of Radiation Oncology, Brigham and Women's/Dana-Farber Cancer Center, Boston, Massachusetts

**Lawrence B. Marks, MD**   Professor and Chairman, Department of Radiation Oncology, University of North Carolina, Chapel Hill, North Carolina

**Peter J. Rossi, MD**   James C. Kennedy Chair in Prostate Cancer, Associate Professor and Medical Director, Department of Radiation Oncology, Winship Cancer Institute at Emory Saint Joseph's Hospital, Atlanta, Georgia

**Ron Shiloh, MD**   Clinical Instructor, Department of Radiation Oncology, Brigham and Women's/Dana-Farber Cancer Center, Boston, Massachusetts

**Sophia K. Smith, PhD, MSW**   Associate Professor, Duke University School of Nursing, Durham, North Carolina

**Denise Spector, PhD, MPH, MSN, ANP-BC**   Clinical Director, Duke Cancer Survivorship Program, Duke Cancer Institute; Assistant Consulting Professor, Duke University School of Nursing, Durham, North Carolina

**Alfredo I. Urdaneta, MD**   Assistant Professor, Department of Radiation Oncology, Virginia Commonwealth University Medical Center, Richmond, Virginia

**Akila N. Viswanathan, MD, MPH**   Professor and Executive Vice Chair, Department of Radiation Oncology and Molecular Radiation Sciences, Johns Hopkins Medicine, Baltimore, Maryland

**Abraham Wu, MD**   Assistant Attending Radiation Oncologist, Memorial Sloan Kettering Cancer Center, New York, New York

**Torunn I. Yock, MD, MCH**   Associate Professor, Harvard Medical School; Director, Pediatric Radiation Oncology, Quality Improvement Chair, Department of Radiation Oncology, Massachusetts General Hospital, Francis H. Burr Proton Therapy Center, Harvard University, Boston, Massachusetts

**Sue S. Yom, MD, PhD, MAS**   Associate Professor, Department of Radiation Oncology, University of California, San Francisco, California

**Timothy M. Zagar, MD**   Assistant Professor, Departments of Neurosurgery and Radiation Oncology, Director, CyberKnife Radiosurgery Program, University of North Carolina, Chapel Hill, North Carolina

**Sherry Zhao, MD**   Resident Physician, Department of Radiation Oncology, Virginia Commonwealth University Medical Center, Richmond, Virginia

# Preface

Cancer affects 1.7 million new lives each year. Over 60% of those diagnosed with cancer will undergo radiation therapy (RT) at some point in their disease process—whether for curative intent or for palliation. Radiation is highly effective as a tumoricidal agent, and for some cancers it is the primary definitive therapy (consider anal and prostate cancers as examples). In fact, some would argue that RT was instrumental in a paradigm shift in the approach to cancer treatment that cure was possible. Radiation was applied to Hodgkin lymphoma as early as 1901 (only six years after the discovery of x-rays) resulting in dramatic responses. However, Hodgkin lymphoma is also an exemplar for the other side of radiation—the late effects which can be devastating for cancer survivors.

Radiation oncologists today take great care both to accurately target tumor and minimize normal tissue irradiation. Our technology aids in this effort. However, no tumor is treated ex vivo; thus, in all cases there is some normal tissue affected. Thus the effects of radiation persist in cancer survivors.

This handbook provides a concise summary of the presentation and management of both acute and late radiation side effects. The ability to effectively manage the acute effects on patients undergoing treatment is critical for radiation oncology professionals as well as other medical fields, as patients are nearly always treated in multidisciplinary fashion. Fortunately, most late-appearing effects from radiation are uncommon, and therein lies an important aspect of this handbook: a collection of the experience of disease site experts who see and treat both the acute and late effects with frequency. Their summarized evidence-based practice provides guidance to anyone whose practice touches cancer patients and survivors. This handbook would not be possible without the time and effort put forth by the esteemed authors; we hope you find it a useful and practical guide to your practice, whether it be daily management or as a reference for the occasional patient with a history of radiation.

*Bridget F. Koontz, MD*

# 1
# Radiation Therapy Effects on the Central Nervous System

*Christina K. Cramer, Michael D. Chan, and John P. Kirkpatrick*

## OVERVIEW
- Radiation injury to the central nervous system (CNS) can dramatically impact daily functioning and quality of life (QOL).
- The brain and spinal cord are late-responding tissues and care must be taken to avoid delayed and permanent radiation toxicity.
- Brain tissue can tolerate high doses when given to small volumes (except for a few critical structures), but low doses to large volume causes late effects.
- Spinal cord tolerance is driven by maximum dose because of its lack of redundancy and long axonal tracts.

Understanding the consequences of radiation on any normal tissue is essential for the delivery of safe therapeutic radiation, but it is especially critical for the nervous system because severe and permanent radiation injury can dramatically impact QOL and daily functioning. Ambulation, sensory processing, language, and cognition are all dependent on the integrity of the CNS and are processes highly prioritized by cancer patients (1–3). The CNS consists of the brain and the spinal cord. The cranial nerves and 31 spinal nerves are considered part of the peripheral nervous system, except for cranial nerve II (optic nerve).

Both the brain and the spinal cord are considered late-reacting tissues with a low alpha/beta ratio given the limited cellular regeneration in the adult nervous system. While the redundant circuitry and plasticity of the brain allows for some adaptation in the face of disruption by tumor, surgery, or radiation, the organization of the spinal cord with less redundancy and long fiber tracts means an extreme injury at one level of the spinal cord can prevent the transmission of neural impulses beyond that point. In considering the effect of dose volume parameters on the risk of radiation-associated dysfunction, traditional dogma has described the brain as an organ comprising functional subunits organized as a parallel circuit because there is a large effect of volume on dose tolerance. Thus, small volumes of brain tissue can receive high doses with little change in function (depending on the location within the brain), while treating the whole brain to even quite low doses can have a major negative impact. Conversely, the spinal cord is described as a series circuit where there is a more pronounced volume effect; maximum dose is most relevant to predicting normal tissue injury, and strict adherence to spinal cord dose constraints are recommended. Although describing the brain and spinal cord as parallel and series circuits guides general principles of radiation treatment design, in reality, this is an oversimplification. Small, eloquent regions of the brain are functionally serial subunits where severe injury of a single functional subunit can have devastating consequences. Conversely, a small, localized injury to spinal cord gray matter (as opposed to the ascending or descending tracts) may be more analogous to injury of a parallel organ.

The two most important clinical references for tissue tolerances to radiation are the Emami publication (4) and Quantitative Analyses of Normal Tissue Effects in the Clinic (QUANTEC) (5). Both are a valuable resource when considering dose-tolerance levels for the nervous system, but clinical judgment must be exercised in applying these findings. While Emami used expert consensus in the pre-3D planning era to develop tables specifying the tolerated dose for a 5% rate of radionecrosis at 5 years (TD5/5) and 50% risk of injury at 5 years (TD50/5) for 26 normal tissues for specific endpoints, the QUANTEC report provides tables that specify doses/volume constraints for tissues and endpoints supported by published data.

## BRAIN

- Acute radiation injury is driven by demyelination and edema.
- Late effects include neuronal loss and white matter changes.
- Radiation fatigue is common after brain radiation therapy (RT) and is likely due to transient demyelination. Radiation fatigue peaks 4 to 8 weeks after treatment and typically recovers from weeks 8 to 12. Somnolence syndrome consisting of fatigue, lethargy, clumsiness, and cognitive decline is a severe form of this side effect.
- Cognitive decline after whole brain RT is common and bothersome late effect.
- Radiation increases the risk for stroke and secondary brain tumors in long-term survivors.
- Radiation necrosis can be symptomatic depending on the location and volume. Treatment initially is with steroids but in severe cases or when there is concern for tumor progression can escalate to resection, resection with laser interstitial thermal therapy (LITT), anti-angiogenic therapy with bevacizumab or hyperbaric oxygen.
- Both fractionated external beam treatment and stereotactic radiosurgery (SRS) can result in transient edema and inflammation, which can be difficult to distinguish from tumor progression.

### Whole-Organ and Non–Site-Specific Effects

*Cerebrovascular Syndrome*

Nuclear disasters, such as the atomic bomb explosions in Hiroshima and Nagasaki, reveal that a single, total body exposure to a high dose of ionizing radiation (10 Gy or more) is acutely lethal. *Cerebrovascular syndrome* occurs within hours to days of such an exposure. Vascular injury mediates extreme cerebral edema causing headache, nausea, seizures, herniation, and ultimately death. Supportive care with steroids and antiepileptics is recommended. In contrast, fractionated whole-brain radiation treatment to doses of 30 Gy for brain metastases is well tolerated in the short term but acutely produces fatigue and alopecia. Late effects of fractionated whole-brain RT include white matter changes on imaging, poorer attention span, and short-term recall.

## *Radiation-Induced White Matter Changes and Radiation-Induced Cognitive Decline*

Despite the tremendous benefit of therapeutic brain irradiation in many situations, there are drawbacks—particularly, the adverse impact on cognitive functioning. Studying radiation-induced cognitive decline (RICD) and identifying risk-reduction strategies has proved to be incredibly challenging. These challenges include acquiring an accurate pretreatment baseline, patient participation in neurocognitive testing, attrition due to disease progression, confounding medications including steroids, antiepileptic medications, and chemotherapeutics, and confounding comorbid conditions including depression/anxiety. In pediatric patients, whole-brain radiation therapy (WBRT) to 24 Gy is associated with significant IQ decline over time in a dose-dependent manner (6–8). Younger age at time of irradiation, female gender, NF-1 mutant positive status, use of intrathecal methotrexate, and volume of brain irradiated are all factors associated with greater RICD. In adults, the picture is much less clear; in 2010, when QUANTEC was published, the data for RICD in adults was considered weak with some studies showing a decline in scores on objective neurocognitive tests compared to preradiation baseline scores and some studies showing no difference.

In general, adult studies use less comprehensive cognitive batteries and follow-up is shorter. In addition, tumor progression can cause neurocognitive decline as well, so WBRT may be partially protective of neurocognitive function in patients with a high tumor burden (9). However, WBRT likely contributes to subtle/early or profound/late neurocognitive decline in verbal learning and memory in longer-term survivors (10–13).

Since 2010, additional data from the European Organisation for Research and Treatment of Cancer (EORTC) 22952-26001 and Alliance N0574 trials both showed no survival advantage to the addition of WBRT to SRS for a limited number of brain metastases and lower neurocognitive functioning (NCF) scores and QOL scores in patients receiving WBRT (14–16). Although NCF measurements were still challenged in these trials by the confounding factors previously discussed, the data were convincing enough that American Society for Radiation Oncology's (ASTRO) 2014 Choosing Wisely campaign recommended that WBRT should not be routinely given for a limited number of metastases with a preference for radiosurgery alone (reserving WBRT for salvage). Notably, RICD is also a late effect seen in an estimated 30% of glioma patients treated with partial-brain irradiation (17). Elderly patients with primary CNS lymphoma seem to be particularly vulnerable to more severe cases of RICD and for this reason, upfront WBRT is generally deferred for patients over 60 years who are eligible for high-dose methotrexate (18,19). When WBRT is required, then lower total doses (23.4 Gy at 1.8 Gy daily [20] rather than 40–45 Gy at 2–1.8 Gy daily) are preferred for patients over 60 years.

Radiation-induced white matter changes have been documented as a late effect of RT since the 1980s and early 1990s, and is classically described as increased T1 and T2 signal in white matter tracts within radiation ports, and particularly in the periventricular regions (21–24). Correlating imaging changes with neurocognitive function after radiation, however, has proven challenging often because the most affected white matter tracts are adjacent to a tumor which itself alters white matter microstructure. Yet, despite knowing that posttreatment white matter changes are common, evidence of how to interpret this information relative to a patient's clinical functioning is sparse. One recent large cohort study from the Netherlands has shown that cognitive performance does in fact correlate with white matter microstructure (25). Interpreting the significance of white matter changes in relation to cognitive changes is an area of great interest for many neuroradiologists, neurooncologists, and radiation oncologists, and is a field that will likely develop rapidly in the next decade.

A variety of mitigating medications including memantine, donepezil, methylphenidate, gingko biloba, methylphenidate, and armodafinil have been tested with varying degrees of success (26–31). Currently, management of cognitive decline is highly variable between institutions and is patient specific. Neurocognitive rehabilitation and a trial of donepezil for persistent deficits is a more common strategy. For cognitive deficits suspected to be fatigue related, a trial of methylphenidate or armodafinil may be appropriate.

## *Somnolence Syndrome*

The subacute constellation of fatigue, lethargy, clumsiness, and cognitive decline is termed *somnolence syndrome*. Radiation-related fatigue for patients receiving treatment to the brain is common. The reported incidence varies widely and is confounded by an existing high rate of reported fatigue postsurgery and preradiation for patients with primary brain tumors (3). The etiology is believed to be related to a transient demyelination in response to radiation. In patients receiving 6 weeks of radiation for primary brain tumors, patient-reported scores of fatigue begin to increase roughly halfway through the treatment and peak at the end of treatment, staying elevated for roughly 2 weeks posttreatment before beginning to improve. QOL scores nadir roughly at 6 weeks after treatment (32). The Littman somnolence syndrome scale is the most widely utilized grading system for fatigue (see Table 1.1). Managing treatment-related fatigue generally involves counseling patients that fatigue is expected and encouraging patients to stay physically active during and after x-ray therapy (XRT). In patients with greater baseline fatigue or very bothersome fatigue, armodafinil or methylphenidate may be helpful.

## *Stroke*

It has been long known that radiation treatment accelerates atherosclerosis and intimal thickening in small, medium, and large blood vessels thus increasing the risk of a cerebrovascular accident (CVA). It is thought that reactive oxygen species generated during treatment initiate a proinflammatory cascade ultimately leading to arterial stenosis (33). The clinical consequences of this late effect are best illustrated in long-term survivors of craniopharyngioma, where high doses of radiation are delivered to the circle of Willis. In a large retrospective review of 123 patients treated for

Table 1.1 Non-Site-Specific Effects

| Side effect | Clinical signs and symptoms | Timing | Etiology | Management |
|---|---|---|---|---|
| Cerebrovascular syndrome | Headache, nausea, vomiting, seizures | Acute | Vascular injury leading to cerebral edema | Steroids (dexamethasone 8 mg IV 4x daily)<br>Antiepileptics<br>Antiemetics<br>Supportive care |
| Cognitive decline | Decreased short-term memory and attention | Late | Multifactorial (inflammatory, white matter damage) | Memantine (20 mg daily during radiation continuing for 6 months after as tolerated)<br>Donepezil (5–10 mg daily)<br>Cognitive rehabilitation |
| Fatigue and somnolence syndrome | Fatigue, lethargy, clumsiness, apathy, cognitive decline | Subacute | Transient demyelination | Armodafinil (150 mg daily)<br>Methylphenidate (5 mg twice a day starting dose, up to 15 mg twice a day)<br>Physical therapy |
| Posttreatment tumor edema | Headache, nausea, focal neurologic symptoms, seizures. Increased T2 or FLAIR signal around treated lesion | Subacute | Vascular disruption | Steroids (slow dexamethasone taper to as low a dose as tolerates)<br>Observation with serial imaging |

*(continued)*

**Table 1.1 Non–Site-Specific Effects** (continued)

| Side effect | Clinical signs and symptoms | Timing | Etiology | Management |
|---|---|---|---|---|
| Radiation necrosis | Headache, nausea, focal neurologic symptoms, seizures | Late | Inflammatory reaction to normal tissue injury | Steroids<br>Bevacizumab<br>LITT<br>Resection |
| Ischemic stroke | Acute focal neurologic symptoms with corresponding imaging | Late | Progressive vascular | Acute stroke management and rehabilitation<br>Consider antiplatelet therapy |

FLAIR, fluid attenuation inverse response; LITT, laser interstitial thermal therapy.

craniopharyngioma in Vancouver, British Columbia, Lo et al report an 11% rate of CVA after long-term follow-up (34). The risk is compounded by hypopituitarism in many of these patients as low growth hormone (GH) is associated with higher rates of cerebrovascular disease (CVD) (33,35). Cohort studies of Japanese atomic bomb and Chernobyl survivors show elevated risk ratios for cerebrovascular events which were dependent on total dose and exposure time. Preventative strategies include minimizing irradiation volume and appropriate management of comorbid CVA risk factors, such as hypertension.

### Secondary Malignancy

Meningiomas and gliomas are the most common secondary malignancies after RT to the brain, with radiation-induced meningioma being the most common (36). The likelihood of a radiation-induced meningioma is approximately 25% at 25 years. Risk factors for decreased latency in development of radiation-induced meningioma are young age at exposure, increased total dose, and larger volume of brain treated.

### Radiation-Induced Edema and Radionecrosis

Radiation necrosis is a late effect of radiation thought to be a consequence of direct damage to vascular endothelial cells and glial cells resulting in a local inflammatory cascade involving hypoxia-inducible factor 1-alpha (HIF1-alpha). In fact, the dead tissue in the center of a radionecrotic lesion is relatively inert and the symptoms associated with radionecrosis are the result of the hyperinflammatory conditions at the margin of the lesion and normal brain parenchyma. The classic description on MRI is a "soap bubble" or "swiss cheese" appearance, but in reality, distinguishing radiation necrosis from tumor progression is extremely challenging. On diffusion mapping, radiation necrosis tends to exhibit increased diffusion while tumor progression is associated with diffusion restriction (37). Magnetic resonance (MR) perfusion can also be used and in general, increased regional cerebral blood volume (rCBV) is associated with tumor recurrence (38). Often, none of these techniques demonstrate sufficient specificity and sensitivity to make the diagnosis in and of themselves. Surgical resection or biopsy remains the gold standard. Radiographic stabilization with conservative treatment allows a clinician to conclude that the prior changes were necrosis rather than progression, but this is a retrospective diagnosis.

Radiation necrosis is virtually never seen in patients treated solely with fractionated whole-brain radiation at the doses commonly used now in clinical practice. For partial-brain irradiation, a dose-toxicity relationship is evident as well. Unlike whole-brain radiation, partial-brain irradiation usually employs higher doses (between 45 and 60 Gy) for primary brain tumors rather than secondary metastatic disease. Radiation necrosis in this setting is possible although still rare.

The Emami publication (4,5) predates the 3D planning era but estimated a TD5/5 of 45 Gy to the whole brain and a TD5/5 of 60 Gy to one-third of the brain. A dose of 60 Gy to the whole brain was estimated to result in a 50% risk of necrosis within 5 years (TD 50/5). The QUANTEC report concluded that this estimate was overly conservative, instead estimating that an EQD2 of 72 Gy in 2-Gy fractions results in a 5% risk of radiation necrosis. A dose of 90 Gy in 2-Gy fractions has been predicted to yield a 10% risk of necrosis (39). Notably, hyperfractionated twice-daily radiation in this setting results in greater toxicity (40) and the normal tissue complication curve is unpredictable with fraction sizes above 2.5 Gy.

The risk of radiation necrosis in patients receiving radiosurgery is dependent on dose, target location, and the treated volume. Radiation Therapy Oncology Group (RTOG) 95-05 was a dose-escalation study including patients with either primary or metastatic brain tumors having previously received partial- or whole-brain radiation. The maximum tolerated dose (MTD) for targets 31 to 40 mm in diameter (equivalent to a uniform sphere with volume 15.5–33.3 mL) was 15 Gy, and for targets 21 to 30 mm in diameter (4.3–14.4 mL) 18 Gy. For targets smaller than 20 mm (<4.2 mL equivalent sphere volume), the MTD was never reached but escalation stopped at 24 Gy (41).

Radiation necrosis is ideally addressed through prevention, by optimizing dose delivered and volume treated. Current treatment technologies utilizing MRI delineation of tumor and image guidance have improved the ability to reduce the overall volume of irradiated healthy brain. Bevacizumab at the time of radiosurgery in the setting of reirradiation can reduce the risk of radiation necrosis and radiation-induced edema (42). Management of radiation necrosis generally includes initial conservative management with steroids and serial imaging. In the setting of expanding radiographic enhancement concerning either progressive disease or necrosis, options include resection, resection with LITT, and antiangiogenic therapy with bevacizumab or hyperbaric oxygen.

More common than radiation necrosis is transient, treatment-related edema and inflammation that can mask lesion progression. In glioma patients, immediate posttreatment enlargement of T1 contrast enhancement without clinical decline and with subsequent radiographic stabilization, is termed *pseudoprogression*. This is estimated to happen in up to 35% of patients treated for malignant glioma (43). Evaluation of the MRI by a neuroradiologist, serial scans, and rarely biopsy may be needed to differentiate between radiation treatment effect and tumor progression.

### Site-Specific Effects

- Lesions in the brainstem are treated with conservative doses because of its essential function.
- Optic nerve and chiasm tolerate fractionated doses up to 55 Gy and single doses up to 8 Gy. Higher doses are associated with increasing risk of vision loss, with minimally effective treatment once it occurs. Direct radiation to the lens commonly causes cataracts.
- Fractionated doses above 45 Gy or single doses over 14 Gy increase the risk for hearing loss.
- Radiation to the hypothalamus/pituitary gland can cause hormonal deficits. Endocrinology consultation for monitoring and replacement as needed is recommended for high-risk patients.
- Radiation dose to the hippocampus may contribute to radiation-related memory loss, and dose avoidance strategies are currently under study.

## Brainstem

Radiation damage to the brainstem can have devastating effects resulting in permanent cranial neuropathies, motor or sensory deficits, and even disruption of essential cardiorespiratory function (Table 1.2). The Emami tables estimate that the TD5/5 for necrosis/infarct with treatment of the whole brainstem is 50 Gy, the T5/5 for treating two-thirds of the brainstem, and the T5/5 for treating one-third is 60 Gy. These are likely overly conservative and the QUANTEC analysis recommends that small doses (1–10 mL) can be treated to a maximum dose of 59 Gy and that the whole brainstem can tolerate 54 Gy. In a single fraction, the maximum recommended dose per QUANTEC is 12.5 Gy, which yields a less than 5% risk of necrosis. Higher doses of 15 to 20 Gy can be used safely to small volumes for patients with a limited life expectancy and therefore a lower chance of experiencing late toxicity of higher doses (44). In the acute setting and at lower doses (30–35 Gy in standard fractionation) radiation to the brainstem can result in central nausea.

## Optic Structures (Optic Nerves and Optic Chiasm)

Radiation-induced optic neuropathy (RION) is a rare but devastating complication of intracranial radiation adjacent to the optic nerves or chiasm characterized by permanent partial or complete visual field loss. Damage to an optic nerve can result in monocular vision loss in the ipsilateral eye. Damage to the entire optic chiasm can result in bilateral vision loss while damage to the central portion with only the decussating fibers from each eye results in bitemporal hemianopsia. Damage to a single optic tract causes homonymous hemianopsia of the contralateral visual field (ie, damage to the left optic tract results in right visual field loss, which is comprised of input from the temporal side of the retina in the left eye and the medial retina on the right eye). The optic apparatus is generally between 2 and 5 mm in thickness so thin-cut MRI and scrupulous image registration are essential for accurate contouring. Care should be taken to contour the optic apparatus in continuity and not to overcontour any portion. These errors can lead to exceeding dose constraints to the nonvisualized portion of the optic nerve or underdosing the perioptic nerve area.

The initial Emami tables quoted a TD5/5 of 50 Gy and TD50/5 of 65 Gy. The QUANTEC reanalysis of available dose-volume information supplanted these (45). QUANTEC concluded that Dmax volumes above 60 Gy in the setting of fractionated treatment or a Dmax above 12 Gy in single treatment radiosurgery were both associated with a steep rise in toxicity. Although most studies included in this analysis reported Dmax, greater mean dose is associated with greater risk of RION independent of max dose—hinting that some volume effect likely exists (46). Fractionation effects have also been documented, with fraction doses greater than or equal to 1.9 Gy associated with greater risk (47). QUANTEC concluded that fractionated doses of 55 Gy or less were associated with near-zero rates of RION, doses between 55 and 60 Gy associated with a 3% to 7% risk and doses of 60 Gy or above associated with a risk between 7% and 20%. For patients with pituitary adenoma, however, tolerance of the chiasm appears to be less with RION occurring at doses as low as 46 Gy. In single-fraction radiosurgery, RION is rare with doses less than 8 Gy and infrequent with doses less than

**Table 1.2 Site Specific Effects**

| Side effect | Clinical signs and symptoms | Etiology | Management |
|---|---|---|---|
| Central nausea | Vomiting, anorexia | Disruption of the area postrema | Ondansetron<br>Dexamethasone (same) |
| Optic neuropathy | Visual field deficits | Damage of white matter tracts/fibers | Dexamethasone<br>Bevacizumab<br>Hyperbaric oxygen<br>Pentoxifylline/vitamin E |
| Other cranial neuropathies | V: numbness<br>VII: facial weakness<br>XII: dysphagia | Damage of white matter tracts/fibers | As noted in the previous entry, Optic neuropathy |
| Cataracts | Cloudy or blurry vision | ROS cause abnormal accumulation of lens proteins | Lens replacement |
| Retinopathy | Visual blurring or vision loss | Neovascularization | Bevacizumab |
| Hearing loss | Decreased performance on auditory tests | Sensorineural hearing loss via damage to the inner hair cells of the cochlea or CN VIII | Cochlear implants<br>Auditory brainstem implant |
| Hypopituitarism | Infertility, delayed growth, hypocortisolism, hypothyroidism | Direct cellular damage to hypothalamic and/or pituitary cells | Hormone replacement therapy |

CN, cranial nerve; ROS, reactive oxygen species.

10 Gy. Doses higher than 12 Gy are associated with a greater than 10% risk, which is considered unacceptable. Treatment options for RION are limited. Trials of dexamethasone, pentoxifylline, vitamin E, and bevacizumab are all reasonable options but have been used with limited success.

Lens

Radiation-induced cataracts are typical posterior subcapsular cataracts and can be identified as radiation related by a skilled ophthalmologist. They are postulated to be a consequence of reactive oxygen species creating abnormal aggregation of lens proteins and damaged lens fiber cells. Historically, cataract formation was considered a deterministic event (implying that cataract formation is associated with a threshold dose and higher exposure levels are associated with more severe cataracts). The threshold was thought to be 2 Gy. Subsequent evaluation of cataract formation in workers with occupational exposures as well as reanalysis of survivors of the atomic bomb and Chernobyl, suggested a much lower threshold. In 2011, the International Commission on Radiological Protection (ICRP) concluded that the threshold dose for cataracts was 0.5 Gy (a dose estimated to produce a 1% incidence of vision-impairing cataracts over 20 years) and reduced the occupational equivalent dose limit for the lens from 150 mSv per year to 20 mSv per year (48–52). Some subsequent data have even suggested that cataract formation is a stochastic event (ie, no threshold dose and while increased exposure increases the probability of cataract formation, it does not predict cataract severity).

Retina

Radiation-induced retinopathy can result either from external beam RT for brain or head and neck cancer or from eye plaque brachytherapy for choroidal melanomas. The mechanism is believed to be initial radiation–related vascular damage which induces neovascularization (53). Treatment options include steroids, bevacizumab, laser coagulation, and hyperbaric oxygen. The TD5/5 from the Emami estimates for radiation-induced retinopathy is 45 Gy with a TD50/5 of 65 Gy. The patients most at risk for radiation-induced retinopathy are patients receiving eye plaque brachytherapy. Long-term follow-up of patients receiving brachytherapy indicate that a very high proportion (68%) who had good vision at the time of brachytherapy had poor vision (worse than 20/100 visual acuity) at 10 years (54). Tumor size, proximity to the fovea, and tumor recurrence were all predictors of vision decline.

*Cochlea*

Radiation damage typically results in high-frequency hearing loss. QUANTEC states that a mean of 45 Gy is associated with a 30% rate of hearing loss (55). Loss of serviceable hearing (often defined by the Gardner Robertson scale) occurs as a result of direct and indirect damage to the inner hair cells of the cochlea, which serve as mechanoreceptors transducing pressure variants in the air into neural-electrical impulses (56). Concurrent platinum-based chemotherapy agents can act synergistically and render patients more vulnerable to radiation-related hearing loss, and a mean cochlear dose below 35 Gy may be indicated in this setting. For single-fraction radiosurgery, keeping the dose below 4 Gy keeps the rate of hearing loss at or below 25% (57). Treatment options can include cochlear implants (although if cranial nerve [CN] VIII is damaged cochlear implants will be of minimal use) or auditory brainstem implants (which bypass both the cochlea and CN VIII).

## *Hypothalamic-Pituitary Axis*

Endocrine abnormalities are not uncommon after whole-brain irradiation, radiation to the nasopharynx or base of skull, or total body irradiation. The hypothalamus is more radiosensitive than the pituitary. GH is the most vulnerable anterior pituitary hormone to irradiation, followed by gonadotropin, corticotropin, and thyrotropin deficiency. Isolated GH deficiency can occur in some pediatric patients receiving 10 to 12 Gy of cranial irradiation, approximately 50% in patients receiving 18 to 24 Gy, and occurs in most patients receiving 30 Gy or more (50). Precocious puberty with impaired pubertal growth (due to a relative GH insufficiency compared to gonadotropins). Higher fractionated doses (50–60 Gy) can result in pan-hypopituitarism and hyperprolactinemia owing to a release of hypothalamic inhibition. Children receiving 18 to 24 Gy of whole-brain irradiation for acute lymphoblastic leukemia (ALL) are more likely to be overweight or obese compared to their peers (likely a multifactorial phenomenon but reduced leptin sensitivity has been implicated). At higher doses (>50 Gy), damage to the ventromedial nucleus of the hypothalamus may result in hyperphagia and subsequent obesity. Cranial irradiation to doses less than 24 Gy can be associated with precocious puberty and subsequent gonadotrophin deficiency. Doses higher than 24 Gy more often results in delayed puberty. Treatment for hypothalamic-pituitary-adrenal (HPA) axis dysfunction after radiation includes hormone replacement therapy managed by endocrinology. Close attention should be given to patients with hypocortisolism during acute illnesses as they require stress-dose steroids to assist their body in appropriately mounting a response. Endocrinology consultation for serial hormonal monitoring is recommended for high-risk patients.

## *Hippocampus*

The hippocampus has long been recognized as a key anatomic location for declarative memory. Because the hippocampal subgranular and subventricular zones are repositories of adult neural stem cells and normal tissue toxicity is often mediated via stem cell death in other sites of the body, much of the corresponding preclinical rodent research looking at the effect of radiation on the hippocampus has focused on decreased neurogenesis after radiation. This has been shown to be dose dependent and fractionation dependent, with the irradiated neural stem cells preferentially maturing to a glial rather than neural fate (58). Moreover, human autopsy studies have shown decreased numbers of hippocampal stem cells compared with control patients (59). Preclinical rodent data indicates that radiation disrupts the function of mature hippocampal cells by interfering with experience-dependent upregulation of proteins important in synaptic architecture (60), by changing ion channel subunit composition, reducing the number of readily releasable synaptic vesicles, changing dendritic spine architecture (61), and decreasing spontaneous neural discharges. Only recently have retrospective dosimetric reviews of prospective trials with neurocognitive data been published. One study found that the V55Gy of the hippocampus is associated with post-XRT cognitive impairment. A V55Gy of 25% was associated with a 45.9% impairment rate and a V55Gy of 50% was associated with an 80.6% impairment rate (62). Collectively the preclinical and retrospective research has spawned the idea of selectively avoiding the hippocampus during WBRT to try to mitigate the cognitive side effects.

## SPINE

- Radiation myelopathy is rare but can present as peripheral sensory or motor deficits in the absence of tumor progression.
- Children and those receiving concurrent chemotherapy may be more sensitive to radiation. When possible, most practitioners try not to have radiation to the spine administered on the same day as chemotherapy.
- Radiation myelopathy is considered an irreversible side effect, although steroids are used to treat symptoms and hyperbaric oxygen has been used to promote tissue repair.
- Prevention is paramount with a number of studies providing single dose and fractionated dose recommendations.

Radiation myelopathy is rare but can be a devastating complication of radiation causing pain, paresthesia, sensory deficits, paralysis, Brown-Sequard syndrome, and bowel/bladder incontinence. It is defined as symptomatic, peripheral sensory or motor deficits caused by radiation treatment in the absence of tumor progression. Many studies use complete motor paralysis as their endpoint. The vast majority of radiation myelopathy cases occur between 6 months and 3 years after RT. The mechanism of injury is believed to be vascular and endothelial cell damage as well as glial cell damage.

Irradiated volume has a large impact on dose tolerance in the spinal cord making maximum dose the most widely used constraint. Per the QUANTEC analysis, in the de novo setting, doses of 54 Gy and 61 Gy in 2 Gy per fraction are thought to be associated with a less than 1% and approximately 10% risk of myelopathy, respectively (63). In the setting of SRS, a max dose of 13 Gy in a single fraction to the cord or 20 Gy in three fractions is associated with a less than 1% risk of myelopathy. For reirradiation after standard fractionation and using standard fractionation in the second course, cord tolerance appears to increase at least 25% at 6 months after the initial course of RT.

The dose tolerance is lowest when the full thickness of the cord is irradiated, and increases with partial cord irradiation (63,66). There are also local-regional differences in radiosensitivity within the spinal cord—the dose-response curve is more right shifted with irradiation of the central gray matter compared with irradiation of the long, white matter tracts. The difference has been attributed both to differences in vascularization, distribution of oligodendrocyte progenitors, and functional differences between the regions (white matter tracts versus gray matter cell bodies).

Normal tissue repair allows for partial recovery of dose tolerance over time. In primate studies, an initial course of 44 Gy was given followed by a second course of either 57 Gy or 66 Gy after a period of recovery time. Collating this data with additional prior data led to estimates of tolerance recovery of 34 Gy (76%), 38 Gy (85%), and 45 Gy (101%) at 1, 2, and 3 years, respectively (64). An initial BED of 100 Gy to the spinal cord appears to be safe. Accounting for time since initial course, one can allow for 25%, 33%, and 50% at 6 months, 1 year, and 2 years, respectively, and calculate an allowable BED for a second course (65). It is important to note that patients receiving chemotherapy may be more sensitive and so the rates of myelopathy may be higher than predicted in these populations.

Treatment for radiation myelopathy can include steroids, pentoxifylline, and hyperbaric oxygen. Unfortunately, in cases of true radiation myelopathy, it is unlikely that these treatments will substantially reverse the consequences of radiation damage.

# REFERENCES

1. Li J, Bentzen SM, Li J, et al. 2008. Relationship between neurocognitive function and quality of life after whole-brain radiotherapy in patients with brain metastasis. *Int J Radiat Oncol Biol Phys.* 2008;71(1):64–70.
2. Blakeley JO, Coons SJ, Corboy JR, et al. Clinical outcome assessment in malignant glioma trials: measuring signs, symptoms, and functional limitations. *Neuro Oncol.* 2016;18(Suppl 2):ii13–ii20.
3. Armstrong TS, Bishof AM, Brown PD, et al. Determining priority signs and symptoms for use as clinical outcomes assessments in trials including patients with malignant gliomas: Panel 1 Report. *Neuro Oncol.* 2016;18(Suppl 2):ii1–ii12.
4. Emami B, Lyman J, Brown A, et al. Tolerance of normal tissue to therapeutic irradiation. *Int J Radiat Oncol Biol Phys.* 1991;21(1):109–122.
5. Marks LB, Ten Haken RK, Martel MK. 2010. Guest editor's introduction to QUANTEC: a users guide. *Int J Radiat Oncol Biol Phys.* 2010;76(3):S1–S2.
6. Moore IM, Kramer JH, Wara W, et al. Cognitive function in children with leukemia. Effect of radiation dose and time since irradiation. *Cancer.* 1991;68(9):1913–1917.
7. Hill JM, Kornblith AB, Dana J, et al. A comparative study of the long term psychosocial functioning of childhood Acute Lymphoblastic Leukemia survivors treated by Intrathecal Methotrexate with or without Cranial Radiation. *Cancer.* 1998;82(1):208–218.
8. Smibert E, Anderson V, Godber T, Ekert H. Risk factors for intellectual and educational sequelae of cranial irradiation in Childhood Acute Lymphoblastic Leukaemia. *Br J Cancer.* 1996;73(6):825–830.
9. Meyers CA. Neurocognitive function and progression in patients with brain metastases treated with whole-brain radiation and motexafin gadolinium: results of a randomized Phase III trial. *J Clin Oncol.* 2003;22(1):157–165.
10. Aoyama H, Shirato H, Tago M, et al. Stereotactic radiosurgery plus whole-brain radiation therapy vs stereotactic radiosurgery alone for treatment of brain metastases: a randomized controlled trial. *JAMA.* 2006;295(21):2483–2491.
11. Chang EL, Wefel JS, Hess KR, et al. Neurocognition in patients with brain metastases treated with radiosurgery or radiosurgery plus whole-brain irradiation: a randomised controlled trial. *Lancet Oncol.* 2009;10(11):1037–1044.
12. Welzel G, Grit W, Katharina F, et al. Memory function before and after whole brain radiotherapy in patients with and without brain metastases. *Int J Radiat Oncol Biol Phys.* 2008;72(5):1311–1318.

13. Bosma I, Vos MJ, Heimans JJ, et al. The course of neurocognitive functioning in high-grade glioma patients. *Neuro Oncol.* 2007;9(1):53–62.
14. Brown PD, Jaeckle K, Ballman KV, et al. Effect of radiosurgery alone vs radiosurgery with whole brain radiation therapy on cognitive function in patients with 1 to 3 brain metastases: a randomized clinical trial. *JAMA.* 2016;316(4):401–409.
15. Kocher M, Soffietti R, Abacioglu U, et al. Adjuvant whole-brain radiotherapy versus observation after radiosurgery or surgical resection of one to three cerebral metastases: results of the EORTC 22952-26001 study. *J Clin Oncol.* 2011;29(2):134–341.
16. Soffietti R, Kocher M, Abacioglu UM, et al. A European organisation for research and treatment of cancer phase III trial of adjuvant whole-brain radiotherapy versus observation in patients with one to three brain metastases from solid tumors after surgical resection or radiosurgery: quality-of-life results. *J Clin Oncol.* 2013;31(1):65–72.
17. Greene-Schloesser D, Dana G-S, Robbins ME, et al. Radiation-induced brain injury: a review. *Front Oncol.* 2012;2. doi:10.3389/fonc.2012.00073
18. Shah AC, Kelly DR, Nabors LB, et al. Treatment of primary CNS lymphoma with high-dose methotrexate in immunocompetent pediatric patients. *Pediatr Blood Cancer.* 2010;55(6):1227–1230.
19. Shah GD, Yahalom J, Correa DD, et al. Combined immunochemotherapy with reduced whole-brain radiotherapy for newly diagnosed primary CNS lymphoma. *J Clin Oncol.* 2007;25(30):4730–4735.
20. Morris PG, Correa DD, Yahalom J, et al. Rituximab, methotrexate, procarbazine, and vincristine followed by consolidation reduced-dose whole-brain radiotherapy and cytarabine in newly diagnosed primary CNS lymphoma: final results and long-term outcome. *J Clin Oncol.* 2013;31:3971–3979.
21. Wang YJ, King AD, Hua Z, et al. Evolution of radiation-induced brain injury: MR imaging–based study. *Radiology.* 2010;254(1):210–218.
22. Curran WJ, Charles H-L, Luis S, et al. Magnetic resonance imaging of cranial radiation lesions. *Int J Radiat Oncol Biol Phys.* 1987;13(7):1093–1098.
23. Corn BW, Yousem DM, Scott CB, et al. White matter changes are correlated significantly with radiation dose. Observations from a randomized dose-escalation trial for malignant glioma (Radiation Therapy Oncology Group 83-02). *Cancer.* 1994;74(10):2828–2835.
24. Constine LS, Konski A, Ekholm S, et al. Adverse effects of brain irradiation correlated with MR and CT imaging. *Int J Radiat Oncol Biol Phys.* 1988;15(2):319–330.
25. Cremers LGM, de Groot M, Hofman A, et al. Altered tract-specific white matter microstructure is related to poorer cognitive performance: the rotterdam study. *Neurobiol Aging.* 2016;39:108–117.
26. Brown PD, Shook S, Laack NN, et al. Memantine for the prevention of cognitive dysfunction in patients receiving whole-brain radiation therapy (WBRT): first report of RTOG 0614, a placebo-controlled, double-blind, randomized trial. *Int J Radiat Oncol Biol Phys.* 2012;84(3):S1–S2.
27. Butler JM, Case D, Atkins J, et al. A phase III, double blind, placebo-controlled prospective randomized clinical trial of effect of d-threo-methylphenidate HCl (d-MPH) on quality of life in brain tumor patients receiving radiation therapy. *Int J Radiat Oncol Biol Phys.* 2005;63:S80.
28. Attia A, Albert A, Rapp SR, et al. Phase II study of ginkgo biloba in irradiated brain tumor patients: effect on cognitive function, quality of life, and mood. *J Neurooncol.* 2012;109(2):357–363.

29. Rapp SR, Case LD, Peiffer A, et al. Donepezil for irradiated brain tumor survivors: a Phase III randomized placebo-controlled clinical trial. *J Clin Oncol.* 2015;33(15):1653–1659.
30. Page BR, Shaw EG, Lu L, et al. 2015. Phase II double-blind placebo-controlled randomized study of armodafinil for brain radiation-induced fatigue. *Neuro Oncol.* 17(10):1393–1401.
31. Shaw EG. Phase II study of donepezil in irradiated brain tumor patients: effect on cognitive function, mood, and quality of life. *J Clin Oncol.* 2006;24(9):1415–1420.
32. Powell C, Guerrero D, Sardell S, et al. Somnolence syndrome in patients receiving radical radiotherapy for primary brain tumours: a prospective study. *Radiother Oncol.* 2011;100(1):131–136.
33. Weintraub NL, Jones WK, Manka D. Understanding radiation-induced vascular disease. *J Am Coll Cardiol.* 2010;55(12):1237–1239.
34. Lo AC, Howard AF, Nichol A, et al. Long-term outcomes and complications in patients with craniopharyngioma: the british columbia cancer agency experience. *Int J Radiat Oncol Biol Phys.* 2014;88(5):1011–1018.
35. Lo AC, Howard AF, Nichol A, et al. A cross-sectional cohort study of cerebrovascular disease and late effects after radiation therapy for craniopharyngioma. *Pediatr Blood Cancer.* 2016;63(5):786–793.
36. Yamanaka R, Hayano A, Kanayama T. Radiation-induced gliomas: a comprehensive review and meta-analysis. *Neurosurg Rev.* 2016. doi:10.1007/s10143-016-0786-8
37. White NS, McDonald C, McDonald CR, et al. Diffusion-weighted imaging in cancer: physical foundations and applications of restriction spectrum imaging. *Cancer Res.* 2014;74(17):4638–4652.
38. Barajas RF, Chang JS, Sneed PK, et al. Distinguishing recurrent intra-axial metastatic tumor from radiation necrosis following gamma knife radiosurgery using dynamic susceptibility-weighted contrast-enhanced perfusion MR imaging. *AJNR Am J Neuroradiol.* 2009;30(2):367–372.
39. Lawrence YR, Li XA, el Naqa I, et al. Radiation dose–volume effects in the brain. *Int J Radiat Oncol Biol Phys.* 2010;76(3):S20–S27.
40. Murray KJ, Scott C, Greenberg HM, et al. A randomized phase III study of accelerated hyperfractionation versus standard in patients with unresected brain metastases: a report of the Radiation Therapy Oncology Group (RTOG) 9104. *Int J Radiat Oncol Biol Phys.* 1997;39(3):571–574.
41. Shaw E, Charles S, Luis S, et al. Single dose radiosurgical treatment of recurrent previously irradiated primary brain tumors and brain metastases: final report of RTOG protocol 90-05. *Int J Radiat Oncol Biol Phys.* 2000;47(2):291–298.
42. Cuneo KC, Vredenburgh J, Desjardins A, et al. Impact of concurrent and adjuvant bevacizumab on the risk of radiation necrosis following radiosurgery for recurrent glioma. *Int J Radiat Oncol Biol Phys.* 2012;84(3):S7.
43. Brandsma D, Stalpers L, Taal W, et al. Clinical features, mechanisms, and management of pseudoprogression in malignant gliomas. *Lancet Oncol.* 2008;9(5):453–461.
44. Mayo C, Charles M, Ellen Y, Merchant TE. Radiation associated brainstem injury. *Int J Radiat Oncol Biol Phys.* 2010;76(3):S36–S41.
45. Mayo C, Martel MK, Marks LB, et al. Radiation dose-volume effects of optic nerves and chiasm. *Int J Radiat Oncol Biol Phys.* 2010;76(3, Suppl):S28–S35.
46. Martel MK, Sandler HM, Cornblath WT, et al. Dose-volume complication analysis for visual pathway structures of patients with advanced paranasal sinus tumors. *Int J Radiat Oncol Biol Phys.* 1997;38(2):273–284.

47. Parsons JT, Bova FJ, Fitzgerald CR, et al. Radiation optic neuropathy after megavoltage external-beam irradiation: analysis of time-dose factors. *Int J Radiat Oncol Biol Phys*. 1994;30(4):755–763.

48. Barnard SG, Ainsbury EA, Quinlan RA, Bouffler SD. Radiation protection of the eye lens in medical workers—basis and impact of the ICRP recommendations. *Br J Radiol*. 2016;89(1060):20151034. doi:10.1259/bjr.20151034

49. Phipps AW, Silk TJ, Fell TP. The impact of recent ICRP recommendations of dose coefficients, annual limits on intake, and monitoring programmes for thorium. *Radiat Prot Dosimetry*. 1998;79(1):115–118.

50. Stewart FA, Akleyev AV, Hauer-Jensen M, et al. ICRP publication 118: ICRP statement on tissue reactions and early and late effects of radiation in normal tissues and organs – threshold doses for tissue reactions in a radiation protection context. *Ann ICRP*. 2012;41(1–2):1–322.

51. Bouffler S, Ainsbury E, Gilvin P, Harrison J. Radiation-induced cataracts: the health protection agency's response to the ICRP statement on tissue reactions and recommendation on the dose limit for the eye lens. *J Radiol Prot*. 2012;32(4):479–488.

52. Gilvin P, Tanner R, Bouffler S, et al. Footnote to 'radiation-induced cataracts: the health protection agency's response to the icrp statement on tissue reactions and recommendation on the dose limit for the eye lens'. *J Radiol Prot*. 2013;33(3):704–705.

53. Reichstein D. Current treatments and preventive strategies for radiation retinopathy. *Current Opinion in Ophthalmology*. 2015;26(3):157–166.

54. Shields CL, Shields JA, Cater J, et al. Plaque radiotherapy for uveal melanoma: long-term visual outcome in 1106 consecutive patients. *Archives Ophthalmol*. 2000;118(9):1219–1228.

55. Bhandare N, Jackson A, Eisbruch A, et al. Radiation therapy and hearing loss. *Int J Radiat Oncol Biol Phys*. 2010;76(3):S50–S57.

56. Mujica-Mota MA, Lehnert S, Devic S, et al. Mechanisms of radiation-induced sensorineural hearing loss and radioprotection. *Hearing Research*. 2014;312:60–68.

57. Massager N, Nissim O, Delbrouck C, et al. Irradiation of cochlear structures during vestibular schwannoma radiosurgery and associated hearing outcome. *J Neurosurg*. 2007;107(4):733–739.

58. Roman DD, Sperduto PW. Neuropsychological effects of cranial radiation: current knowledge and future directions. *Int J Radiat Oncol Biol Phys*. 1995;31(4):983–998.

59. Nagai R, Tsunoda S, Hori Y, Asada H. Selective vulnerability to radiation in the hippocampal dentate granule cells. *Surgical Neurol*. 2000;53(5):503–507.

60. Shi, L, Adams MM, Long A, et al. Spatial learning and memory deficits after whole-brain irradiation are associated with changes in NMDA receptor subunits in the hippocampus. *Radiation Research*. 166(6):892–899.

61. Park M-K, Kim S, Jung U, et al. Effect of acute and fractionated irradiation on hippocampal neurogenesis. *Molecules*. 2012;17(8):9462–9468.

62. Okoukoni C, McTyre E, Peiffer AM, et al. Hippocampal dosimetry predicts for cancer-related cognitive impairment in patients treated with cranial radiation therapy: dosimetric results of a prospective clinical trial. *Int J Radiat Oncol Biol Phys*. 2016;96(2):S90–S91.

63. Kirkpatrick JP, van der Kogel AJ, Schultheiss TE. Radiation dose–volume effects in the spinal cord. *Int J Radiat Oncol Biol Phys*. 2010.76(3):S42–S49.

64. Ang KK, Jiang GL, Feng Y, et al. Extent and kinetics of recovery of occult spinal cord injury. *Int J Radiat Oncol Biol Phys*. 2001;50(4):1013–1020.
65. Nelson JW, Yoo DS, Sampson JH, et al. Stereotactic body radiotherapy for lesions of the spine and paraspinal regions. *Int J Radiat Oncol Biol Phys*. 2009;73(5):1369–1375.
66. Schultheiss TE. The radiation dose–response of the human spinal cord. *Int J Radiat Oncol Biol Phys*. 2008;71(5):1455–1459.

# Radiation Therapy Effects in Head and Neck Cancer

*Thomas J. Galloway and Sue S. Yom*

## OVERVIEW
- Radiation therapy (RT) can cure patients with head and neck cancer. However, this cure can come with significant acute and late toxicity.
- Supportive management is essential during radiation treatment.
- Patient education and specialist utilization, as needed, aid in management of late toxicity.

While some radiation side effects, such as dermatitis and mucositis, are temporary effects which will resolve with supportive care, others occur months to years after RT (hypothyroidism, fibrosis). However, some effects can begin during RT but persist long after treatment has ended. Examples include xerostomia, fatigue, and depression. In this chapter, we categorize toxicities, but recognize that symptoms may persist beyond the acute therapy period.

## ACUTE TOXICITY
Table 2.1 provides a summary of acute toxicity conditions discussed in this section.

### Dermatitis
*Definition*
- Acute radiation dermatitis results from injury to the rapidly dividing cells of the dermis, epidermis, and feeding vasculature.
- The condition is characterized by erythema, edema, dry and wet desquamation, blistering and bleeding, and erosion and ulceration of the skin.
- There may be visible tanning or darkening of the skin preceding desquamation and slough.

*Timing*
- Prodromal changes to skin begin within 24 hours of radiation exposure (1).
- Visible reaction starts around 10 to 14 days after radiation course begins (2).
- Dry desquamation can be expected at dosages over 30 Gy (3).
- Moist desquamation can be expected at dosages over 40 Gy (3).

**Table 2.1** Acute Toxicity Related to Head and Neck Cancer RT

| Organ | Ailment | Usual timing | Mild | Moderate/severe | Preventative strategies |
|---|---|---|---|---|---|
| Skin | Dermatitis | 14 days | • Emollients | • Debridement of peel and slough<br>• Nonadherent or special wound dressings prn<br>• Antibiotic cream prn<br>• Pain management | • Lubrication/emollients<br>• Good hygiene |
| Salivary glands | Xerostomia | 7+ days<br>Peaks at 4 weeks<br>May persist long term | • Salivary substitutes<br>  ○ Hyetellose, hyprolose, or caramellose<br>• Salivary stimulants<br>  ○ Citrus cough drops, xylitol | • Parasympathetic stimulants<br>  ○ Bethanechol, pilocarpine, cevimeline<br>• Acupuncture | • Radiation dose reduction to parotid/submandibular glands |
| Taste buds | Dysgeusia | 4–6+ weeks | • Treat xerostomia<br>• Dietary counseling | • Zinc supplementation | • Radiation dose reduction to oral cavity |
| Mucosa | Mucositis | 2+ weeks | • Oratect gel and Gelclair<br>• Benzylamine or phenol<br>• Viscous lidocaine<br>• Doxepin | • Low energy helium-neon laser treatment<br>• Opioids<br>• Gabapentin | • Good oral hygiene<br>• Baking soda rinses<br>• Supersaturated calcium phosphate solutions (Caphosol, NeutraSal, SalivaMAX) |

*(continued)*

**Table 2.1** Acute Toxicity Related to Head and Neck Cancer RT (*continued*)

| Organ | Ailment | Usual timing | Mild | Moderate/severe | Preventative strategies |
|---|---|---|---|---|---|
| | Nausea | 3+ weeks | • Ginger | • Antihistamines (diphenhydramine, meclizine)<br>• Anticholinergics (scopolamine)<br>• Benzodiazepines (lorazepam)<br>• Dopamine antagonists (metoclopramide, prochlorperazine, promethazine)<br>• 5-HT receptor (serotonin) antagonists (ondansetron, granisetron, palonosetron)<br>• Substance P antagonists (aprepitant, fosaprepitant) | • Radiation dose reduction to posterior brainstem |

(*continued*)

**Table 2.1** Acute Toxicity Related to Head and Neck Cancer RT *(continued)*

| Organ | Ailment | Usual timing | Mild | Moderate/severe | Preventative strategies |
|---|---|---|---|---|---|
| | Fatigue | 7+ days | • Nonbenzodiazepine hyponotics (zolpidem, eszopiclone)<br>  ○ Short-term only<br>• Increased exercise<br>• Strict sleep hygiene and better regulation of the sleep-wake cycle<br>• Psychosocial or cognitive-behavioral interventions (84)<br>• Nutritional counseling<br>• Meditation, yoga, and mindfulness-based stress reduction methods | • Dopamine reuptake inhibitor (methylphenidate, modafinil) | • Sleep hygiene<br>• Manage comorbidities |
| | Depression | At any time | • Psychological or psychiatric services | • SSRIs<br>• SNRIs<br>• TCAs<br>• MAOIs<br>• Unique medications such as mirtazapine and bupropion | • Screening and early identification |
| Hair follicles | Alopecia | 21+ days | • Avoid sun exposure to the scalp<br>• Treat the hair gently using a soft brush and gentle shampoo<br>• Avoid use of heat on the hair, such as hair dryer, hot rollers, or curling irons<br>• Avoid use of bleach or hair dyes or permanent curling solutions<br>• Use a wig or hat | • Reconstructive surgical procedures | • Scalp-sparing radiation techniques |

RT, radiation therapy; SNRIs, serotonin-norepinephrine reuptake inhibitors; SSRIs, selective serotonin reuptake inhibitors; TCAs, tricyclic antidepressants; MAOIs, monoamine oxidase inhibitors.

## Prevention

- Should observe three basic principles at all times:
  - Lubrication and restoration of moisture to the skin;
  - Maintenance of skin integrity;
  - Protection of the skin from environmental stress or exposure.
- Patient education should focus on protecting the skin from trauma and recognizing signs of infection.
- Practical management for patients (4):
  - Unscented, lanolin-free, water-based moisturizing lotion can be applied prophylactically at the beginning of RT.
  - Avoid contact of products to skin that could be irritating:
    - Avoid alcohol- or menthol-containing products;
    - Avoid perfumes, aftershave, or chlorine exposure;
    - Use a mild, nonalkaline, unscented soap;
    - Use an electric razor to avoid cuts to the skin;
    - Wear loose-fitting clothing and avoid scratching or rubbing the skin.
  - Good hygiene and cleanliness is needed; washing the skin with lukewarm water or saline soaks is encouraged.
  - Avoidance of sun exposure or sunscreen when necessary.
  - Topical low-dose steroids are commonly used to soothe local irritation and itching, but have the negative effect of skin atrophy and delayed healing (5).

## Screening

- Physician should be aware of patient-related factors:
  - Anatomic site;
  - Body mass index;
  - Age;
  - Ethnicity;
  - Sun-reactive skin type;
  - Medical comorbidities such as collagen vascular disease and HIV;
  - Smoking;
  - Possible genetic mutations.
- Treatment-related factors may pose increased risk:
  - Volume of skin within the high-dose treatment area;
  - Beam energy;
  - Total dose and fractionation;
  - Use of bolus and its frequency;
  - Use of tangential beams or intensity-modulated radiation;
  - Concurrent or recent use of radiosensitizers, chemotherapy, and targeted therapies.

- Validated common scoring systems to track toxicity:
  - Radiation Therapy Oncology Group (RTOG)/European Organisation for Research and Treatment of Cancer (EORTC)—grades acute and late effects and is most commonly used (6);
  - Late Effects of Normal Tissues/Subjective; Objective; Management; Analytic (LENT/SOMA)—grades only late effects (7);
  - Common Terminology Criteria for Adverse Events (CTCAE)—grades only acute effects (8).
- Lacouture et al have proposed a dermatologic grading scale for effects associated with targeted therapies (estimated glomerular filtration rate [EGFR] inhibition) (9).
- Grading scales that incorporate patient-reported outcomes (PROs):
  - Radiation-Induced Skin Reaction Assessment Scale (RISRAS) (10);
  - Catterall Skin Scoring Profile (11);
  - Skindex-16 (12);
  - Skin Cancer Index (13);
  - Dermatology Life Quality Index (14).
- Grading scales incorporating PROs when using targeted therapies:
  - Functional Assesment of Cancer Therapy Epidermal Growth Factor Receptor Inhibitor (FACT-EGFRI-18) (15);
  - Hand-foot syndrome (HFS-14) (16).

### *Treatment*

- Frequent use of moisturizing lotions or creams.
- Avoid bolus effect of tape or bandages.
- Dry slough should be manually or enzymatically debrided.
- Friction may be reduced with nonstick barrier films or specialized non-adherent dressings.
- Infection should be addressed promptly with topically applied antibiotic medications or dressings.
- Specialized topical dressings should be applied to any areas of friction or open wound.

## Xerostomia

### *Definition*

- A subjective condition;
- A feeling of oral dryness or "dry mouth";
- May be associated with decreased function or loss of function of the salivary glands;
- Results in altered taste, reduced intraoral lubrication, halitosis, dental infections, caries, and speech and eating difficulties.

## 2. RADIATION THERAPY EFFECTS IN HEAD AND NECK CANCER 25

### *Timing*
- Typically peaks in severity in the last two weeks of a radiation treatment course;
- May be perceived by patients as early as the first week of treatment.

### *Prevention*
- Radiation dosage to the parotid and submandibular glands is critical.
- The effects are proportional to the amount of radiation dosage delivered.
- Standard known tolerance levels, if exceeded, will result in very severe effects (17).

### *Screening*
- Patients should be inspected at least weekly for signs of worsening xerostomia.
- All patients receiving more than 2 to 3 weeks of RT to the oral cavity or pharyngeal regions are at risk for severe xerostomia.
- Validated common scoring systems to track toxicity:
  - RTOG/EORTC;
  - LENT/SOMA;
  - CTCAE.

### *Treatment*
- Salivary substitutes that temporarily hydrate the mucosa:
  - Ingredients such as hyetellose, hyprolose, or caramellose.
- Gustatory stimulants:
  - Acidic, bitter, or sweet substances such as citrus flavors or cough drops.
  - Xylitol, a sugar substitute used in gum and lozenges, may have positive effects on dentition.
- Pharmacologic stimulants are generally parasympathomimetic agents:
  - Bethanechol, pilocarpine, and cevimeline comprise this class of medications (18).
  - Common side effects include sweating, dizziness, headache, nausea, flushing, and increased urge to urinate.
- Acupuncture:
  - Found to be effective in some single-institution experiences and uncontrolled trials, but a systematic review failed to identify compelling evidence of efficacy (19).
  - A prospective randomized phase II trial of standardized electronic acupuncture found some evidence of similar efficacy to pilocarpine with fewer side effects (20).

## Dysgeusia

### Definition

- Radiation may cause alterations in taste perception (dysgeusia), ranging from complete (ageusia) to partial (hypogeusia) loss of the sense of taste.
- Alteration of taste may occur in up to 75% of head and neck cancer patients (21).
- Dysgeusia results in anorexia, weight loss, malnutrition, and poor quality of life (QOL) (22).

### Timing

- A longitudinal study found taste alterations in head and neck cancer patients prior to starting RT, with the possibility of preexisting effects due to nerve damage by the cancer or nutritional deficiencies, such as zinc levels (23).
- RT causes a dose-related cytotoxic effect on taste buds which reduces their density, which is linked to taste perception and sensitivity (24,25).
- Dysgeusia correlates with the extent of oral cavity radiated to high doses (50 Gy), with peak incidence of symptoms at 1 month after RT followed by improvement until at least 12 months (26).

### Prevention

- Avoidance of a high mean dose to the oral cavity may be the best form of prevention.
- Studies of zinc supplementation to prevent radiation-induced taste effects have yielded highly conflicting results (27–29).

### Treatment

Reducing effects of xerostomia may help to mitigate some taste alteration.

## Mucositis

### Definition

- Acute mucositis results from progressive vasocongestion and edema of the mucosa accompanied by erosion and denudation of the surface epithelium.
- It may affect the mouth, pharynx, esophagus, or other gastrointestinal organs.
- Severe cases progress to ulceration with pseudomembrane formation and constant pain.
- Mucositis increases the risk of infection due to disruption of the mucosal barrier.
- The resultant pain and dysphagia affect oral intake and nutrition (30).

### Timing

- Typically begins at 2 to 3 weeks after start of RT and plateaus at the 4th week (31);
- May persist for weeks to months after discontinuation of an extended radiation treatment course.

## Prevention

- Patient risk factors include (32,33):
  - Radiated subsite of the oral cavity or oropharynx;
  - Age;
  - Smoking;
  - Alcoholism;
  - Poor oral health;
  - Poor nutritional status;
  - HIV status;
  - Concurrent or recent exposure to radiosensitizers, chemotherapy, and targeted therapies.
- Treatment-related factors include (34–36):
  - The volume of mucosa included in the high-dose areas of radiation;
  - Total dosage prescribed;
  - Higher dose per fraction;
  - Use of altered fractionation or hyperfractionation;
  - Use of conventional versus intensity-modulated RT (IMRT).

## Screening

- Frequent visual evaluation of the oral cavity;
- Assessment of functional abilities such as dysphagia and odynophagia;
- Clinician-rated grading scales:
  - CTCAE;
  - RTOG/EORTC;
  - LENT/SOMA;
  - WHO Oral Toxicity Scale (37).

## Treatment

- Oral cavity should be kept very clean and free of residue:
  - Rinse thoroughly after meals.
  - Frequent oral cleansing and disinfection with a weak solution of salt and baking soda several times daily.
  - Commercially available supersaturated calcium phosphate solutions (Caphosol, NeutraSal, SalivaMAX) have shown some advantage in head-to-head trials against the standard baking soda and salt solution.
- Injury and irritation to the mucosal surfaces should be avoided:
  - Recommend a soft bland diet that requires minimal chewing.
  - Patients should avoid spicy or acidic foods.
  - Caffeine and alcohol result in irritating or drying the mucosa.
  - Extra-soft toothbrush minimizes trauma.

- Soothing and lubricating the mucosal surfaces of the mouth and throat may help to prevent and heal mucositis:
  - Oratect gel and Gelclair are mucosal adhesive, water-soluble films that provide a protective barrier (38).
  - Sucralfate is a mucosal coating agent designed to protect the mucosa, but there may be no difference when compared to saline rinses (39).
  - Small pilot studies using glutamine have demonstrated a reduction in severity and length of mucositis and pain (40,41).
  - Randomized trials and a meta-analysis of honey have shown promising results (42–44).
  - The conclusiveness of most mucositis prevention studies is limited due to small patient numbers, the use of objective or unvalidated measures, and the lack of a placebo control.
- Pharmacologic preventive interventions:
  - Results of clinical trials for amifostine, a radioprotectant, are conflicting:
    - Some evidence suggests it may improve the patient-reported experience (45).
    - Side effects include hypotension and potentially severe nausea.
  - Granulocyte macrophage colony stimulating factor (GM-CSF) given either subcutaneously or orally showed promising results in some in pilot studies, but subsequent randomized trials have yet to clearly confirm these results (46).
  - Palifermin is a novel keratinocyte growth factor and has demonstrated efficacy in the acceleration of epithelial restoration in stem cell transplant patients although the benefit in a head and neck cancer trial was not significant (47,48).
- Topical short-acting pain control is important to maintain oral intake and relieve pain:
  - Topical analgesic solutions such as benzylamine or phenol are frequently used, although these only treat the symptoms and not the underlying condition.
  - Viscous lidocaine is frequently combined with an antihistamine (diphenhydramine, eg, Benadryl) and antacid (magnesium hydroxide/aluminum hydroxide, eg, Maalox) +/- antifungal medication (nystatin) and does show efficacy against pain, but systemic absorption and lack of true efficacy against the underlying condition is a concern (49–51).
  - In a small study, morphine mouthwash appeared to provide further reduction in mucositis and superior patient satisfaction to lidocaine-based solution (52).
  - Doxepin mouthrinse was shown to produce overall benefits superior to placebo and equivalent to lidocaine-based preparations and may be longer acting (49,53).
  - Low-energy helium-neon laser treatment was associated with a reduction in the frequency of grade 3 mucositis and pain compared to placebo, but this is not widely available (54).

- If pain is continuous and refractory to topical approaches, blocking pain responses centrally is important for patient well-being:
  - Opioid analgesics (55);
  - Gabapentin has shown to produce improved analgesia and reduce opioid requirements (56).

## Oral Infection

### Definition
Bacterial, fungal, or viral infections can occur, especially in areas of injury within the oral or pharyngeal regions.

### Timing
Typically, infections begin to arise coincident with mucositis (57).

### Prevention
- Excellent oral hygiene promotes control over microbial flora.
  - Frequent rinsing and gargling of the mouth and throat will reduce the overall pathogenic load.
  - Use of a water-pik, extra-soft toothbrush, or oral swab may be useful in removing debris and residue that adheres to mucosal surfaces.

### Screening
- Patients should be examined at least weekly to check for signs of mucosal injury and infection.
- Fungal infection is extremely common and should be anticipated in the majority of patients receiving radiation to the mouth or throat (58).

### Treatment
- The majority of oral infections in patients with mucositis are due to *Candida albicans* but other *Candida* species are often present (59):
  - Typically whitish, cottony appearance.
  - May be easily confused with early mucositis or pseudomembrane formation.
  - Commonly treated either topically or systemically:
    - Nystatin rinse;
    - Clotrimazole troche;
    - Fluconazole is an effective drug of choice in many cases (60).
  - Fluconazole interacts with many drugs and may be contraindicated in some patients; nystatin is systemically absorbed to a much lesser extent but has the disadvantage of a bad taste contained in a heavily sugared solution which may cause gastrointestinal upset (61).
  - One small study showed a reduction in severe mucositis with fluconazole prophylaxis (62).

- In the less than 10% of cases of infection refractory to fluconazole, lesions should be cultured to ascertain species and sensitivity; alternative azoles may be required (63).
- Herpes simplex virus (HSV) accounts for most other severe infections, especially in transplant patients.
  - May occur in over one-fourth of patients with ulcerative radiation mucositis (64).
  - Treated effectively with acyclovir or valacyclovir.
- For intraoral bacterial infections, minocycline or tetracycline have shown efficacy when added to dental rinse solutions (65–67).

## Nausea

### Definition

- Nausea consists of gastrointestinal discomfort and a sensation of wanting to vomit which may precede actual vomiting.
- Nausea is a common side effect in patients undergoing any cancer therapy.

### Timing

- May occur in patients who have received more than 3 weeks of radiation treatment;
- Often related to timing of radiation and/or chemotherapy administration.

### Prevention

- The best treatment of nausea is prevention.
- Fifty percent to 80% of patients undergoing radiation and all patients undergoing systemic therapy treatments should be considered at some level of risk (68).
- Preventive medications should be prescribed in advance of the anticipated symptoms, to a level concordant with the risk associated with the specific regimen (69).

### Screening

- Patient factors that increase the risk of nausea:
  - Prior nausea reactions;
  - Younger patient age;
  - Female gender (70,71);
  - Recent or current exposure to emetogenic systemic therapy agents (72).
- The characteristics of the RT strongly influence the likelihood of experiencing nausea or vomiting:
  - Large-scale mucosal irradiation increases the risk of inflammatory secretions and tissue edema which worsen the sensation of nausea.
  - Brain and skull base irradiation may affect the physiologic vomiting center in the medulla or the chemoreceptor trigger zone in the base of the fourth ventricle.

- Patients receiving concurrent radiosensitizing chemotherapy that is emetogenic experience combined effects (73).
  - Cisplatin is the most emetogenic chemotherapy agent in common use.
  - Any patient receiving any form of systemic therapy is considered at increased risk for nausea.

*Treatment*

- Major classes of antinausea agents (73):
  - Antihistamines (diphenhydramine, meclizine);
  - Anticholinergics (scopolamine);
  - Benzodiazepines (lorazepam);
  - Steroids (dexamethasone, methylprednisolone);
  - Dopamine antagonists (metoclopramide, prochlorperazine, promethazine);
  - 5-HT receptor (serotonin) antagonists (ondansetron, granisetron, palonosetron);
  - Substance P antagonists (aprepitant, fosaprepitant);
- Evolving treatment paradigms:
  - An antipsychotic medication, olanzapine, was recently found to be more effective than metoclopramide, and as effective as aprepitant in combination with 5-HT antagonists (74–76).
  - Dronabinol, a synthetic form of the active ingredient in cannabis, is approved for refractory chemotherapy–induced nausea and vomiting (77–79).
  - The efficacy of ginger is supported by only limited data (80).
- Patients at high risk for nausea should take a 5-HT antagonist with consideration of around-the-clock scheduled use and may also require short preparatory or pulsed courses of dexamethasone.
- Substance P antagonists are not yet clearly indicated for RT-induced nausea, but are highly effective in patients who take chemotherapy.
- Patients experiencing nausea may find it difficult to ingest oral medications, and effective management may require intravenous or transdermal administration of antinausea medications.

## Fatigue

*Definition*

- Fatigue is a "distressing, persistent, subjective sense of physical, emotional and/or cognitive tiredness or exhaustion related to cancer or cancer treatment that is not proportional to recent activity and interferes with usual functioning" (81).
- Causes are very uncertain, with theories related to (82):
  - Inflammatory mediators released during treatment;
  - Stress of transportation to daily radiation treatment;
  - The emotional stress of cancer;

- Effects due to circulating cancer cells or the malignant cancer mass itself;
- Sleep disturbance related to treatments;
- The very common usage of steroids during cancer therapy;
- A combination of all of these factors.

## *Timing*

- The onset may occur after as little as a week of exposure to RT.
- Effects may linger for a few to several months or even years.

## *Prevention*

- Avoid excessive use of steroids at night if possible.
- Encourage excellent sleep hygiene:
  - Avoidance of alcohol or late meals in the evening;
  - Reduced emotional and physical stimulation prior to sleep time;
  - Removal of light sources and noise from the room.
- Address any potential medical causes of fatigue such as:
  - Medication effects;
  - Uncontrolled pain;
  - Anemia;
  - Malnutrition;
  - Psychological or psychiatric disorder;
  - Physiologic reasons for sleep disturbance such as obesity or altered airway;
  - Renal, cardiac, or pulmonary dysfunction;
  - Endocrine dysfunction such as hypothyroidism or hypogonadism.

## *Screening*

- Almost all patients undergoing large-scale RT complain of some level of fatigue.
- The National Comprehensive Cancer Network (NCCN) guidelines recommend assessing fatigue with the question, "How would you rate your fatigue on a scale of 0 to 10 over the past 7 days?" (81).

## *Treatment*

- Short-acting benzodiazepines are not recommended for addressing sleep disturbance in elderly adults due to side effects:
  - Tolerance and addiction;
  - Rebound insomnia;
  - Reduced deep sleep;
  - Daytime fatigue and cognitive impairment;
  - Increased risk for vehicular accidents and falls.

- Nonbenzodiazepine hypnotics (zolpidem, eszopiclone):
  - May produce less tolerance and rebound effect than benzodiazepines;
  - Use for more than a few weeks is discouraged due to similar long-term effects.
- Nonpharmacologic interventions include:
  - Increased exercise;
  - Strict sleep hygiene and better regulation of the sleep-wake cycle;
  - Psychosocial or cognitive-behavioral interventions (83);
  - Nutritional counseling;
  - Meditation, yoga, and mindfulness-based stress reduction methods (84,85).
- Stimulants (methylphenidate, modafinil) (86,87):
  - Have been used to combat daytime fatigue;
  - In randomized trials, showed no improved effect over placebo (88).

## Depression

### Definition

- Depression is a mood disorder characterized by:
  - Persistent feelings of sadness and/or anxiety;
  - Loss of interest or pleasure in hobbies and activities;
  - Decreased energy;
  - Feelings of hopelessness, helplessness, and irritability.
- Patients may have difficulty concentrating, remembering things, or making decisions.
- Patients may have sleep disturbances, such as oversleeping, not wanting to wake up, or waking up in the middle of the night.
- Patients may have appetite or weight changes.

### Timing

- It may be coincident with cancer diagnosis or may be of long-standing nature that preceded the cancer diagnosis and is exacerbated by it.
- Exacerbation of underlying mood disorder may become acutely apparent during any phase of the process of cancer workup and treatment.
- Among patients with head and neck cancer, the incidence of major depressive disorder is 15% to 50% (89,90).

### Prevention

- While prevention of depression is not possible, its detrimental effects on the quality of care can be prevented with screening, identification, and prompt referral to a qualified mental health specialist.

*Screening*

- Screening for depression is recommended for head and neck cancer patients in the NCCN guidelines; practitioners are referred to the NCCN guidelines in "distress management."
  - Specific details of screening tools or recommendations for action when depression is identified are limited, due to a wide variety in the availability of mental health services and approaches to management of depression.
- Suicidality, with a specific plan to harm oneself, or psychosis, is an indication for urgent hospitalization.
  - A 24-hour, toll-free National Suicide Prevention Lifeline is accessible at 1-800-273-TALK (8255) or www.suicidepreventionlifeline.org.

*Treatment*

- Management of pain and other physical symptoms should be instituted before or with initiation of antidepressant treatment.
- Pharmacologic intervention (91):
  - Should be considered for moderate to severe major depression;
  - Should be combined with psychosocial interventions.
- Major classes of antidepressant medications include:
  - Selective serotonin reuptake inhibitors (SSRI);
  - Serotonin and norepinephrine reuptake inhibitors (SNRI);
  - Tricyclic antidepressants (TCA);
  - Monoamine oxidase inhibitors (MAOI);
  - Unique medications such as mirtazapine and bupropion.
- All antidepressants carry a U.S. Food and Drug Administration (FDA)-mandated black box warning:
  - In some cases, children, teenagers, and young adults under age 25 years may experience an increase in suicidal thoughts or behavior when taking antidepressants.
  - This is especially in the first few weeks of starting a new antidepressant or changing a dose of medication.
  - Patients of all ages taking antidepressants should be watched closely.
  - Prompt referral to a qualified mental health specialist is mandatory.

## Alopecia

*Definition*

- Alopecia, or epilation of the hair-bearing skin, is due to the high susceptibility of the growing hair follicles to ionizing radiation.

*Timing*

- Hair loss is related to the radiation dose received to the hair follicles in the hair-bearing regions of the skin.

- At 3 Gy, there is early reversible alopecia, while some degree of permanent alopecia begins to occur at doses above 7 Gy to 8 Gy (92).
- Complete hair regrowth will occur by 2 to 4 months after the occurrence of reversible radiation-induced alopecia.

### Prevention

- Exiting radiation beams can be assessed to predict where the greatest areas of hair loss will occur (93).
- Dosimetric protection of hair-bearing areas (such as used in the "scalp sparing technique") is effective at reducing hair loss (94,95).
- Preventives under study include nitroxides (Tempol), vitamin $D_3$, or prostaglandins (96–98).

### Treatment

- To reduce hair loss and encourage regrowth, patients may be counseled to:
  - Avoid sun exposure to the scalp.
  - Treat the hair gently using a soft brush and gentle shampoo.
  - Avoid use of heat on the hair, such as hair dryer, hot rollers, or curling irons.
  - Avoid use of bleach or hair dyes or permanent curling solutions.
  - Use a wig or hat.
- Reconstructive surgical procedures such as scalp tissue expansion and hair transplantation can address permanent alopecia (99).

## Pain

### Timing

- In head and neck oncology, pain is often a tumor-revealing problem—approximately 50% of cancer patients have pain at diagnosis (100).
- A majority of patients will develop pain during treatment.
- Approximately one-third of patients will note posttreatment pain months after completion of therapy.
- The presentation of worsening pain in the head and neck cancer survivor is a strong indicator of tumor recurrence. A diagnosis of chronic pain is made only after tumor recurrence has been ruled out with physical examination, imaging, and/or biopsy.

### Prevention

- Posttreatment chronic pain is a complex, multifactorial problem.
- Chronic pain may result from permanent damage to the oral soft tissues, including epithelial atrophy, submucosal fibrosis, and/or neuropathy.
- Avoidance of mouth irritants can help minimize/prevent posttreatment pain: tobacco smoke, harsh mouthwash, alcohol (101).
- Prior to the initiation of radiation, patients should have a comprehensive oral assessment with extraction of nonrestorable teeth.

*Screening*

All evaluations in the follow-up setting should record pain on a 1 to 10 scale.

*Treatment*
- Physical therapy/massage therapy
  - Although frequently prescribed, investigations into the efficacy of posttreatment physical therapy are incomplete.
  - Progressive resistance exercise training (PRET) significantly reduced shoulder pain when compared to standard therapeutic exercises for patients managed with a head and neck operation (102).
- Acupuncture
  - A randomized trial of acupuncture once a week for 4 weeks versus usual care demonstrated a significant amelioration of symptoms related to shoulder pain from a neck dissection among head and neck cancer survivors (103).
- Topical and nonnarcotic agents
  - In the setting of radiation mucositis during treatment, patients may develop protracted mucosal sensitivity.
  - Topical rinses (magic mouthwash and mucosal lidocaine) can provide temporary mucosal relief.
  - Anti-inflammatory medications are often prescribed, although little data is available to ascertain the degree of relief that these medications provide.
- Narcotic pain medications
  - If nonnarcotic attempts to ameliorate pain are unsuccessful, narcotic pain medications can be employed.

## LATE TOXICITY
### External Lymphedema/Fibrosis
*Definition*

External lymphedema describes symptoms pertaining to the skin and subcutaneous/deep soft tissues of the face, neck, and shoulders. It may result in swelling, tightness, and decreased range of motion with associated limited range of motion and discomfort.

*Timing*
- Can be appreciated as early as 3 months after completion of head and neck therapy (104).
- Severity can increase with time, as lymphedema results when the lymphatic load exceeds the transport capacity of the lymphatic system secondary to tumor and/or surgery and/or radiation (105).

*Prevention*
- For many patients secondary lymphedema may be unavoidable.
- Avoidance of bilateral neck dissections (106) if an oncologically safe alternative is available.

## Screening

- External lymphedema/fibrosis occurs in approximately 50% of head and neck cancer patients.
- Patients note many symptoms consistent with fibrosis on routine follow-up ("stiffness," "tightness," "pain").
- Tape measurement, useful in other areas of lymphedema (eg, extremity) is not useful secondary to no consistent and reproducible reference points.
- A preliminary evaluation of a 65-item PRO tool has been reported (107); however, it is unclear how this PRO will be handled in addition to the many PROs utilized in the management of head and neck cancer survivors.
- There is no validated, reliable, clinically useful tool for clinicians to monitor external lymphedema in the head and neck cancer patients.
- Major discrepancies exist between physician-based and patient based assessments of fibrosis (108).

## Treatment

- Complete decongestive therapy (CDT) has four components:
  - Manual lymph drainage (MLD);
  - Use of compression garments and pads;
  - Skin care;
  - Basic face, neck, and oral cavity exercises.
- CDT improves head and neck lymphedema in 60% of patients (109).
- Outpatient CDT seems to be more successful than patient-directed CDT at home.
- Pentoxifylline + vitamin E can be effective in the management of radiation induced fibrosis (110):
  - Pentoxifylline dose is 800 mg/day;
  - Vitamin E dose is 1000 IU/day;
  - Duration of therapy can be long (at least 6 months).
- Early physical therapy after neck dissection is associated with increased range of motion of the shoulder (111).

## Evidence

Mucosal head and neck squamous cancer has a proclivity to metastasize to lymph nodes, and is frequently regionally advanced at diagnosis (often requiring multimodality therapy to the neck)—therefore, secondary lymphedema/fibrosis is often unavoidable. It is therefore not surprising that an estimated 50% of patients treated for head and neck cancer develop this symptom. Although the current understanding suggests that lymphedema and fibrosis have different underlying mechanisms (112), and certain patients will develop only one and not the other (eg, fibrosis in absence of lymphedema), they share common inflammatory components and are therefore typically evaluated together (113).

Some component of prevention is possible with judicious treatment choices during initial management. Bilateral neck dissections as initial therapy should be avoided when an oncologically safe alternative is available secondary to high rates of posttreatment lymphedema (106). Postradiation bilateral neck dissections should be avoided as the practice is associated with higher rates of posttreatment complications than unilateral neck dissections (114), and observation of an initially involved but post (chemo) radiation "low risk" hemi-neck seems safe (115). In a similar vein, multimodality therapy should be avoided when single modality therapy will suffice as the incidence of external fibrosis increases with an increasing number of treatment modalities used in the pursuit of cure. Single modality treatment has a lower risk of external lymphedema than either surgery + postop RT or chemoRT.

## Pharynx: Dysphagia

### Definition

Difficulty swallowing, often described as food hanging up or getting stuck, increased choking. Posttreatment dysphagia is a recognized but incompletely understood complication of head and neck cancer therapy.

### Timing

- Certain patients will present with pretreatment dysphagia due to local effects of the primary tumor.
- Most patients will be swallowing worse than baseline at 3 months after head and neck (chemo)radiation—regardless of eventual long-term swallowing function (116).
- Development of dysphagia manifested as aspiration pneumonia and/or gastrostomy tube placement can occur more than 5 years after completion of treatment (117).

### Prevention

- Avoid unnecessary irradiation to the uninvolved larynx (118).
  - Mean larynx dose to be less than 35 Gy.
- Avoid unnecessary irradiation to the uninvolved pharyngeal constrictors. This does not impair tumor control and is associated with a low rate of dysphagia at 1 year posttreatment (119).
  - Mean dose to the uninvolved pharynx to be less than 40 Gy;
  - Pharyngeal constrictor avoidance is contraindicated in the following situations
    - Grossly positive retropharyngeal lymph node(s);
    - Tumor involvement of the posterior pharyngeal wall.
- Avoid transoral surgery for T4 base-of-tongue tumors (120).
- The consequences of prophylactic gastrostomy tube placement are controversial and subject to institutional bias. Avoidance of gastrostomy tube placement has been reported as a means to prevent long-term dysphagia.

- "Pharyngocise"
  - A small randomized controlled trial suggested that active swallowing exercises during chemoradiation improved swallowing outcomes when compared to both "usual care" and a sham intervention (121).

## Screening

- All patients (even those who report no swallowing difficulty) should be evaluated by a speech language pathologist (SLP) for a formal swallowing evaluation prior to the initiation of head and neck radiation.
  - Patients can be instructed to do a series of exercises during treatment to promote strength and mobility of key swallowing musculature.
- All patients should be evaluated by the SLP after the completion of head and neck radiation.
- Every follow-up examination for a head and neck cancer survivor should include screening questions to ascertain if swallowing is worsening.
- Any history of "pneumonia" reported by the head and neck cancer survivor should be evaluated with a formal swallowing evaluation by an SLP to ascertain if aspiration is occurring.

## Treatment

- Appropriate swallowing rehabilitation can eliminate aspiration, decrease the risk of pneumonia, and successfully return more than 75% of select patients who aspirate to oral intake years after treatment (122).
- Serial esophageal dilation can open radiation-related esophageal strictures even in cases of complete or near-complete closure (123).

## Evidence

There are four components to a normal swallow—the oral preparatory phase, the oral phase, the pharyngeal phase, and the esophageal phase. Depending on the location of a primary tumor and the treatment modalities employed to eradicate, head and neck cancer treatment can affect one or more phases of a normal swallow, resulting in dysphagia for head and neck cancer patients.

Prevention starts with treatment planning. The supraglottic and glottic larynx should be contoured as an organ at risk (124) and incorporated into the treatment planning algorithm (125). A mean dose level of less than 35 Gy to the uninvolved larynx is recommended in the setting of bilateral neck radiation; for unilateral neck radiation a lower mean dose level is often achievable. Given that the dose to the larynx is thought to be a continuous function, less dose to the organ below established guidelines that does not compromise target coverage should be pursued.

It is extremely important that radiation oncologists be aware of the potential for swallowing difficulties in head and neck cancer patients. Prior to treatment, clinical evaluation alone cannot detect silent aspirators (126). After chemoradiation, it is estimated that as many as 50% of patients silently aspirate (127). Whether it is before the initiation of (chemo)radiation or during follow-up, a low threshold should exist to refer patients for a speech and swallowing evaluation. This is useful for both diagnosis of speech and swallowing dysfunction and institution of appropriate swallowing rehabilitation.

Appropriate swallowing rehabilitation is encouragingly successful—even years after treatment. Practitioners with head and neck practices should be familiar with frequent referrals to an SLP and/or speech/swallowing center.

## Dental Issues and Osteoradionecrosis (ORN) of the Jaw

*Dental QOL*

Dental status has a significant impact on the QOL of head and neck cancer survivors. Many patients have poor dentition at diagnosis, and poor dentition posttreatment increases the risk of ORN and infection.

The reduced quantity and altered composition of saliva that is encountered after radiation treatment to the head and neck is known to increase the incidence of dental caries. Patients should meet with a dentist prior the initiation of RT (in general, an evaluation within the past month is desired). Long-term fluoride and diligent oral hygiene are a must after the completion of therapy

### Osteoradionecrosis

*Definition*

Exposed, irradiated bone in the absence of recurrent or residual tumor. It is a complication of radiation resulting from obliterative endarteritis and decreased vascular supply in irradiated bone—leading to hypoxic areas in the bone that are less able to tolerate an injury (surgery, dental extractions, etc.) (128). The mandible is the most commonly affected bone. This is likely due to the fact that a larger part of the mandible is typically exposed to high doses of radiation than the maxilla (129) and has a poorer blood supply than the maxilla (130).

*Timing*

- Wide variation in onset;
- Can be diagnosed anytime from shortly after the completion of radiation to many years posttreatment during survivorship (129).

*Prevention*

- Pretreatment dental evaluation—all nonrestorable teeth should be extracted prior to the initiation of radiation (131).
- Postradiation fluoride prophylaxis—fluoride gel applied for 5 minutes per day in custom trays reduces caries by 92% in irradiated head and neck cancer patients, provided that compliance exceeds 70% (132).
- Conformal radiation
  - Limiting high-dose regions to the mandible/maxilla with highly conformal radiation plans along strict dental hygiene results in a low risk of ORN (133). However, some reports suggest that the use of IMRT does not significantly decrease the risk of ORN when compared to 3D conformal RT (3DCRT) (134).

- Reduced radiation dose to the parotid gland with IMRT results in both increased salivary output and increased recovery when compared to 3DCRT (135).
  - Mean dose to contralateral parotid to be less than 20 Gy;
  - Mean dose to bilateral parotid composite contour to be less than 26 Gy (17).
- Reduced radiation dose to the parotid leads to better posttreatment salivation and avoidance of posttreatment dental caries, although the patient-reported QOL benefit to parotid avoidance is unclear (136).
- Reduced radiation dose to the submandibular gland results in increased mucin-containing resting saliva (137).
- Reduced dose to the oral cavity is associated with improved patient-reported QOL, likely secondary to better posttreatment salivation (138).
- Preradiation extractions of healthy teeth do **not** seem to decrease the incidence of ORN (139).

### *Screening*

- Every patient who has received external beam radiation that delivers dose to either the oral cavity or a major salivary gland should be considered a "high-risk" dental patient for the remainder of their life.
  - From a practical standpoint, this is almost all mucosal squamous cell carcinoma of the head and neck except the T1-2 true vocal cord patient.
- High-risk dental patients should see a dentist at least every 3 to 6 months for routine cleaning and surveillance.
- Posttreatment tumor surveillance follow-up should include a detailed oral cavity examination for evaluation of recurrence/second primary and surveillance for ORN.
- A panoramic scanning dental x-ray of the upper and lower jaw obtained in the dentist office (panorex) that demonstrates bone loss should be evaluated further.
- Any CT that images the mandible that is interpreted as osteomyelitis in a head and neck cancer survivor should be evaluated for concomitant ORN.

### *Treatment*

- Good oral hygiene
  - Regular rinses, brushing, and flossing.
  - Rinses should be either nonacidic fluoride preparations or bicarbonate preparations.
  - Brushing and flossing should be gentle and thorough.
- Antibiotics and conservative debridement for early and limited ORN
  - There is no standard antibiotic regimen for ORN (140).
  - Antibiotic therapy should either be based on gram stain results or empiric to cover oral microbes.

- Conservative debridement (141).
  - Local wound irrigation;
  - Curettage;
  - Debridement;
  - Sequestrectomy.
- Hyperbaric oxygen
  - Hyperbaric oxygen is used by many medical centers to prevent/treat ORN.
  - It is a time-consuming process requiring 30 to 40 treatment "dives," generally once daily for 6 to 8 weeks. Each dive takes 90 to 120 minutes.
  - The most common side effects are myopia (reversible) and barotrauma.
  - Prevention using hyperbaric oxygen:
    - This refers to the situation where trauma to an irradiated mandible/maxilla is planned, but there is no exposed bone or symptoms. Most commonly this is a mandibular extraction.
    - Teeth that received a dose higher than 50 Gy have a higher rate of ORN and generally trigger a recommendation of hyperbaric oxygen.
    - A randomized controlled trial suggests that the incidence of ORN after planned extractions is significantly lower with prophylactic hyperbaric oxygen (142).
    - The rate of ORN in the arm without hyperbaric oxygen is much higher (30%) than that of patients managed without hyperbaric oxygen in more modern series (143).
    - In general, hyperbaric oxygen is still recommended for patients needing extractions on the basis of weak evidence.
  - Treatment of overt ORN using hyperbaric oxygen:
    - This refers to the situation where a patient has signs and/or symptoms of ORN:
      - Pain;
      - Dysesthesia in the inferior alveolar nerve distribution;
      - Areas of bone exposure visible on exam;
      - Trismus;
      - Fistula.
    - A randomized trial comparing hyperbaric oxygen versus placebo suggested that hyperbaric oxygen was associated with worse outcomes than placebo (144):
      - The trial was stopped early secondary to early data demonstrating no benefit to the intervention.
      - It is unclear why one-third of the patients randomized to the placebo arm improved (10% recovery was expected).
    - A retrospective questionnaire administered to patients after the completion of hyperbaric oxygen reported that a majority of patients noted that their symptoms were improved after hyperbaric oxygen (145).

- Pentoxifylline and tocopherol +/− clodronate
  - Pentoxifylline is a methylxanthine derivative that exerts an antitumor necrosis factor (TNF)-alpha effect, increases erythrocyte flexibility, vasodilates, inhibits inflammatory reactions in vivo, and inhibits human dermal fibroblast proliferation.
  - PENTOCLO regimen demonstrates a high rate of success in poor-prognosis ORN (146).
  - PENTOCLO regimen
    - Five days a week:
      - Pentoxifylline 800 mg;
      - Vitamin E 1000 IU;
      - Clodronate 1600 mg.
    - Two others days weekly:
      - Prednisone 20 mg;
      - Ciprofloxacin 1000 mg.
  - The PENTOCLO regimen is designed to be taken long term
    - Median treatment was 16 ± 9 months.
- Resection
  - Resection and immediate microvascular reconstruction can remedy refractory ORN (147).

## Hearing Loss

### Timing

- Interval between completion of RT and development of persistent sensorineural hearing loss (SNHL) is 1 to 2 years.
- Range of development of SNHL is 0.5 to 6 years.
- Late hearing loss is likely multifactorial.
- Latency between completion of radiation and development of SNHL does not seem to be influenced by increasing radiation dose and/or concomitant cisplatin (148).

### Prevention

- Given the known ototoxicity of cisplatin, all patients scheduled to receive cisplatin require a baseline audiogram prior to the start of therapy (even if the patient professes that hearing is not difficult).
- Sensorineural hearing loss
  - Cisplatin is highly ototoxic.
    - Use of concurrent cisplatin should be limited to patients for whom there is a definite benefit.
      - Definitive chemoradiation
        - Stage III to IV (T1-2 N2-3 and/or T3-4).
      - Adjuvant chemoradiation
        - Positive margins;
        - Extracapsular spread.

- Related to radiation dose to the cochlea/middle ear.
  - The cochlea/middle ear should be contoured as an avoidance structure (149).
  - Because the volume is small (often <0.5 cc if the cochlea alone is contoured), it should be evaluated as a mean dose function.
  - The radiation dose limit recommendations are lower when cisplatin is used concurrently (150).
    - RT alone: Cochlea dose to be less than 40 Gy;
    - ChemoRT: Cochlea dose to be less than 10 Gy.
- Conductive hearing loss
  - Related to radiation dose to the Eustachian tube/middle ear;
  - Pathogenesis is unclear, but seems related to the following:
    - Direct radiation irritation to the middle ear causing inflammation and tissue fluid increase, obstructing recirculation;
    - Direct radiation damage to the cartilage, cilium, and tensor veli palatine, decreasing normal functions of the Eustachian tube.
  - The ear canal can be considered an avoidance structure when oncologically safe
    - Median dose to develop middle ear complications
      - 60 Gy (45–80 Gy) (148).

## Screening

- Any patient complaining of hearing loss to any member of the head and neck team or any physician should be referred for a screening audiogram.
- Should the audiogram demonstrate dysfunction or worsening in ability from the pretreatment screening evaluation, a referral to an otologist is indicated.
- In absence of symptoms/patient complaint, routine hearing screening is not indicated.

## Treatment

- Sensorineural hearing loss
  - Hearing aids.
- Conductive hearing loss
  - Most instances of radiation-induced serous effusion resolve spontaneously.
  - For cases that do not respond spontaneously, management by an otolaryngologist is recommended.
    - Tympanostomy + aspiration (may need to be repeated, ultimate success rate 30%–50%);
    - Myringotomy + grommet insertion (151).

## Voice Dysfunction

*Definition*

Often presents as hoarseness, but can include garbled speech and any difficulty with pitch, quality, and clarity. Fluent and coherent speech is the result of a complex process that involves not only the glottic larynx, but the oral cavity and pharynx in combination with adequate lubrication from functioning salivary glands. Therefore, damage to any components of the upper aerodigestive tract can manifest as problems with speech. However, it is important to understand that difficulty with speech may be a presenting symptom of tumor recurrence. Only after recurrence/second primary tumor has been ruled out should a diagnosis of late radiation toxicity be assigned for voice dysfunction in head and neck cancer survivors. Dysphonia is an underappreciated long-term side effect of head and neck cancer treatment.

*Timing*

- Many tumors can cause speech dysfunction at diagnosis.
- Many patients present with an acquired speech problem as a result of head and neck surgery.
- Direct radiation effects to the upper aerodigestive tract can cause speech problems during a course of radiation (152).
- Late radiation cranial nerve (ie, CN X or XII) dysfunction can appear many years after the completion of therapy, causing speech difficulties (153).

*Prevention*

- All patients should see an SLP prior to the initiation of head and neck cancer treatment for speech exercise training that will continue through a course of head and neck radiation.
  - Tongue range of motion exercises.
- Dose avoidance to the glottic larynx and supraglottic larynx:
  - Mean dose of less than 35 Gy is typically recommended (125).
  - However, data demonstrates worse patient-reported outcomes as dose increases over 20 Gy (154)—dose to larynx should be as low as possible while still covering target.

*Screening*

- All patients should be evaluated by the SLP after the completion of head and neck radiation.
- All patients should specifically be asked if they are satisfied with their voice quality during posttreatment evaluation.
  - Patients' perceived changes in voice and speech quality post-versus pretreatment correlate weakly with expert judgment (155).

*Treatment*

- Voice therapy
  - Patients who receive voice rehabilitation posttreatment report better self-rated voice function (156).
- Injection laryngoplasty
  - Vocal fold medicalization can improve speech outcomes for patients with unilateral vocal cord paralysis after radiation (157).

## Peripheral Neuropathy

*Definition*

Neuropathic pain or weakness. Lhermitte's syndrome is a relatively common occurrence presenting as an electrical-type sharp pain running from the neck down to the upper extremities. The brachial plexus is a network of nerves formed by the anterior rami of the four most inferior cervical nerves (C5, C6, C7, C8) and the most superior thoracic nerve (T1). It passes inferiomedially between the anterior and middle scalene muscles to the subclavian artery and laterally beneath the clavicle and into the axilla. From a head and neck cancer perspective, the brachial plexus is in the low neck (level 4 and the supraclavicular fossa). It is responsible for the cutaneous and muscular innervation of the upper limb. A brachial plexus injury from a single course of radiation is rare.

*Timing*

- Median time to development of a brachial plexus injury is more than 2 years (158).
- Earliest reported injury is at 6 months.
- Injuries are known to develop after 6 years since the completion of radiation.

*Prevention*

- Brachial plexopathy is a radiation dose–related phenomenon.
- The brachial plexus should be contoured as an avoidance structure (159).
- Dose limit: V70 higher than 10% (158).
- Unclear if other aggravating factors can predispose to development of symptoms at a lower dose level (cisplatin chemotherapy, surgical manipulation, diabetes).

*Screening*

- Most common symptom is pain.
- Formal brachial plexopathy (pain, numbness, tingling, and weakness) is rare, even at high doses of radiation.
- Nerve conduction analyses of patients with suspected brachial plexus injury can confirm:
  - Demyelination resulting in reduced sensory conduction;
  - Differences in latency and amplitude between affected and unaffected arm;
  - Reduced motor conduction nerve velocity.

### Treatment
- Hyperbaric oxygen does not seem to reverse the symptoms of radiation-induced brachial plexopathy (160).
- There is no data that pentoxifylline reverses the symptoms of radiation-induced brachial plexopathy.

## Psychosocial/Economic Effects
### Definition
Anxiety, mood disorders, fatigue, and depression are common in head and neck cancer survivors, although these important symptoms are sometimes overlooked. In addition, facial disfigurement, loss of function precluding normal social function (eg, eating in a restaurant), and lack of employment impact the posttreatment QOL.

### Timing
- Many patients report psychosocial problems at diagnosis (ie, prior to treatment).
- Patient issues with body disfigurement and limitations with speech/swallowing/other normal daily functions are thought to improve over time (161) with the patience and compassion of family and friends.
- The economic impact of head and neck cancer is immediate. Attendance to daily radiation treatments is often impossible to reconcile with a work schedule, and often requires a leave of absence. Returning to work may take months after treatment is complete. The treatment itself is expensive, even in the setting of single modality therapy (162).

### Prevention
Encourage support group participation—many centers have support groups comprising of head and neck cancer patients, caregivers, and family with a facilitator (generally a SLP and/or counselor and/or social worker).

### Screening
- Patients with body image changing operations should be evaluated for consequences of the operation, even many years later.
- Factors that predict for depression (163):
  - Tracheostomy and/or laryngeal stoma;
  - Gastrostomy tube dependence;
  - Continued smoking.

### Treatment
- Improvement of functional aspects of the head and neck damaged by tumors and/or treatment can improve psychosocial outlook.
- Reports suggest that mental health services are severely underutilized among head and neck cancer survivors (163). Appropriate referrals are indicated.
- Many patients reported symptom improvement over time, but the interval to improvement may be 12 to 18 months from the completion of radiation.

# REFERENCES

1. Simonen P, Hamilton C, Ferguson S, et al. Do inflammatory processes contribute to radiation induced erythema observed in the skin of humans? *Radiother Oncol.* 1998;46(1):73–82.
2. Schmuth M, Sztankay A, Weinlich G, et al. Permeability barrier function of skin exposed to ionizing radiation. *Arch Dermatol.* 2001;137(8):1019–1023.
3. Fowble B. *Skin care in radiation oncology: a practical guide.* New York, NY: Springer Science+Business Media; 2016.
4. McQuestion M. Evidence-based skin care management in radiation therapy: clinical update. *Seminars in oncology nursing.* 2011;27(2):e1–e17.
5. Fisher DA. Adverse effects of topical corticosteroid use. *West J Med.* 1995;162(2):123–126.
6. Cox JD, Stetz J, Pajak TF. Toxicity criteria of the Radiation Therapy Oncology Group (RTOG) and the European Organization for Research and Treatment of Cancer (EORTC). *Int J Radiat Oncol Biol Phys.* 1995;31(5):1341–1346.
7. LENT SOMA scales for all anatomic sites. *Int J Radiat Oncol Biol Phys.* 1995;31(5):1049–1091.
8. National Cancer Institute. Common Terminology Criteria for Adverse Events. http://ctep.cancer.gov/protocolDevelopment/electronic_applications/ctc.htm. Updated November 14, 2016.
9. Lacouture ME, Maitland ML, Segaert S, et al. A proposed EGFR inhibitor dermatologic adverse event-specific grading scale from the MASCC skin toxicity study group. *Support Care Cancer.* 2010;18(4):509–522.
10. Noble-Adams R. Radiation-induced skin reactions. 3: Evaluating the RISRAS. *Br J Nurs.* 1999;8(19):1305–1312.
11. Catterall M, Rogers C, Thomlinson RH, Field SB. An investigation into the clinical effects of fast neutrons. Methods and early observations. *Br J Radiol.* 1971;44(524):603–611.
12. Chren MM, Lasek RJ, Quinn LM, et al. Skindex, a quality-of-life measure for patients with skin disease: reliability, validity, and responsiveness. *J Invest Dermatol.* 1996;107(5):707–713.
13. Rhee JS, Matthews BA, Neuburg M, et al. The skin cancer index: clinical responsiveness and predictors of quality of life. *Laryngoscope.* 2007;117(3):399–405.
14. Lewis V, Finlay AY. 10 years experience of the Dermatology Life Quality Index (DLQI). *J Investig Dermatol Symp Proc.* 2004;9(2):169–180.
15. Wagner LI, Berg SR, Gandhi M, et al. The development of a Functional Assessment of Cancer Therapy (FACT) questionnaire to assess dermatologic symptoms associated with epidermal growth factor receptor inhibitors (FACT-EGFRI-18). *Support Care Cancer.* 2013;21(4):1033–1041.
16. Sibaud V, Dalenc F, Chevreau C, et al. HFS-14, a specific quality of life scale developed for patients suffering from hand-foot syndrome. *Oncologist.* 2011;16(10):1469–1478.
17. Deasy JO, Moiseenko V, Marks L, et al. Radiotherapy dose-volume effects on salivary gland function. *Int J Radiat Oncol Biol Phys.* 2010;76(3, Suppl):S58–S63.
18. Johnson JT, Ferretti GA, Nethery WJ, et al. Oral pilocarpine for post-irradiation xerostomia in patients with head and neck cancer. *N Engl J Med.* 1993;329(6):390–395.
19. Zhuang L, Yang Z, Zeng X, et al. The preventive and therapeutic effect of acupuncture for radiation-induced xerostomia in patients with head and neck cancer: a systematic review. *Integr Cancer Ther.* 2013;12(3):197–205.

20. Wong R, Major P, Sagar S. Phase 2 study of acupuncture-like transcutaneous nerve stimulation for chemotherapy-induced peripheral neuropathy. *Integr Cancer Ther.* 2016;15(2):153–164.

21. Mossman K, Shatzman A, Chencharick J. Long-term effects of radiotherapy on taste and salivary function in man. *Int J Radiat Oncol Biol Phys.* 1982;8(6): 991–997.

22. Irune E, Dwivedi RC, Nutting CM, Harrington KJ. Treatment-related dysgeusia in head and neck cancer patients. *Cancer Treat Rev.* 2014;40(9):1106–1117.

23. Mirza N, Machtay M, Devine PA, et al. Gustatory impairment in patients undergoing head and neck irradiation. *Laryngoscope.* 2008;118(1):24–31.

24. Conger AD. Loss and recovery of taste acuity in patients irradiated to the oral cavity. *Radiat Res.* 1973;53(2):338–347.

25. Shatzman AR, Mossman KL. Radiation effects on bovine taste bud membranes. *Radiat Res.* 1982;92(2):353–358.

26. Sapir E, Tao Y, Feng F, et al. Predictors of dysgeusia in patients with oropharyngeal cancer treated with chemotherapy and intensity modulated radiation therapy. *Int J Radiat Oncol Biol Phys.* 2016;96(2):354–361.

27. Halyard MY, Jatoi A, Sloan JA, et al. Does zinc sulfate prevent therapy-induced taste alterations in head and neck cancer patients? Results of phase III double-blind, placebo-controlled trial from the North Central Cancer Treatment Group (N01C4). *Int J Radiat Oncol Biol Phys.* 2007;67(5):1318–1322.

28. Ripamonti C, Zecca E, Brunelli C, et al. A randomized, controlled clinical trial to evaluate the effects of zinc sulfate on cancer patients with taste alterations caused by head and neck irradiation. *Cancer.* 1998;82(10):1938–1945.

29. Najafizade N, Hemati S, Gookizade A, et al. Preventive effects of zinc sulfate on taste alterations in patients under irradiation for head and neck cancers: A randomized placebo-controlled trial. *J Res Med Sci.* 2013;18(2):123–126.

30. Cawley MM, Benson LM. Current trends in managing oral mucositis. *Clinical journal of oncology nursing.* 2005;9(5):584–592.

31. Trotti A, Bellm LA, Epstein JB, et al. Mucositis incidence, severity and associated outcomes in patients with head and neck cancer receiving radiotherapy with or without chemotherapy: a systematic literature review. *Radiother Oncol.* 2003;66(3):253–262.

32. Eilers J. Nursing interventions and supportive care for the prevention and treatment of oral mucositis associated with cancer treatment. *Oncol Nurs Forum.* 2004;31(4, Suppl):13–23.

33. Kostler WJ, Hejna M, Wenzel C, Zielinski CC. Oral mucositis complicating chemotherapy and/or radiotherapy: options for prevention and treatment. *CA Cancer J Clin.* 2001;51(5):290–315.

34. Elting LS, Cooksley CD, Chambers MS, Garden AS. Risk, outcomes, and costs of radiation-induced oral mucositis among patients with head-and-neck malignancies. *Int J Radiat Oncol Biol Phys.* 2007;68(4):1110–1120.

35. Rubenstein EB, Peterson DE, Schubert M, et al. Clinical practice guidelines for the prevention and treatment of cancer therapy-induced oral and gastrointestinal mucositis. *Cancer.* 2004;100(9, Suppl):2026–2046.

36. Sonis ST. Oral mucositis in cancer therapy. *The journal of supportive oncology.* 2004;2(6, Suppl 3):3–8.

37. *Oral toxicity scale.* Geneva: World Health Organization; 2004.

38. Smith T. Gelclair: managing the symptoms of oral mucositis. *Hosp Med.* 2001;62(10):623–626.
39. Carter DL, Hebert ME, Smink K, et al. Double blind randomized trial of sucralfate vs placebo during radical radiotherapy for head and neck cancers. *Head Neck.* 1999;21(8):760–766.
40. Huang EY, Leung SW, Wang CJ, et al. Oral glutamine to alleviate radiation-induced oral mucositis: a pilot randomized trial. *Int J Radiat Oncol Biol Phys.* 2000;46(3):535–539.
41. Cerchietti LC, Navigante AH, Lutteral MA, et al. Double-blinded, placebo-controlled trial on intravenous L-alanyl-L-glutamine in the incidence of oral mucositis following chemoradiotherapy in patients with head-and-neck cancer. *Int J Radiat Oncol Biol Phys.* 2006;65(5):1330–1337.
42. Biswal BM, Zakaria A, Ahmad NM. Topical application of honey in the management of radiation mucositis: a preliminary study. *Support Care Cancer.* 2003;11(4):242–248.
43. Motallebnejad M, Akram S, Moghadamnia A, et al. The effect of topical application of pure honey on radiation-induced mucositis: a randomized clinical trial. *The journal of contemporary dental practice.* 2008;9(3):40–47.
44. Xu JL, Xia R, Sun ZH, et al. Effects of honey use on the management of radio/chemotherapy-induced mucositis: a meta-analysis of randomized controlled trials. *Int J Oral Maxillofac Surg.* 2016;45(12):1618–1625.
45. Brizel DM, Wasserman TH, Henke M, et al. Phase III randomized trial of amifostine as a radioprotector in head and neck cancer. *J Clin Oncol.* 2000;18(19):3339–3345.
46. Su YB, Vickers AJ, Zelefsky MJ, et al. Double-blind, placebo-controlled, randomized trial of granulocyte-colony stimulating factor during postoperative radiotherapy for squamous head and neck cancer. *Cancer Journal.* 2006;12(3):182–188.
47. Spielberger R, Stiff P, Bensinger W, et al. Palifermin for oral mucositis after intensive therapy for hematologic cancers. *N Engl J Med.* 2004;351(25):2590–2598.
48. Le QT, Kim HE, Schneider CJ, et al. Palifermin reduces severe mucositis in definitive chemoradiotherapy of locally advanced head and neck cancer: a randomized, placebo-controlled study. *J Clin Oncol.* 2011;29(20):2808–2814.
49. Miller RC, Le-Rademacher J, Sio TTW, et al. A phase III, randomized double-blind study of doxepin rinse versus Magic Mouthwash versus placebo in the treatment of acute oral mucositis pain in patients receiving head and neck radiotherapy with or without chemotherapy (Alliance A221304). *Int J Radiat Oncol Biol Phys.* 2016;96(5):938. doi:10.1016/j.ijrobp.2016.09.047
50. Silva FC, Marto JM, Salgado A, et al. Nystatin and lidocaine pastilles for the local treatment of oral mucositis. *Pharm Dev Technol.* 2017;22(2):266–274. doi:10.1080/10837450.2016.1221424
51. Worthington HV, Clarkson JE, Bryan G, et al. Interventions for preventing oral mucositis for patients with cancer receiving treatment. *Cochrane Database Syst Rev.* 2011(4):CD000978. doi:10.1002/14651858.CD000978.pub5
52. Sarvizadeh M, Hemati S, Meidani M, et al. Morphine mouthwash for the management of oral mucositis in patients with head and neck cancer. *Adv Biomed Res.* 2015;4:44. doi:10.4103/2277-9175.151254

53. Leenstra JL, Miller RC, Qin R, et al. Doxepin rinse versus placebo in the treatment of acute oral mucositis pain in patients receiving head and neck radiotherapy with or without chemotherapy: a phase III, randomized, double-blind trial (NCCTG-N09C6 [Alliance]). *J Clin Oncol.* 2014;32(15):1571–1577.
54. Bensadoun RJ, Franquin JC, Ciais G, et al. Low-energy He/Ne laser in the prevention of radiation-induced mucositis. A multicenter phase III randomized study in patients with head and neck cancer. *Support Care Cancer.* 1999;7(4):244–252.
55. Papas AS, Clark RE, Martuscelli G, et al. A prospective, randomized trial for the prevention of mucositis in patients undergoing hematopoietic stem cell transplantation. *Bone marrow transplantation.* 2003;31(8):705–712.
56. Bar Ad V, Weinstein G, Dutta PR, et al. Gabapentin for the treatment of pain syndrome related to radiation-induced mucositis in patients with head and neck cancer treated with concurrent chemoradiotherapy. *Cancer.* 2010;116(17):4206–4213.
57. Folwaczny M, Hickel R. Control of bacterial infection for effective treatment of oral mucositis. *Lancet.* 2002;360(9332):574.
58. da Silva AR, de Andrade Neto JB, da Silva CR, et al. Berberine antifungal activity in fluconazole-resistant pathogenic yeasts: action mechanism evaluated by flow cytometry and biofilm growth inhibition in *Candida* spp. *Antimicrob Agents Chemother.* 2016;60(6):3551–3557.
59. Thaweboon S, Thaweboon B, Srithavaj T, Choonharuangdej S. Oral colonization of *Candida* species in patients receiving radiotherapy in the head and neck area. *Quintessence Int.* 2008;39(2):e52–e57.
60. Garcia-Cuesta C, Sarrion-Perez MG, Bagan JV. Current treatment of oral candidiasis: A literature review. *J Clin Exp Dent.* 2014;6(5):e576–e582.
61. Lyu X, Zhao C, Yan ZM, Hua H. Efficacy of nystatin for the treatment of oral candidiasis: a systematic review and meta-analysis. *Drug Des Devel Ther.* 2016;10:1161–1171.
62. Nicolatou-Galitis O, Velegraki A, Sotiropoulou-Lontou A, et al. Effect of fluconazole antifungal prophylaxis on oral mucositis in head and neck cancer patients receiving radiotherapy. *Support Care Cancer.* 2006;14(1):44–51.
63. Marin Martinez EM, Aller Garcia AI, Martin-Mazuelos E. [Epidemiology, risk factors and in vitro susceptibility in candidaemia due to non-*Candida albicans* species]. *Rev Iberoam Micol.* 2016;33(4):248–252.
64. Nicolatou-Galitis O, Athanassiadou P, Kouloulias V, et al. Herpes simplex virus-1 (HSV-1) infection in radiation-induced oral mucositis. *Support Care Cancer.* 2006;14(7):753–762.
65. Rothwell BR, Spektor WS. Palliation of radiation-related mucositis. *Spec Care Dentist.* 1990;10(1):21–25.
66. Huang TY, Chu HC, Lin YL, et al. Minocycline attenuates 5-fluorouracil-induced small intestinal mucositis in mouse model. *Biochem Biophys Res Commun.* 2009;389(4):634–639.
67. Schenk G, Flemmig TF, Betz T, et al. Controlled local delivery of tetracycline HCl in the treatment of periimplant mucosal hyperplasia and mucositis. A controlled case series. *Clin Oral Implants Res.* 1997;8(5):427–433.
68. Feyer PC, Maranzano E, Molassiotis A, et al. Radiotherapy-induced nausea and vomiting (RINV): MASCC/ESMO guideline for antiemetics in radiotherapy: update 2009. *Support Care Cancer.* 2011;19(Suppl 1):S5–S14.

69. Roila F, Herrstedt J, Aapro M, et al. Guideline update for MASCC and ESMO in the prevention of chemotherapy- and radiotherapy-induced nausea and vomiting: results of the Perugia consensus conference. *Ann Oncol*. 2010;21(Suppl 5): v232–v243.

70. Hesketh PJ, Grunberg SM, Herrstedt J, et al. Combined data from two phase III trials of the NK1 antagonist aprepitant plus a 5HT 3 antagonist and a corticosteroid for prevention of chemotherapy-induced nausea and vomiting: effect of gender on treatment response. *Support Care Cancer*. 2006;14(4):354–360.

71. Roila F, Boschetti E, Tonato M, et al. Predictive factors of delayed emesis in cisplatin-treated patients and antiemetic activity and tolerability of metoclopramide or dexamethasone. A randomized single-blind study. *Am J Clin Oncol*. 1991;14(3):238–242.

72. Ingle RJ, Burish TG, Wallston KA. Conditionability of cancer chemotherapy patients. *Oncol Nurs Forum*. 1984;11(4):97–102.

73. Herrstedt J. Antiemetics: an update and the MASCC guidelines applied in clinical practice. *Nat Clin Pract Oncol*. 2008;5(1):32–43.

74. Navari RM, Nagy CK, Gray SE. The use of olanzapine versus metoclopramide for the treatment of breakthrough chemotherapy-induced nausea and vomiting in patients receiving highly emetogenic chemotherapy. *Support Care Cancer*. 2013;21(6):1655–1663.

75. Navari RM, Nagy CK, Le-Rademacher J, Loprinzi CL. Olanzapine versus fosaprepitant for the prevention of concurrent chemotherapy radiotherapy-induced nausea and vomiting. *J Community Support Oncol*. 2016;14(4):141–147.

76. Navari RM, Qin R, Ruddy KJ, et al. Olanzapine for the prevention of chemotherapy-induced nausea and vomiting. *N Engl J Med*. 2016;375(2):134–142.

77. Lane M, Vogel CL, Ferguson J, et al. Dronabinol and prochlorperazine in combination for treatment of cancer chemotherapy-induced nausea and vomiting. *J Pain Symptom Manage*. 1991;6(6):352–359.

78. Meiri E, Jhangiani H, Vredenburgh JJ, et al. Efficacy of dronabinol alone and in combination with ondansetron versus ondansetron alone for delayed chemotherapy-induced nausea and vomiting. *Curr Med Res Opin*. 2007;23(3): 533–543.

79. Cotter J. Efficacy of crude marijuana and synthetic delta-9-tetrahydrocannabinol as treatment for chemotherapy-induced nausea and vomiting: a systematic literature review. *Oncol Nurs Forum*. 2009;36(3):345–352.

80. Bossi P, Cortinovis D, Cossu Rocca M, et al. Searching for evidence to support the use of ginger in the prevention of chemotherapy-induced nausea and vomiting. *J Altern Complement Med*. 2016;22(6):486–488.

81. Berger AM, Mooney K, Alvarez-Perez A, et al. Cancer-related fatigue, version 2.2015. *J Natl Compr Canc Netw*. 2015;13(8):1012–1039.

82. Wang XS. Pathophysiology of cancer-related fatigue. *Clinical journal of oncology nursing*. 2008;12(5, Suppl):11–20.

83. Breitbart W, Poppito S, Rosenfeld B, et al. Pilot randomized controlled trial of individual meaning-centered psychotherapy for patients with advanced cancer. *J Clin Oncol*. 2012;30(12):1304–1309.

84. Mustian KM, Sprod LK, Janelsins M, et al. Multicenter, randomized controlled trial of yoga for sleep quality among cancer survivors. *J Clin Oncol*. 2013;31(26): 3233–3241.

85. Andersen SR, Wurtzen H, Steding-Jessen M, et al. Effect of mindfulness-based stress reduction on sleep quality: results of a randomized trial among Danish breast cancer patients. *Acta oncologica*. 2013;52(2):336–344.
86. Bruera E, Valero V, Driver L, et al. Patient-controlled methylphenidate for cancer fatigue: a double-blind, randomized, placebo-controlled trial. *J Clin Oncol*. 2006;24(13):2073–2078.
87. Caraceni A, Simonetti F. Psychostimulants: new concepts for palliative care from the modafinil experience? *J Pain Symptom Manage*. 2004;28(2):97–99.
88. Spathis A, Fife K, Blackhall F, et al. Modafinil for the treatment of fatigue in lung cancer: results of a placebo-controlled, double-blind, randomized trial. *J Clin Oncol*. 2014;32(18):1882–1888.
89. Lydiatt WM, Moran J, Burke WJ. A review of depression in the head and neck cancer patient. *Clin Adv Hematol Oncol*. 2009;7(6):397–403.
90. Rieke K, Boilesen E, Lydiatt W, et al. Population-based retrospective study to investigate preexisting and new depression diagnosis among head and neck cancer patients. *Cancer Epidemiol*. 2016;43:42–48.
91. Rodin G, Katz M, Lloyd N, et al. Treatment of depression in cancer patients. *Current oncology*. 2007;14(5):180–188.
92. Malkinson FD, Keane JT. Radiobiology of the skin: review of some effects on epidermis and hair. *J Invest Dermatol*. 1981;77(1):133–138.
93. Rosenthal DI, Chambers MS, Fuller CD, et al. Beam path toxicities to non-target structures during intensity-modulated radiation therapy for head and neck cancer. *Int J Radiat Oncol Biol Phys*. 2008;72(3):747–755.
94. Kao J, Darakchiev B, Conboy L, et al. Tumor directed, scalp sparing intensity modulated whole brain radiotherapy for brain metastases. *Technol Cancer Res Treat*. 2015;14(5):547–555.
95. Welsh JS, Mehta MP, Mackie TR, et al. Helical tomotherapy as a means of delivering scalp-sparing whole brain radiation therapy. *Technol Cancer Res Treat*. 2005;4(6):661–662; author reply 662.
96. Metz JM, Smith D, Mick R, et al. A phase I study of topical Tempol for the prevention of alopecia induced by whole brain radiotherapy. *Clin Cancer Res*. 2004;10(19):6411–6417.
97. Baltalarli B, Bir F, Demirkan N, Abban G. The preventive effect of vitamin D3 on radiation-induced hair toxicity in a rat model. *Life Sci*. 2006;78(14):1646–1651.
98. Hanson WR, Pelka AE, Nelson AK, Malkinson FD. Subcutaneous or topical administration of 16,16 dimethyl prostaglandin E2 protects from radiation-induced alopecia in mice. *Int J Radiat Oncol Biol Phys*. 1992;23(2):333–337.
99. Rannan-Eliya YF, Rannan-Eliya S, Graham K, et al. Surgical interventions for the treatment of radiation-induced alopecia in pediatric practice. *Pediatr Blood Cancer*. 2007;49(5):731–736.
100. Epstein JB, Hong C, Logan RM, et al. A systematic review of orofacial pain in patients receiving cancer therapy. *Support Care Cancer*. 2010;18(8):1023–1031.
101. Cooperstein E, Gilbert J, Epstein JB, et al. Vanderbilt Head and Neck Symptom Survey version 2.0: report of the development and initial testing of a subscale for assessment of oral health. *Head Neck*. 2012;34(6):797–804.
102. McNeely ML, Parliament MB, Seikaly H, et al. Effect of exercise on upper extremity pain and dysfunction in head and neck cancer survivors: a randomized controlled trial. *Cancer*. 2008;113(1):214–222.

103. Pfister DG, Cassileth BR, Deng GE, et al. Acupuncture for pain and dysfunction after neck dissection: results of a randomized controlled trial. *J Clin Oncol.* 2010;28(15):2565–2570.

104. Deng J, Ridner SH, Dietrich MS, et al. Factors associated with external and internal lymphedema in patients with head-and-neck cancer. *Int J Radiat Oncol Biol Phys.* 2012;84(3):e319–e328.

105. Smith BG, Lewin JS. Lymphedema management in head and neck cancer. *Current opinion in otolaryngology & head and neck surgery.* 2010;18(3):153–158.

106. Ahn C, Sindelar WF. Bilateral radical neck dissection: report of results in 55 patients. *J Surg Oncol.* 1989;40(4):252–255.

107. Deng J, Ridner SH, Murphy BA, Dietrich MS. Preliminary development of a lymphedema symptom assessment scale for patients with head and neck cancer. *Support Care Cancer.* 2012;20(8):1911–1918.

108. Yang X, Yoshida E, Cassidy RJ, et al. Quantitative ultrasonic Nakagami imaging of neck fibrosis after head and neck radiation therapy. *Int J Radiat Oncol Biol Phys.* 2015;92(2):407–414.

109. Smith BG, Hutcheson KA, Little LG, et al. Lymphedema outcomes in patients with head and neck cancer. *Otolaryngol Head Neck Surg.* 2015;152(2):284–291.

110. Delanian S, Balla-Mekias S, Lefaix JL. Striking regression of chronic radiotherapy damage in a clinical trial of combined pentoxifylline and tocopherol. *J Clin Oncol.* 1999;17(10):3283–3290.

111. McGarvey AC, Hoffman GR, Osmotherly PG, Chiarelli PE. Maximizing shoulder function after accessory nerve injury and neck dissection surgery: a multicenter randomized controlled trial. *Head Neck.* 2015;37(7):1022–1031.

112. Avraham T, Zampell JC, Yan A, et al. Th2 differentiation is necessary for soft tissue fibrosis and lymphatic dysfunction resulting from lymphedema. *Fed Am Soc Exp Biol.* 2013;27(3):1114–1126.

113. Deng J, Ridner SH, Wells N, et al. Development and preliminary testing of head and neck cancer related external lymphedema and fibrosis assessment criteria. *Eur J Oncol Nurs.* 2015;19(1):75–80.

114. Somerset JD, Mendenhall WM, Amdur RJ, et al. Planned postradiotherapy bilateral neck dissection for head and neck cancer. *Am J Otolaryngol.* 2001;22(6):383–386.

115. Fried D, Weissler M, Shores C, et al. Incidence of nodal disease after nonsurgical therapy in head and neck squamous cell carcinoma patients with bilateral neck disease: can a bilateral neck dissection be avoided? *Am J Clin Oncol.* 2013;36(2):188–191.

116. Frowen J, Cotton S, Corry J, Perry A. Impact of demographics, tumor characteristics, and treatment factors on swallowing after (chemo)radiotherapy for head and neck cancer. *Head Neck.* 2010;32(4):513–528.

117. Ward MC, Adelstein DJ, Bhateja P, et al. Severe late dysphagia and cause of death after concurrent chemoradiation for larynx cancer in patients eligible for RTOG 91–11. *Oral oncology.* 2016;57:21–26.

118. Galloway TJ, Amdur RJ, Liu C, et al. Revisiting unnecessary larynx irradiation with whole-neck IMRT. *Practical radiation oncology.* 2011;1(1):27–32.

119. Feng FY, Kim HM, Lyden TH, et al. Intensity-modulated chemoradiotherapy aiming to reduce dysphagia in patients with oropharyngeal cancer: clinical and functional results. *J Clin Oncol.* 2010;28(16):2732–2738.

120. Rich JT, Liu J, Haughey BH. Swallowing function after transoral laser microsurgery (TLM) +/- adjuvant therapy for advanced-stage oropharyngeal cancer. *Laryngoscope.* 2011;121(11):2381–2390.

121. Carnaby-Mann G, Crary MA, Schmalfuss I, Amdur R. "Pharyngocise": randomized controlled trial of preventative exercises to maintain muscle structure and swallowing function during head-and-neck chemoradiotherapy. *Int J Radiat Oncol Biol Phys.* 2012;83(1):210–219.

122. Logemann JA, Pauloski BR, Rademaker AW, Colangelo LA. Super-supraglottic swallow in irradiated head and neck cancer patients. *Head Neck.* 1997;19(6):535–540.

123. Francis DO, Hall E, Dang JH, et al. Outcomes of serial dilation for high-grade radiation-related esophageal strictures in head and neck cancer patients. *Laryngoscope.* 2015;125(4):856–862.

124. Kumar A, Soares HP, Balducci L, et al. Treatment tolerance and efficacy in geriatric oncology: a systematic review of phase III randomized trials conducted by five National Cancer Institute-sponsored cooperative groups. *J Clin Oncol.* 2007;25(10):1272–1276.

125. Rancati T, Schwarz M, Allen AM, et al. Radiation dose-volume effects in the larynx and pharynx. *Int J Radiat Oncol Biol Phys.* 2010;76(3, Suppl):S64–S69.

126. Rosen A, Rhee TH, Kaufman R. Prediction of aspiration in patients with newly diagnosed untreated advanced head and neck cancer. *Arch Otolaryngol Head Neck Surg.* 2001;127(8):975–979.

127. Eisbruch A, Lyden T, Bradford CR, et al. Objective assessment of swallowing dysfunction and aspiration after radiation concurrent with chemotherapy for head-and-neck cancer. *Int J Radiat Oncol Biol Phys.* 2002;53(1):23–28.

128. Marx RE. Osteoradionecrosis: a new concept of its pathophysiology. *J Oral Maxillofac Surg.* 1983;41(5):283–288.

129. Chopra S, Kamdar D, Ugur OE, et al. Factors predictive of severity of osteoradionecrosis of the mandible. *Head Neck.* 2011;33(11):1600–1605.

130. Beumer J, Harrison R, Sanders B, Kurrasch M. Osteoradionecrosis: predisposing factors and outcomes of therapy. *Head Neck surgery.* 1984;6(4):819–827.

131. Vissink A, Burlage FR, Spijkervet FK, et al. Prevention and treatment of the consequences of head and neck radiotherapy. *Crit Rev Oral Biol Med.* 2003;14(3):213–225.

132. Dreizen S, Brown LR, Daly TE, Drane JB. Prevention of xerostomia-related dental caries in irradiated cancer patients. *J Dent Res.* 1977;56(2):99–104.

133. Ben-David MA, Diamante M, Radawski JD, et al. Lack of osteoradionecrosis of the mandible after intensity-modulated radiotherapy for head and neck cancer: likely contributions of both dental care and improved dose distributions. *Int J Radiat Oncol Biol Phys.* 2007;68(2):396–402.

134. Maesschalck T, Dulguerov N, Caparrotti F, et al. Comparison of the incidence of osteoradionecrosis with conventional radiotherapy and intensity-modulated radiotherapy. *Head Neck.* 2016; 38:1695–1702.

135. Eisbruch A, Kim HM, Terrell JE, et al. Xerostomia and its predictors following parotid-sparing irradiation of head-and-neck cancer. *Int J Radiat Oncol Biol Phys.* 2001;50(3):695–704.

136. Kam MK, Leung SF, Zee B, et al. Prospective randomized study of intensity-modulated radiotherapy on salivary gland function in early-stage nasopharyngeal carcinoma patients. *J Clin Oncol.* 2007;25(31):4873–4879.

137. Murdoch-Kinch CA, Kim HM, Vineberg KA, et al. Dose-effect relationships for the submandibular salivary glands and implications for their sparing by intensity modulated radiotherapy. *Int J Radiat Oncol Biol Phys*. 2008;72(2):373–382.

138. Little M, Schipper M, Feng FY, et al. Reducing xerostomia after chemo-IMRT for head-and-neck cancer: beyond sparing the parotid glands. *Int J Radiat Oncol Biol Phys*. 2012;83(3):1007–1014.

139. Chang DT, Sandow PR, Morris CG, et al. Do pre-irradiation dental extractions reduce the risk of osteoradionecrosis of the mandible? *Head Neck*. 2007;29:528–536.

140. Wahl MJ. Osteoradionecrosis prevention myths. *Int J Radiat Oncol Biol Phys*. 2006;64(3):661–669.

141. Pitak-Arnnop P, Sader R, Dhanuthai K, et al. Management of osteoradionecrosis of the jaws: an analysis of evidence. *Eur J Surg Oncol*. 2008;34(10):1123–1134.

142. Marx RE, Johnson RP, Kline SN. Prevention of osteoradionecrosis: a randomized prospective clinical trial of hyperbaric oxygen versus penicillin. *Journal of the American Dental Association*. 1985;111(1):49–54.

143. Nabil S, Samman N. Incidence and prevention of osteoradionecrosis after dental extraction in irradiated patients: a systematic review. *Int J Oral Maxillofac Surg*. 2011;40(3):229–243.

144. Annane D, Depondt J, Aubert P, et al. Hyperbaric oxygen therapy for radionecrosis of the jaw: a randomized, placebo-controlled, double-blind trial from the ORN96 study group. *J Clin Oncol*. 2004;22(24):4893–4900.

145. Bui QC, Lieber M, Withers HR, et al. The efficacy of hyperbaric oxygen therapy in the treatment of radiation-induced late side effects. *Int J Radiat Oncol Biol Phys*. 2004;60(3):871–878.

146. Delanian S, Chatel C, Porcher R, et al. Complete restoration of refractory mandibular osteoradionecrosis by prolonged treatment with a pentoxifylline-tocopherol-clodronate combination (PENTOCLO): a phase II trial. *Int J Radiat Oncol Biol Phys*. 2011;80(3):832–839.

147. Shaha AR, Cordeiro PG, Hidalgo DA, et al. Resection and immediate microvascular reconstruction in the management of osteoradionecrosis of the mandible. *Head Neck*. 1997;19(5):406–411.

148. Bhandare N, Antonelli PJ, Morris CG, et al. Ototoxicity after radiotherapy for head and neck tumors. *Int J Radiat Oncol Biol Phys*. 2007;67(2):469–479.

149. Pacholke HD, Amdur RJ, Schmalfuss IM, et al. Contouring the middle and inner ear on radiotherapy planning scans. *Am J Clin Oncol*. 2005;28(2):143–147.

150. Hitchcock YJ, Tward JD, Szabo A, et al. Relative contributions of radiation and cisplatin-based chemotherapy to sensorineural hearing loss in head-and-neck cancer patients. *Int J Radiat Oncol Biol Phys*. 2009;73(3):779–788.

151. Xu YD, Ou YK, Zheng YQ, et al. The treatment for postirradiation otitis media with effusion: a study of three methods. *Laryngoscope*. 2008;118(11):2040–2043.

152. Jacobi I, van der Molen L, Huiskens H, et al. Voice and speech outcomes of chemoradiation for advanced head and neck cancer: a systematic review. *Eur Arch Otorhinolaryngol*. 2010;267(10):1495–1505.

153. Awan MJ, Mohamed AS, Lewin JS, et al. Late radiation-associated dysphagia (late-RAD) with lower cranial neuropathy after oropharyngeal radiotherapy: a preliminary dosimetric comparison. *Oral oncology*. 2014;50(8):746–752.

154. Vainshtein JM, Griffith KA, Feng FY, et al. Patient-reported voice and speech outcomes after whole-neck intensity modulated radiation therapy and chemotherapy for oropharyngeal cancer: prospective longitudinal study. *Int J Radiat Oncol Biol Phys*. 2014;89(5):973–980.

155. van der Molen L, van Rossum MA, Jacobi I, et al. Pre- and posttreatment voice and speech outcomes in patients with advanced head and neck cancer treated with chemoradiotherapy: expert listeners' and patient's perception. *J Voice*. 2012;26(5):664.e25–664.e33.

156. Tuomi L, Andrell P, Finizia C. Effects of voice rehabilitation after radiation therapy for laryngeal cancer: a randomized controlled study. *Int J Radiat Oncol Biol Phys*. 2014;89(5):964–972.

157. Chang J, Courey MS, Al-Jurf SA, et al. Injection laryngoplasty outcomes in irradiated and nonirradiated unilateral vocal fold paralysis. *Laryngoscope*. 2014;124(8):1895–1899.

158. Chen AM, Wang PC, Daly ME, et al. Dose–volume modeling of brachial plexus-associated neuropathy after radiation therapy for head-and-neck cancer: findings from a prospective screening protocol. *Int J Radiat Oncol Biol Phys*. 2014;88(4):771–777.

159. Hall WH, Guiou M, Lee NY, et al. Development and validation of a standardized method for contouring the brachial plexus: preliminary dosimetric analysis among patients treated with IMRT for head-and-neck cancer. *Int J Radiat Oncol Biol Phys*. 2008;72(5):1362–1367.

160. Pritchard J, Anand P, Broome J, et al. Double-blind randomized phase II study of hyperbaric oxygen in patients with radiation-induced brachial plexopathy. *Radiother Oncol*. 2001;58(3):279–286.

161. Bjordal K, Ahlner-Elmqvist M, Hammerlid E, et al. A prospective study of quality of life in head and neck cancer patients. Part II: longitudinal data. *Laryngoscope*. 2001;111(8):1440–1452.

162. Kim K, Amonkar MM, Hogberg D, Kasteng F. Economic burden of resected squamous cell carcinoma of the head and neck in an incident cohort of patients in the UK. *Head Neck Oncol*. 2011;3:47. doi:10.1186/1758-3284-3-47

163. Chen AM, Daly ME, Vazquez E, et al. Depression among long-term survivors of head and neck cancer treated with radiation therapy. *JAMA Otolaryngol Head Neck Surg*. 2013;139(9):885–889.

# 3

# Radiation Therapy Effects on the Thorax

*Orit Kaidar-Person, Timothy M. Zagar, and Lawrence B. Marks*

## OVERVIEW

- Radiation to the thorax is common and can cause both acute and late toxicity to the esophagus, lungs, heart, spinal cord, and chest wall.
- The risk of radiation therapy (RT) toxicity is related to factors such as the patient, tumor, and other treatments received.

Primary and metastatic cancers in and around the thorax are common (eg, primaries of the lung, breast, esophagus; metastases to the lungs, axillary lymph nodes) and RT plays an important role in their treatment. Thoracic RT can cause clinically meaningful acute and late normal tissue effects involving a variety of organs, most notably the esophagus, lungs, heart, spinal cord, and chest wall. The risk factors for RT-associated toxicity may be patient related (eg, age, gender, comorbidities, tobacco use), tumor related (eg, size, location), and treatment related (eg, RT technique, dose/volume parameters, chemotherapy, surgery).

RT doses and treatment volumes should be carefully determined based on these factors as well as the indication(s) for therapy (eg, cure versus palliation). There are numerous techniques available, (eg, three-dimensional conformal radiation therapy [3DCRT], intensity-modulated radiation therapy [IMRT], arc therapy, and stereotactic body radiation therapy [SBRT]) and the selection of the optimal approach should consider these same factors, as well as things such as availability, local expertise/experience, and cost.

It is important to recognize that due to the physics of therapeutic radiation, incidental dose to normal tissue is unavoidable, irrespective of technique. Thus, the selection of different techniques, and indeed the selection of competing treatment plans within a given technique, is essentially a balancing act (eg, "is it better to deliver X dose to . . . or Y dose to . . ."). Further, different organs have different anatomic substructures (eg, "parallel" or "series" architecture; analogous to electrical circuits), and different inherent sensitivities to radiation, resulting in different dose/volume/outcome relationships. For example, high doses to small volumes are well tolerated in "parallel" organs such as the lung, but not well tolerated by organs arranged in series, such as the bronchus or spinal cord. Common RT fractionation schemes used in the thorax and recommended dose/volume constraints are summarized in Tables 3.1 to 3.3.

This chapter focuses on the common toxicities of the lung and esophagus.

**Table 3.1 Common Tumor Types and RT Fractionation Used in the Thorax**

| Tumor type | Commonly used RT treatments | Comments |
|---|---|---|
| Lung cancer | • CRT to definitive RT doses<br>200 cGy × 30–33 fx = 6,000 to 6,600 cGy daily fractionation for non-small cell, or<br>150 cGy × 30 fx = 4,500 cGy at 1.5 Gy twice a day for small cell<br>• Postoperative:<br>180 cGy × 25 fx = 4,500 cGy<br>180 cGy × 28 fx = 5,040 cGy<br>180 cGy × 30 fx = 5,400 cGy<br>• Palliation:<br>300 cGy × 10 fx = 3,000 cGy<br>• SBRT:<br>Peripherally located tumors<br>1,200 cGy × 4 fx = 4,800 cGy<br>1,800 cGy × 3 fx = 5,400 cGy<br>2,000 cGy × 3 fx = 6,000 cGy<br>Central located tumors<br>1,000 cGy × 5 fx = 5,000 cGy | • Metabolic PET volume is often used for delineation<br>• Postoperative RT dose is often dependent on the indication for RT (eg, positive margins, nodal disease)<br>• Similar clinical outcomes for early stage NSCLC with SBRT versus surgery (1)<br>• SBRT for lesions >3 cm is associated with increased toxicity (2)<br>• SBRT: preferably fx that will result in $BED_{10}$ Gy >100 Gy<br>• SBRT also used for lung oligometastatic disease<br>• SBRT for central located lung lesions await maturation of data from the RTOG 0813 trial (3) |
| Esophageal cancer | • Preoperative, CRT:<br>180 cGy × 23 fx = 4,140 cGy[a]<br>180 cGy × 25 fx = 4,500 cGy<br>200 cGy × 25 fx = 5,000 cGy | • In the postoperative setting in cases of gross residual disease, a boost to a total 500–900 cGy may be considered |

*(continued)*

**Table 3.1** Common Tumor Types and RT Fractionation Used in the Thorax *(continued)*

| Tumor type | Commonly used RT treatments | Comments |
|---|---|---|
| | • Definitive, CRT: <br> 200 cGy × 25 fx = 5,000 cGy <br> 180 cGy × 28 fx = 5,040 cGy <br> • Postoperative <br> 180 cGy × 25 fx = 4,500 cGy <br> 180 cGy × 28 fx = 5,040 cGy | |
| Lymphoma | • 200 cGy × 10–20 fx = 2,000–4,000 cGy | • Current protocols aim to minimize the RT dose and field size as clinically permitting (ie, total dose according to response to chemotherapy, involved site field RT, metabolic PET volume used for delineation) (4) |

[a]Cross trial protocol (5).
BED, biologically effective dose; CRT, concomitant chemoradiation therapy; NSCLC, non-small cell lung cancer; RT, radiation therapy; RTOG, Radiation Therapy Oncology Group; SBRT, stereotactic body radiation therapy.

**Table 3.2 QUANTEC Recommendations for Conventional Fractionation**

| Structure | Volume (mL) | Total dose (Gy) | Endpoint | Comments |
|---|---|---|---|---|
| Lung[a] | 30% | <20 | Clinical pneumonitis <20% | QUANTEC constraints are for whole lung volume. Some trials report toxicity for lung minus PTV or lung minus GTV |
| Lung | Mean | <20 | Clinical pneumonitis <20% | QUANTEC constraints are for whole lung volume. Some trials report toxicity for lung minus PTV or lung minus GTV |
| Esophagus | Mean | <34 | Grade ≥3 acute esophagitis 5%–20% | Appears to be a dose volume response. Recommended to avoid circumferential RT |

[a]Based on 3DCRT.
GTV, gross tumor volume; PTV, planning tumor volume; QUANTEC, quantitative analyses of normal tissue effects in the clinic.
*Source:* From Ref. (4). Pinnix CC, Smith GL, Milgrom S, et al. Predictors of radiation pneumonitis in patients receiving intensity modulated radiation therapy for Hodgkin and non-Hodgkin lymphoma. *Int J Radiat Oncol Biol Phys.* 2015;92(1):175–182.

## ACUTE TOXICITY

### Lung

*Radiation Pneumonitis*

- *Timing:* 1 to 6 months after completion of RT (80% within 10 months).
- *Increased risk:* female sex and low performance status (7). The risk of radiation pneumonitis (RP) with concurrent chemotherapy depends on the chemotherapy protocol: concomitant carboplatin/paclitaxel has been associated with an increased risk of RP compared to etoposide/cisplatin (8). Induction carboplatin/gemcitabine and concomitant gemcitabine has been associated with increased rate of RP and other lung toxicities (eg, adult respiratory distress syndrome) compared to carboplatin/paclitaxel (9). There is conflicting evidence whether decreased baseline lung function or smoking increases the risk for RP (7). Risk factors for lung toxicity with SBRT have been suggested to include older age and larger tumor size (2).
- *Clinical presentation:* shortness of breath, dry cough (or productive sometimes of thick white sputum), and occasionally low-grade fever. Patients often have a normal physical exam. In more severe cases, patients may be tachypneic, exhibit labored breathing, and have audible rales. Blood

**Table 3.3 TG101 Recommendations for SBRT According to Fractionation**[a]

| Structure | 1 Fraction | | | 3 Fractions | | | 5 Fractions | | | End point (Grade ≥3) | Comments |
|---|---|---|---|---|---|---|---|---|---|---|---|
| | Max critical volume above threshold (mL) | Threshold dose (Gy) | Max dose point[b] (Gy) | | Threshold dose (Gy) | Max dose point[b] (Gy) | | Threshold dose (Gy) | Max dose point[b] (Gy) | | |
| Lung (RT&LT) | 1500 | 7 | — | | 11.6 (2 Gy/fx) | — | | 12.5 (2.5 Gy/fx) | — | Basic lung function | Parallel organ: volume–dose constraints |
| Lung (RT&LT) | 1000 | 7.4 | — | | 12.4 (3.1 Gy/fx) | — | | 13.5 (2.7 Gy/fx) | — | Pneumonitis | Parallel organ: volume–dose constraints |
| Esophagus | <5 | 11.9 | 15.4 | | 17.7 (5.9 Gy/fx) | 25.2 (8.4 Gy/fx) | | 19.5 (3.9 Gy/fx) | 35 (7 Gy/fx) | Stenosis/fistula | Serial tissue: volume–dose constraints and max dose point Avoid circumferential RT |

(*continued*)

**Table 3.3 TG101 Recommendations for SBRT According to Fractionation[a]** *(continued)*

| Structure | 1 Fraction | | | 3 Fractions | | | 5 Fractions | | | End point (Grade ≥3) | Comments |
|---|---|---|---|---|---|---|---|---|---|---|---|
| | Max critical volume above threshold (mL) | Threshold dose (Gy) | Max dose point[b] (Gy) | | Threshold dose (Gy) | Max dose point[b] (Gy) | | Threshold dose (Gy) | Max dose point[b] (Gy) | | |
| Trachea/large bronchus | <4 | 10.5 | 20.2 | | 15 (5 Gy/fx) | 30 (10 Gy/fx) | | 16.5 (3.3 Gy/fx) | 40 (8 Gy/fx) | Stenosis/fistula | Serial tissue: volume-dose constraints and max dose point Avoid circumferential RT |
| Bronchus, smaller airways | <0.5 | 12.4 | 13.3 | | 18.9 (6.3 Gy/fx) | 23.1 (7.7 Gy/fx) | | 21 (4.2 Gy/fx) | 33 (6.6 Gy/fx) | Stenosis with atelectasis | — |
| Rib | <1 | 22 | 30 | | 28.8 (9.6 Gy/fx) | 36.9 (12.3 Gy/fx) | | 35 (7 Gy/fx) | 43 (8.6 Gy/fx) | Pain or fracture | — |

[a]A recent meta-analysis suggests that higher mean lung dose (MLD), higher $V_{20}$ are associated with increased risk for RT-associated lung toxicity; however, current data do not provide a safe limit for MLD (ipsilateral, both) or $V_{20(2)}$.
[b]"Point" defined ≤0.035.
RT, radiation therapy; RT&LT, right & left; SBRT, stereotactic body radiation therapy.
*Source:* From Ref. (6). Benedict SH, Yenice KM, Followill D, et al. Stereotactic body radiation therapy: the report of AAPM Task Group 101. *Med Phys.* 2010;37(8):4078–4101.

counts are usually normal. Radiographs (eg, chest x-ray or CT scan) *may* show infiltrates in the distribution of RT portals (diffuse haze, patchy infiltrates, ground glass opacification). As these radiologic findings are often *not* present, their absence thus does not rule out pneumonitis. Further, these radiologic findings are not specific for pneumonitis as they are often also present in asymptomatic patients (ie, asymptomatic inflammation within the RT field). Up to 10% of the patients could have immune-mediated hypersensitivity pneumonitis with infiltrates extending to involve unirradiated regions of the lung (10).

- *Differential diagnosis*: exacerbation of chronic obstructive pulmonary disorder, pulmonary embolism, infection, drug-induced pneumonitis (eg, bleomycin, cyclophosphamide, methotrexate), tumor recurrence.
- *Preventive measures*: adherence to RT dose/volume constraints (Tables 3.2 and 3.3), fractionation, RT techniques, and pharmaceutical prevention (Table 3.4).
  - ○ *RT dose/volume constraints* are aimed to minimize the potential risk for RP (Tables 3.2 and 3.3) (1). Most of the dose/volume/outcome data are derived from patients treated with conventional fractionation *and* a limited number of fields (eg, anterior-posterior opposed, off cord oblique opposed), and most of the irradiated lung received ≈ 180 to 200 cGy per fraction. Thus, the use of altered fractionation (27), and/or alternative RT techniques (eg, multifield IMRT or helical tomotherapy [HT]) impact how one interprets the associated dose volume histogram (DVH). Techniques such as arcs and multifield IMRT tend to *reduce* the fraction size received by the incidentally irradiated lung relative to the prescription dose but the volume of lung exposed to lower doses is generally increased (28,29). On the other hand, accelerated fractionation schemes (eg, with multifield radiosurgery) will tend to increase the fraction size received by the incidentally irradiated lung (relative to conventional approaches).

    The ability of some organs to tolerate a low dose being delivered to a large volume is sometimes unknown, so care should be taken when prescribing dose distributions that are of a different character than those used to define the dose/volume constraints (eg, evaluating an IMRT plan based on constraints defined from the "routine 3D era"). Presently, based on available data, it is recommended that the lung $V_{5Gy}$ be less than 55% to 60% when using IMRT techniques.
  - ○ Other RT techniques that may help mitigate lung toxicity include respiratory gating (eg, with machine-based gating or breath-hold techniques). With this technique, the RT delivery is restricted to a specific portion of the respiratory cycle thereby reducing the field size that is needed. Motion tracking (eg, moving the treatment beam in synchrony with the respiratory cycle) is another method that allows using lesser margins, thus reducing the irradiated volume.
  - ○ *Pharmaceutical agents* for prevention or mitigation of RP are not routinely used. None of the agents are listed by the FDA/EMA for prevention/mitigation of RP; however, pre-clinical or clinical data suggest their potential role in reducing the risk of RP (Table 3.4). Amifostine is one of the more-highly studied agents. Several studies

**Table 3.4 Pharmaceutical Experimental Agents Suggested to Reduce the Rates of RT-Associated Thoracic Toxicities**

| Drug | Doses used in trials | Common side effects[a] | Type of RT toxicity |
|---|---|---|---|
| Amifostine[b] | IV 340 mg/m$^2$, over 10 minutes, given daily 15 minutes prior to RT (11). SC or IV push 500 mg, given daily prior to RT. Additional dose of IV 500 mg once a week prior to chemotherapy (12,13–15). | Nausea, vomiting, skin reaction, hypotension (most common cause of drug-associated cardiac toxicity) Certain side effects are less encountered via SC administration (eg, hypotension) | *Lung:* RP: 0%–30% in amifostine arm vs 16%–67% in control arm *Esophagus:* Esophagitis: 16%–39% in amifostine arm vs 35%–84% in control Less treatment breaks because of esophagitis (11) |
| Captopril (ACEi) | RCT aimed dose: per os captopril 50 mg three times a day (16)[c] | Cough, flushing, hypersensitivity reaction, hypotension, hyperkalemia | *Lung:* Reported to reduce and to mitigate risk of RP Data from preclinical (17) and retrospective clinical studies (18,19) |
| Palifermin[d] | IV 180 mcg/kg 3 days before CRT, thereafter once weekly (total seven doses) (20) | Hypersensitivity reaction, fever, joint pain, rush, proteinuria, hypertension | *Lung:* Data from preclinical in vivo studies, given intratracheal to reduce early (RP) and late (fibrosis) RT-associated lung toxicity (21,22) *Esophagus:* Esophagitis: Dysphagia grade ≥2: 61% versus 70% in control arm, $P = .36$ Dysphagia grade ≥3 22% versus 28% in control arm, $P = .50$ |

*(continued)*

**Table 3.4** Pharmaceutical Experimental Agents Suggested to Reduce the Rates of RT-Associated Thoracic Toxicities (*continued*)

| Drug | Doses used in trials | Common side effects[a] | Type of RT toxicity |
|---|---|---|---|
| Pentoxifylline[e] | per os 400 mg three times a day during RT course with/without vitamin E[f] 300 mg twice a day | Hypersensitivity, nausea, vomiting, diarrhea, blurred vision, elevation of liver enzymes | *Lung:* Reduce acute (RP) and late (fibrosis) lung toxicity (23–25) |

[a]Side effects: for complete information please refer to product-specific recommendation.
[b]Amifostine = WR-2721; Ethyol, Medimmune Inc, Gaithersburg, MD.
[c]NRG Oncology Radiation Therapy Oncology Group (RTOG) 0123 phase II RCT: final aimed dose after gradual increment, starting at first day after RT. Initial test dose of 6.25 mg, gradual increment over weeks while monitoring blood pressure (16).
[d]Palifermin = recombinant human keratinocyte growth factor (rHuKGF), Kepivance, Amgen Inc. Palifermin is also used for head and neck CRT to reduce the risk of mucositis.
[e]Pentoxifylline = Ethyl xanthine derivative, Trental, Sanofi aventis, Bridgewater, NJ.
[f]Vitamin E = alpha-tocopherol.
ACEi, angiotensin converting enzyme inhibitor; NRG, National surgical adjuvant breast and bowel project, Radiation therapy oncology group, Gynecology oncology group; RCT, randomized controlled trial; RT, radiation therapy.

conducted in Greece suggested activity (12), but the larger U.S. study failed to confirm their findings. The U.S. study, however, has been criticized since the amifostine was given with only approximately 40% of the radiation fractions (26). Given the conflicting results, and the logistical/clinical challenges associated with its use (eg, hypotension), this approach has largely fallen out of favor.

- *Treatment:* dependent on the patients' symptoms. Patients with very minor symptoms might be monitored or given antitussives (eg, for cough). Patients with meaningful levels of shortness of breath typically should be treated with prednisone. We have typically found that doses of ≈60 mg per day for 2 weeks initially, followed by a relatively slow taper (eg, reducing total daily dose by 10 mg per 1–2 weeks), or according to symptoms, is usually effective and well tolerated. It is important to taper the dose slowly because of the possibility of rebound pneumonitis, as well as potential onset of adrenal insufficiency. If the patient's symptoms recur during the taper (and this is relatively common), we usually increase the dose slightly (eg, to the prior dose where their symptoms were controlled), maintain that dose for a few weeks, and then attempt an even slower taper. Sometimes chronic steroid use is required to control symptoms.

Radiation pneumonitis should be managed cautiously as some patients may experience a rapid decline necessitating oxygen support. Patients with suspected infectious pneumonia who are treated with antibiotics should be monitored closely for persistent symptoms that might actually be RP. In equivocal cases where the diagnosis of infection versus RP is unclear, patients may be started on antibiotics for possible infection, but then rapidly transitioned to steroids if, after several days, there is no improvement with the antibiotics. The diagnosis of RP is somewhat imprecise with 28% of patients being diagnosed with RP also having other medical conditions that were considered to confound the diagnosis (30).

## Recall RP

In patients who had prior RT in whom the lung was exposed to radiation, symptoms of RP may sometimes appear to be brought on by the subsequent receipt of a systemic agent. This is often referred to as "recall RP." Medications that have been described to be associated with "recall RP" include chemotherapy (eg, etoposide, gemcitabine, Adriamycin, paclitaxel, pemetrexed) (31), tyrosine-kinase inhibitors (TKIs) (eg, sunitinib, erlotinib) (32), BRAF inhibitors (eg, vemurafenib) (33), mTOR inhibitors (eg, everolimus) (34), monoclonal antibody (eg, trastuzumab) (35). Further, symptoms of RP can occur in previously irradiated patients when steroids are discontinued (administered for some reason other than pneumonitis). This phenomenon was described in patients with Hodgkin disease who were treated with "mantle field" RT and later with mustargen, oncovin, procarbazine and prednisone (MOPP) chemotherapy. The rapid discontinuation of high doses of prednisone (as part of the MOPP protocol) appeared to bring on pulmonary symptoms. Further, these symptoms improved when steroids were restarted (36).

- *Timing:* hours to days after initiation of the trigger medication, weeks to months after RT.

- *Management:* in case of suspicion of "recall RP," the trigger medication should be stopped and, if needed, treatment as noted earlier for RP be considered.

## Esophagus

### Acute Esophagitis

- *Timing:* onset is 2 to 3 weeks after initiation of conventionally fractionated RT. The severity of acute esophagitis often peaks *during* the course of RT when using conventional fractionation for definitive lung RT, but can occur *after* the course of RT when using accelerated regimens (eg, two fractions per day).
- *Risk factors:* central thoracic tumors, concurrent chemotherapy (where severe esophagitis has been reported in up to 46% of patients), hyperfractionation (ie, higher total daily doses), higher total dose, longer lengths of irradiated esophagus, full circumferential irradiation (11–15,28,37,38).
- *Clinical presentation:* dysphagia or odynophagia, may lead to weight loss and/or dehydration. In rare cases, perforation or obstruction (5,39). Symptoms of acute esophagitis usually slowly resolve within 2 to 3 weeks after completion of RT.
- *Differential diagnosis:* infection (mostly candidiasis, herpes simplex virus [HSV]), gastroesophageal reflux, and mucosal trauma. Fungal superinfection/HSV should be considered in cases of protracted symptoms.
- *Preventive measures:* Severity of acute esophageal toxicity is associated with increased risk for late toxicity, thus preventive measures and early treatment during the acute phase are recommended. Preventive measures include dietary constraints (eg, avoidance of hard/spicy foods and alcohol that might cause trauma to the esophageal mucosa), behavioral modification (eg, reducing tobacco use), and pharmaceuticals (see Tables 3.5 and 3.6). During treatment planning, it is advised to minimize esophageal exposure as is possible (without compromising target coverage). As the esophagus is sometimes challenging to visualize on axial CT, consideration should be given to the use of dilute oral contrast to help esophageal delineation during RT planning.
- *Pharmaceuticals:* for prevention of esophagitis have been suggested (see Table 3.4).
- *RT techniques:* the esophagus has a long course within the thorax (from the pharynx to the stomach, approximately 25 cm in length), and therefore is often irradiated during RT of thoracic malignancies (and also in cases of vertebral body RT). Planning should include appropriate delineation (which is often challenging, oral contrast is advised), avoidance of hotspots in the area of the esophagus, and limiting the volume of esophagus contained within the irradiated volume (38). Sparing part of the circumference should be considered as it may reduce the risk of acute esophagitis and also reduce the risk for stricture (39). IMRT might be an effective way to minimize esophageal exposure (29,38,41). In patients with mediastinal nodal disease, particularly involving the subcarinal area, avoidance of the esophagus is essentially impossible owing to proximity, and in these cases, one typically must accept the likely esophageal reactions as underdosage

**Table 3.5** Dietary Constraints and Behavioral Modifications That Have Been Suggested to Reduce the Rate of Acute Esophagitis

| | Recommendations |
|---|---|
| Dietary constraints | Avoidance of alcohol, citrus fruit juices, hot or cold beverages, spicy food, hard food (eg, crackers, toast), fatty foods (40) <br> Avoid large meals or food that might cause/aggravate gastroesophageal reflux (eg, coffee, chocolate) |
| Behavioral and dietary modification | Advise smoking cessation <br> Patients should be advised to drink between meals and eat small-volume lukewarm semiliquid meals (40) <br> A teaspoon of olive oil prior to every meal (40) <br> Any type of oral medication should be taken in an upright position with adequate volume (25–100 mL, depending on tablet size) of water to avoid transit delay <br> Patients should be instructed to avoid taking oral medication immediately prior to sleeping <br> If possible, avoid medications that might irritate the mucosa (eg, anti-inflammatory drugs, oral bisphosphonates, and certain antibiotics) |
| Pharmaceutical prophylaxis | *Suggested treatment protocol for prophylaxis from a single RCT*[a] *(40):* <br> • Nimesulide—an NSAID, 100 mg per os after dinner <br> • Rantidine—an H2-blocker, 150 mg per os twice a day. <br> • Antacid suspension—100 g of suspension containing: magnesium hydroxide (3.65 g) and aluminum hydroxide (3.25 g) 2–4 teaspoons four times daily, 20–60 min after meals and before sleeping in water or milk <br> • Domperidone—per os 10 mg twice daily <br> • Sodium bicarbonate solution—an alkalinizing agent, per os 3–5 mL every 2 hours <br> Other pharmaceuticals are listed in Table 3.4 |
| Pharmaceutical treatment | • 2% viscus lidocaine <br> • Suspension of 2% viscus lidocaine, 60 mL, sucralfate (1g/mL, 10 mL), antacid (Mylanta®, 30 mL), taken 15–30 mL *per os* PRN (RTOG 0617) <br> • Prokinetic agents (eg, domperidone, metoclopramide), <br> • H2-blockers (rantidine, 150 mg per os twice a day) or proton pump inhibitors <br> • Antifungal medication should be considered in cases of superinfection (ketoconazole 200 mg per os daily or fluconazole 100 mg per os daily <br> • IV hydration |

[a]Data from a small RCT. We do not recommend the routine use of NSAIDs as prophylaxis.
NSAID, nonsteroidal anti-inflammatory drug; RCT, randomized controlled trial; RTOG, Radiation Therapy Oncology Group.

Table 3.6 Summary of RT-Induced Thoracic Toxicity and Potential Treatment

| Organ | Ailment | Usual timing | Mild (first step) | Moderate/severe (second steps) | Preventative strategies |
|---|---|---|---|---|---|
| Lung | Pneumonitis | Weeks to months post-RT | Prednisone | $O_2$, antibiotics and breathing support as indicated per case | RT constraints, reducing irradiated lung volume Amifostine[a] Palifermin[a] Captopril[a] |
|  | Fibrosis | Months to years post-RT | Pentoxifylline and vitamin E[a] | Prednisone $O_2$, antibiotics and breathing support as indicated per case | RT constraints, reducing irradiated lung volume Pentoxifylline +/− vitamin E[a] |
| Esophagus | Esophagitis | During RT Starting from week 2–3 | Topical analgesics, narcotics, antacids suspension, prokinetic agents (eg, metoclopramide, domperidone), H2 blockers or proton pump inhibitors | IV fluids, treatment break, antifungal as indicated | Dietary/behavioral modification RT constraints IMRT sparing Amifostine[a] Palifermin[a] |

*(continued)*

**Table 3.6** Summary of RT-Induced Thoracic Toxicity and Potential Treatment (*continued*)

| Organ | Ailment | Usual timing | Mild (first step) | Moderate/severe (second steps) | Preventative strategies |
|---|---|---|---|---|---|
| | Dysphagia/ Dysmotility | Months to years post-RT[b] | Dietary/behavioral modifications prokinetic agents (eg, metoclopramide, domperidone) Antacids | | |
| | Stricture | Months to years post-RT | Dietary/behavioral modifications prokinetic agents (eg, metoclopramide, domperidone) | Endoscopic dilation[c] | Preventing acute esophagitis Avoiding circumferential RT of esophagus, avoiding hotspots in the esophagus |

[a]Level I evidence is lacking
[b]Acute severe esophagitis might result in chronic/late esophageal complications.
[c]Endoscopic evaluation is mandatory to rule out malignancy. Repeated procedures are often needed.
IMRT, intensity-modulated radiation therapy; RT, radiation therapy.

- *Management:* includes consideration of dietary constraints and behavioral modifications as listed in Tables 3.5 and 3.6, to reduce irritation of the mucosa. Mouthwash composed of topical anesthetics (2% viscous lidocaine), Benadryl elixir, saline, and baking soda can be used prior to meals to reduce pain associated with swallowing. A suspension composed of a topical anesthetic (2% viscous lidocaine, 60 mL), sucralfate (1g/mL, 10 mL), antacids suspension (Mylanta®, 30 mL), taken 15 to 30 mL per os PRN was used to treat esophagitis in the Radiation Therapy Oncology Group (RTOG) 0617. Prokinetic agents (eg, domperidone, metoclopramide), H2-blockers (rantidine, 150 mg per os twice a day), and proton pump inhibitors are also recommended. Antifungal medication should be considered in cases of superinfection (ketoconazole 200 mg per os daily or fluconazole 100 mg per os daily). Treatment breaks and/or feeding tubes can be considered in cases of severe esophagitis, although this is relatively unusual and not preferred. Improvements in symptoms typically begin within several weeks of onset, with gradual continued improvements over time, that can be hastened perhaps by a treatment break. Supportive care such as IV hydration is recommended if oral intake is insufficient, especially for patients who are treated with concomitant chemotherapy and/or other medication that might have nephrotoxic potential. Rarely is nutritional supplementation with feeding tubes (percutaneous endoscopic gastrostomy [PEG], J-tube, dobhoff catheter, etc.) required.

*Hiccups*

Persistent hiccups is an unusual side effect, but can be quite frustrating to the patient in which it occurs. It is likely due to irritation of the diaphragm or phrenic nerve, and can happen with low lying lung or esophageal/gastric cardia fields. There are many different medicines that have been used to treat hiccups, and some include antispasmodics (baclofen), antipsychotics (chlorpromazine), antiemetics (metoclopramide) and proton pump inhibitors (if thought to be GI in origin).

## LATE TOXICITY

### Lung

*Lung Fibrosis*

- *Timing:* months to years after the course of RT. The reported rate of fibrosis varies widely between 4.4% and 80% and is mostly asymptomatic (2,42). After high-dose RT, portions of the irradiated lung will essentially always appear somewhat abnormal on imaging.
- *Preventive measures:* reducing the irradiated lung volume. Experimental pharmaceuticals include amifostine (7), pentoxifylline and vitamin E 500 (43,44) (Table 3.4), but none have been proven to be effective. (See earlier comments about amifostine in the section on Acute lung injury). Preclinical in vivo studies suggest a possible role for melatonin (45), flaxseeds (46,47), and superoxide dismutase (48), although this has not been attempted in humans.

- *Symptoms:* cough, reduced exercise tolerance, and other respiratory symptoms due to reduced lung capacity. The reduced lung reserve leaves patients at increased risk for other pulmonary insults (eg, infection, emboli, cancer progression, and heart failure).
- *Treatment:* no clinically proven effective treatment. Steroids (eg, prednisone) have been suggested as being effective by reducing the inflammatory process. An approved medication for idiopathic lung fibrosis, pirfenidone, was suggested to show activity in reducing RT-associated fibrosis in a small pilot clinical study; however, data of its efficacy in RT-induced lung fibrosis are lacking (49). Supportive measures such as reducing gastroesophageal reflux and vaccination (eg, influenza, pneumococcal pneumonia) are recommended in patients with symptoms of reduced lung capacity. Oxygen supplementation, pulmonary rehabilitation, and supportive care (eg, opioids) should be considered according to severity of symptoms.

**Bronchial strictures** are uncommon after conventional RT (<3%) (50). They are more commonly seen after intrabronchial brachytherapy, high doses of conventionally fractionated RT (eg, >70 Gy) (51), or after lung SBRT for central lesions (eg, within 2 cm of the main bronchial tree, reported in up to 25%) (52,53). Symptomatic patients may need interventions such as bronchoscopic balloon dilatation, endobronchial stent, and surgery.

## Esophagus

### Esophageal Fibrosis/Stricture

- *Timing:* months to years after the course of RT.
- *Prevention*: for acute esophagitis, avoid circumferential esophageal RT (37).
- *Risk factors*: severe acute esophageal toxicity (38), concurrent chemotherapy, intraluminal brachytherapy, hypofractionated RT for central lesions.
- *Clinical manifestation*: dysphagia, dysmotility, stricture, ulceration, and fistula (all are often regarded as late esophagitis). Patients may experience diffuse esophageal spasm, which can present as chest pain and trigger work up for a cardiac event.
- *Differential diagnosis*: malignancy (extrinsic compression or gastroesophageal cancer), infection (eg, candidiasis, HSV), scleroderma, and achalasia.
- *Treatment:* Esophageal dysmotility can be treated with dietary and behavioral modifications to reduce gastroesophageal reflux and to decrease esophageal transit time (similar to recommendations to reduce risk of esophagitis). Some patients may benefit from metoclopramide, which increases the rates of gastric emptying and antacids with/without proton pump inhibitors.

Strictures are often treated with endoscopic dilatation, and this may need to be done repeatedly (54); one study reported repeat endoscopic intervention at a median interval of 5 months (54,55). In cases of refractory stricture, esophageal stenting can be considered but is often *not* successful (54). Areas of stricture or obstruction may be reflective of recurrent tumor and biopsy of suspicious areas should be considered (54). This should be done carefully as there might be some risk of infection or other complications associated with biopsy of a previously irradiated area.

Treatment for esophageal spasm may include antispasmodics, such as calcium channel blockers, nitrates, anticholinergics, or sildenafil. Some patients may benefit from injections of botulinum toxin.

# REFERENCES

1. Zheng X, Schipper M, Kidwell K, et al. Survival outcome after stereotactic body radiation therapy and surgery for stage I non-small cell lung cancer: a meta-analysis. *Int J Radiat Oncol Biol Phys*. 2014;90(3):603–611.
2. Zhao J, Yorke ED, Li L, et al. Simple factors associated with radiation-induced lung toxicity after stereotactic body radiation therapy of the thorax: a pooled analysis of 88 studies. *Int J Radiat Oncol Biol Phys*. 2016;95(5):1357–1366.
3. Chaudhuri AA, Tang C, Binkley MS, et al. Stereotactic ablative radiotherapy (SABR) for treatment of central and ultra-central lung tumors. *Lung Cancer*. 2015;89(1):50–56.
4. Pinnix CC, Smith GL, Milgrom S, et al. Predictors of radiation pneumonitis in patients receiving intensity modulated radiation therapy for Hodgkin and non-Hodgkin lymphoma. *Int J Radiat Oncol Biol Phys*. 2015;92(1):175–182.
5. van Hagen P, Hulshof MC, van Lanschot JJ, et al. Preoperative chemoradiotherapy for esophageal or junctional cancer. *N Engl J Med*. 2012;366(22):2074–2084.
6. Benedict SH, Yenice KM, Followill D, et al. Stereotactic body radiation therapy: the report of AAPM Task Group 101. *Med Phys*. 2010;37(8):4078–4101.
7. Mehta V. Radiation pneumonitis and pulmonary fibrosis in non-small-cell lung cancer: pulmonary function, prediction, and prevention. *Int J Radiat Oncol Biol Phys*. 2005;63(1):5–24.
8. Palma DA, Senan S, Tsujino K, et al. Predicting radiation pneumonitis after chemoradiation therapy for lung cancer: an international individual patient data meta-analysis. *Int J Radiat Oncol Biol Phys*. 2013;85(2):444–450.
9. Salama JK, Stinchcombe TE, Gu L, et al. Pulmonary toxicity in Stage III non-small cell lung cancer patients treated with high-dose (74 Gy) 3-dimensional conformal thoracic radiotherapy and concurrent chemotherapy following induction chemotherapy: a secondary analysis of Cancer and Leukemia Group B (CALGB) trial 30105. *Int J Radiat Oncol Biol Phys*. 2011;81(4):e269–e274.
10. Morgan GW, Breit SN. Radiation and the lung: a reevaluation of the mechanisms mediating pulmonary injury. *Int J Radiat Oncol Biol Phys*. 1995;31(2):361–369.
11. Wynn RB, Mehta V. Reduction of treatment breaks and radiation-induced esophagitis and pneumonitis using amifostine in unresectable non-small cell lung cancer patients receiving definitive concurrent chemotherapy and radiation therapy: a prospective community-based clinical trial. *Semin Oncol*. 2005;32(2, Suppl 3):S99–S104.
12. Koukourakis MI, Romanidis K, Froudarakis M, et al. Concurrent administration of Docetaxel and Stealth liposomal doxorubicin with radiotherapy in non-small cell lung cancer: excellent tolerance using subcutaneous amifostine for cytoprotection. *Br J Cancer*. 2002;87(4):385–392.
13. Komaki R, Lee JS, Kaplan B, Allen P, et al. Randomized phase III study of chemoradiation with or without amifostine for patients with favorable performance status inoperable stage II-III non-small cell lung cancer: preliminary results. *Semin Radiat Oncol*. 2002;12(1, Suppl 1):46–49.

14. Komaki R, Lee JS, Milas L, et al. Effects of amifostine on acute toxicity from concurrent chemotherapy and radiotherapy for inoperable non-small-cell lung cancer: report of a randomized comparative trial. *Int J Radiat Oncol Biol Phys.* 2004;58(5):1369–1377.

15. Sasse AD, Clark LG, Sasse EC, Clark OA. Amifostine reduces side effects and improves complete response rate during radiotherapy: results of a meta-analysis. *Int J Radiat Oncol Biol Phys.* 2006;64(3):784–791.

16. Small W, Jr, James JL, Moore TD, et al. Utility of the ACE inhibitor captopril in mitigating radiation-associated pulmonary toxicity in lung cancer: results from NRG oncology RTOG 0123. *Am J Clin Oncol.* 2016. doi:10.1097/COC.0000000000000289

17. Ghosh SN, Zhang R, Fish BL, et al. Renin-angiotensin system suppression mitigates experimental radiation pneumonitis. *Int J Radiat Oncol Biol Phys.* 2009;75(5):1528–1536.

18. Wang H, Liao Z, Zhuang Y, et al. Do angiotensin-converting enzyme inhibitors reduce the risk of symptomatic radiation pneumonitis in patients with non-small cell lung cancer after definitive radiation therapy? Analysis of a single-institution database. *Int J Radiat Oncol Biol Phys.* 2013;87(5):1071–1077.

19. Kharofa J, Cohen EP, Tomic R, et al. Decreased risk of radiation pneumonitis with incidental concurrent use of angiotensin-converting enzyme inhibitors and thoracic radiation therapy. *Int J Radiat Oncol Biol Phys.* 2012;84(1):238–243.

20. Schuette W, Krzakowski MJ, Massuti B, et al. Randomized phase II study of palifermin for reducing dysphagia in patients receiving concurrent chemoradiotherapy for locally advanced unresectable non-small cell lung cancer. *J Thorac Oncol.* 2012;7(1):157–164.

21. Yi ES, Williams ST, Lee H, et al. Keratinocyte growth factor ameliorates radiation- and bleomycin-induced lung injury and mortality. *Am J Pathol.* 1996;149(6):1963–1970.

22. Meropol NJ, Somer RA, Gutheil J, et al. Randomized phase I trial of recombinant human keratinocyte growth factor plus chemotherapy: potential role as mucosal protectant. *J Clin Oncol.* 2003;21(8):1452–1458.

23. Ozturk B, Egehan I, Atavci S, Kitapci M. Pentoxifylline in prevention of radiation-induced lung toxicity in patients with breast and lung cancer: a double-blind randomized trial. *Int J Radiat Oncol Biol Phys.* 2004;58(1):213–219.

24. Misirlioglu CH, Demirkasimoglu T, Kucukplakci B, et al. Pentoxifylline and alpha-tocopherol in prevention of radiation-induced lung toxicity in patients with lung cancer. *Med Oncol.* 2007;24(3):308–311.

25. Kwon HC, Kim SK, Chung WK, et al. Effect of pentoxifylline on radiation response of non-small cell lung cancer: a phase III randomized multicenter trial. *Radiother Oncol.* 2000;56(2):175–179.

26. Movsas B, Scott C, Langer C, et al. Randomized trial of amifostine in locally advanced non-small-cell lung cancer patients receiving chemotherapy and hyperfractionated radiation: radiation therapy oncology group trial 98-01. *J Clin Oncol.* 2005;23(10):2145–2154.

27. Roach M, 3rd, Gandara DR, Yuo HS, et al. Radiation pneumonitis following combined modality therapy for lung cancer: analysis of prognostic factors. *J Clin Oncol.* 1995;13(10):2606–2612.

28. Bradley JD, Paulus R, Komaki R, et al. Standard-dose versus high-dose conformal radiotherapy with concurrent and consolidation carboplatin plus paclitaxel with or without cetuximab for patients with stage IIIA or IIIB non-small-cell lung cancer (RTOG 0617): a randomised, two-by-two factorial phase 3 study. *Lancet Oncol.* 2015;16(2):187–199.

29. Hu X, He W, Wen S, et al. Is IMRT superior or inferior to 3DCRT in radiotherapy for NSCLC? A meta-analysis. *PLOS ONE*. 2016;11(4):e0151988. doi:10.1371/journal.pone.0151988

30. Kocak Z, Evans ES, Zhou SM, et al. Challenges in defining radiation pneumonitis in patients with lung cancer. *Int J Radiat Oncol Biol Phys*. 2005;62(3):635–638.

31. Shaib W, Lansigan F, Cornfeld D, et al. Gemcitabine-induced pulmonary toxicity during adjuvant therapy in a patient with pancreatic cancer. *JOP*. 2008;9(6):708–714.

32. Onal C, Abali H, Koc Z, Kara S. Radiation recall pneumonitis caused by erlotinib after palliative definitive radiotherapy. *Onkologie*. 2012;35(4):191–194.

33. Forschner A, Zips D, Schraml C, et al. Radiation recall dermatitis and radiation pneumonitis during treatment with vemurafenib. *Melanoma Res*. 2014;24(5):512–516.

34. Clark D, Gauchan D, Ramaekers R, et al. Radiation recall pneumonitis during systemic treatment with everolimus. *Oncol Res*. 2014;22(5–6):321–324.

35. Lee HE, Jeong NJ, Lee Y, et al. Radiation recall dermatitis and pneumonitis induced by trastuzumab (Herceptin(R)). *Int J Dermatol*. 2014;53(3):e159–e160.

36. Castellino RA, Glatstein E, Turbow MM, et al. Latent radiation injury of lungs or heart activated by steroid withdrawal. *Ann Intern Med*. 1974;80(5):593–599.

37. Maguire PD, Sibley GS, Zhou SM, et al. Clinical and dosimetric predictors of radiation-induced esophageal toxicity. *Int J Radiat Oncol Biol Phys*. 1999;45(1):97–103.

38. Grant JD, Shirvani SM, Tang C, et al. Incidence and predictors of severe acute esophagitis and subsequent esophageal stricture in patients treated with accelerated hyperfractionated chemoradiation for limited-stage small cell lung cancer. *Pract Radiat Oncol*. 2015;5(4):e383–e391.

39. Maple JT, Petersen BT, Baron TH, et al. Endoscopic management of radiation-induced complete upper esophageal obstruction with an antegrade-retrograde rendezvous technique. *Gastrointest Endosc*. 2006;64(5):822–828.

40. Sasso FS, Sasso G, Marsiglia HR, et al. Pharmacological and dietary prophylaxis and treatment of acute actinic esophagitis during mediastinal radiotherapy. *Dig Dis Sci*. 2001;46(4):746–749.

41. Kelsey CR, Das S, Gu L, et al. Phase 1 dose escalation study of accelerated radiation therapy with concurrent chemotherapy for locally advanced lung cancer. *Int J Radiat Oncol Biol Phys*. 2015;93(5):997–1004.

42. Poortmans PM, Collette S, Kirkove C, et al. Internal mammary and medial supraclavicular irradiation in breast cancer. *N Engl J Med*. 2015;373(4):317–327.

43. Delanian S, Lefaix JL. Current management for late normal tissue injury: radiation-induced fibrosis and necrosis. *Semin Radiat Oncol*. 2007;17(2):99–107.

44. Delanian S, Balla-Mekias S, Lefaix JL. Striking regression of chronic radiotherapy damage in a clinical trial of combined pentoxifylline and tocopherol. *J Clin Oncol*. 1999;17(10):3283–3290.

45. Jang SS, Kim HG, Lee JS, et al. Melatonin reduces x-ray radiation-induced lung injury in mice by modulating oxidative stress and cytokine expression. *Int J Radiat Biol*. 2013;89(2):97–105.

46. Pietrofesa R, Turowski J, Tyagi S, et al. Radiation mitigating properties of the lignan component in flaxseed. *BMC Cancer*. 2013;13:179. doi:10.1186/1471-2407-13-179

47. Christofidou-Solomidou M, Tyagi S, Tan KS, et al. Dietary flaxseed administered post thoracic radiation treatment improves survival and mitigates radiation-induced pneumonopathy in mice. *BMC Cancer*. 2011;11:269. doi:10.1186/1471-2407-11-269

48. Machtay M, Scherpereel A, Santiago J, et al. Systemic polyethylene glycol-modified (PEGylated) superoxide dismutase and catalase mixture attenuates radiation pulmonary fibrosis in the C57/bl6 mouse. *Radiother Oncol.* 2006;81(2):196–205.
49. Simone NL, Soule BP, Gerber L, et al. Oral pirfenidone in patients with chronic fibrosis resulting from radiotherapy: a pilot study. *Radiat Oncol.* 2007;2:19. doi:10.1186/1748-717X-2-19
50. Marks LB, Bentzen SM, Deasy JO, et al. Radiation dose-volume effects in the lung. *Int J Radiat Oncol Biol Phys.* 2010;76(3, Suppl):S70–S76.
51. Miller KL, Shafman TD, Anscher MS, et al. Bronchial stenosis: an underreported complication of high-dose external beam radiotherapy for lung cancer? *Int J Radiat Oncol Biol Phys.* 2005;61(1):64–69.
52. Song SY, Choi W, Shin SS, et al. Fractionated stereotactic body radiation therapy for medically inoperable stage I lung cancer adjacent to central large bronchus. *Lung Cancer.* 2009;66(1):89–93.
53. Joyner M, Salter BJ, Papanikolaou N, Fuss M. Stereotactic body radiation therapy for centrally located lung lesions. *Acta Oncol.* 2006;45(7):802–807.
54. Committee ASoP, Pasha SF, Acosta RD, et al. The role of endoscopy in the evaluation and management of dysphagia. *Gastrointest Endosc.* 2014;79(2):191–201.
55. O'Rourke IC, Tiver K, Bull C, et al. Swallowing performance after radiation therapy for carcinoma of the esophagus. *Cancer.* 1988;61(10):2022–2026.

Fibrosis - Thickening of scarring of connective tissue
Erythema - superficial redness of the skin, usually in patches
Desquamation - skin peeling

# 4

# Radiation Therapy Effects in Breast Cancer

D. Hunter Boggs and Jennifer De Los Santos

## OVERVIEW

- Radiation therapy (RT) is commonly used as an adjuvant therapy for breast cancer.
- Acute toxicity is typically related to inflammation and dermatitis, while late toxicity is associated with fibrosis and reduced vascularity.

Approximately 1 in 8 women are diagnosed with breast cancer in their lifetimes, and breast cancer represents 30% of all malignancies diagnosed in women in 2016. Breast cancer is the most prevalent malignancy among women and the second most common cause of cancer death in women (1). RT plays a vital role in the prevention of locoregional recurrence both in patients receiving breast conservation surgery and in patients with node-positive or locally advanced breast cancer who undergo mastectomy. In early stage breast cancer, breast conservation therapy (BCT) followed by RT is equivalent to mastectomy in breast cancer outcomes (2). Recent population studies and meta-analyses suggest that BCT followed by RT may indeed be associated with improved survival compared to mastectomy (3). Despite this, mastectomy rates are increasing (4). This is, in part, due to the fear of acute and long-term radiation-induced toxicities instilled in patients and health care providers (5). In order to dispel these fears and to appropriately educate patients and colleagues, it is vital that radiation oncology professionals be knowledgeable of the diagnosis, incidence, and treatment of these toxicities. As treatment techniques have improved with methods such as deep inspiration breath hold to displace the heart from the radiation field and three-dimensional (3D) planning to accurately assess dose homogeneity within the breast and dose distribution to organs at risk, incidence and severity of acute and late toxicities reported in older literature are often much less than they were in the preceding decades (6).

In this chapter we discuss prevention, diagnosis, and management of acute and late toxicities from external beam radiation therapy (EBRT) to the breast in the modern era.

## ACUTE TOXICITY OF THE BREAST (DURING/IMMEDIATELY AFTER TREATMENT)

### Skin

- *Symptoms:* hyperpigmentation, faint erythema, dry desquamation, superficial burning, itching, and mild discomfort

- *Timing:* 0 to 14 days
- *Prevention:* regular cleansing with alkaline soap, emollients, avoiding tight clothing
- *Management:*
  - Grade 1: emollients and protective behavioral strategies
  - Grade 2+: topical barrier agents and analgesics

Acute toxicities in the breast primarily are skin effects. Dermatitis is a common acute effect of radiation, typically first seen within the first few weeks of radiation. Skin recovers quickly after radiation is complete, with symptoms resolving within 2 to 6 weeks, depending on severity.

Two randomized trials demonstrated a decrease in erythema and desquamation in patients who washed with soap and water during RT as opposed to no washing or using water alone. Roy et al found a higher incidence of moist desquamation in the nonwashing group compared to the washing group (33% versus 14%). However, there was no difference in maximal erythema scores (7–9).

Four randomized trials compared topical corticosteroid use to topical emollient (10,11), placebo (12), or no treatment (10), in breast cancer patients receiving contemporary RT. Shukla et al noted a reduction in incidence of grade 2 or higher acute dermatitis (11% versus 37%) and moist desquamation (17% versus 40%) with the use of mometasone furoate 1% twice a week compared to emollient (13). A study by Miller et al failed to show a difference in maximum grade of dermatitis with application of mometasone versus placebo, which was the primary endpoint. However, patient-reported outcomes of pruritus, irritation, burning, and annoyance with skin problems were improved in the corticosteroid group (12). Another study by Schmuth et al found a reduction of grade 4 or higher dermatitis in patients receiving methylprednisolone compared to emollient (11). A recently reported double-blinded phase II trial found a reduction in moist desquamation (45% versus 64.5%) and grade 3 acute skin toxicity (18.8% versus 33.3%) in postmastectomy RT patients receiving mometasone furoate 1% application twice daily for 14 days compared to a topical emollient cream (14). *Taken together, there is sufficient evidence to support prophylactic corticosteroids to prevent severe radiation dermatitis.*

Due to concern for bolus effect, and potential interaction of zinc-based antiperspirants with RT, deodorant use has traditionally been discouraged. This has been disproven by four randomized trials that showed no increase in acute toxicities with nonmetallic (15,16) and aluminum-based (17) deodorant use during radiation treatment. In addition, dosimetric studies revealed that a thickness of more than 0.7 mm for a 10×10 field and more than 1.5 mm for a 1×1 field of skin products during RT is required to significantly alter the dose. *As typical water-based skin applications measure only 0.3 mm on the skin, the recommendation to avoid superficial topical lotions during RT administration is not founded (18).*

*Preventative topical agents such as aloe vera (19), trolamine salicylate (20), sucralfate (21), hyaluronic acid (22), and silver dressing (23) have not been shown to be effective in the prevention of radiation dermatitis.* Heggie et al demonstrated no benefit of aloe vera gel in reducing acute skin reaction compared to a topical aqueous cream. Indeed, the aloe vera arm was associated with worse dry desquamation and pain compared to the control arm (24). Hoopfer et al conducted a randomized trial assessing acute skin erythema in patients receiving aloe vera gel, a placebo cream, or a placebo dry powder. No difference in erythema grade was observed between the arms (25). A randomized trial examining silver sulfadiazine cream found a reduction in total skin injury in the intervention arm compared to general skin care (5.5% versus 7.2%, $P$ <.0001), but further evidence regarding the utility of this intervention is lacking (26). Studies by Mak et al (27) and MacMillan et al (28) found prolonged time of healing in patients receiving hydrogel dressing compared to dry dressing or gentian violet application in patients with moist desquamation, although only MacMillan's study was statistically significant. Conversely, Gollins et al found improvement of moist desquamation healing with hydrocolloid dressing compared to gentian violet (29). In the past, gentian violet was used for wound management due to antibacterial properties, but is rarely used today (30). Table 4.1 summarizes common presentations and recommended treatments for radiation dermatitis.

### Breast Pain

- *Symptoms:* sharp electric shock lasting seconds, dull ache
- *Timing:* 0 to 21 days
- *Prevention:* Not Applicable
- *Management:* Treatment options in order of recommended use/increasing symptom toxicity
  - Analgesics
    - Acetaminophen
  - Anti-inflammatories
    - Ibuprofen 400 mg two or three times a day
    - Naproxen 250 to 500 mg twice a day
  - Opioids (ie, Acetaminophen [APAP]/hydrocodone, oxycodone, etc)
  - Neuropathic pain
    - Duloxetine 60 mg once a day
    - Gabapentin 300 to 1,200 mg three times a day
    - Pregabalin 75 to 150 mg twice a day

Breast pain also can occur from both skin injury and discomfort within deeper soft tissues of the breast. Sharp fleeting breast pain, typically described as an "electric shock," is common after breast conserving surgery and during radiation. Reassurance is often sufficient to comfort the patient. However, more significant pain can also occur within the irradiated breast. Titration of analgesics is appropriate.

**Table 4.1 Recommendations for Acute Skin Management in Order of Recommended Use/Increasing Symptom Toxicity**

| Grade | Symptoms | Timing | Recommendations |
|---|---|---|---|
| Preventative | | | - Maintain irradiated area clean and dry<br>- Wash with lukewarm water and mild unscented alkaline soap<br>- Avoid sun exposure<br>- Avoid tight clothing or clothing that can compromise skin, such as brassieres containing underwires<br>- Water-based moisturizers (unscented, lanolin free, alcohol free) may be applied three or more times per day. Application of moisturizers prior to treatment has more recently been found to be safe, without significant alteration of the distribution of superficial dose<br>- Nonaluminum/aluminum-based deodorant use is allowed during RT<br>- Avoid use of corn starch or baby powder in skin folds<br>- Avoid heating pads or ice packs<br>- Aloe vera, trolamine salicylate, sucralfate, and hyaluronic acid are not recommended for prevention of dermatitis |
| Grade 1 | - Hyperpigmentation<br>- Faint erythema<br>- Dry desquamation<br>- Superficial burning, itching, and mild discomfort | 0–14 days | The previously noted *Preventative Recommendation* measures plus:<br>- Topical corticosteroids for itching or irritation may be applied beginning on the day of RT initiation or at onset of irritative skin symptoms<br>  ○ Hydrocortisone 1% once or twice a day<br>  ○ Methylprednisolone 0.1% once a day<br>  ○ Mometasone furoate 0.1% once a day<br>  ○ Betamethasone 0.1% once a day<br>- Silver sulfadiazine 1% every 8 hours three times a week for 5 weeks (limited data supporting effectiveness) |

(*continued*)

**Table 4.1** Recommendations for Acute Skin Management in Order of Recommended Use/Increasing Symptom Toxicity (*continued*)

| Grade | Symptoms | Timing | Recommendations |
|---|---|---|---|
| Grade 2/3 | Grade 2:<br>• Bright erythema<br>• Moist desquamation<br>• Moderate edema<br>Grade 3:<br>• Confluent moist desquamation<br>• Pitting edema<br>• Blister or vesicle formation<br>• Serous drainage | Grade 2: 10–28 days<br>Grade 3: 10–28 days | • Topical corticosteroids for pruritus and topical irritation (see previous section)<br>• Oral NSAIDs for pain, edema, inflammation<br>  Ibuprofen 200–400 mg up to three times a day<br>  Naproxen 200–500 mg twice a day<br>• Topical lidocaine for superficial pain<br>  Lidocaine 3% cream, small amount applied two or three times a day<br>  May be mixed with topical emollient<br>• Topical therapies for moist desquamation, apply to affected areas only<br>  ○ Beta-glucan cream applied twice a day<br>  ○ Silver sulfadiazine 1% cream once to twice a day (especially if concern for infection)<br>• Absorbent silicone foam bandages or hydrocolloid dressings changed daily may promote reepithelization of denuded tissue. Evidence supporting their use is controversial<br>• Topical or systemic antibiotics for infection<br>  ○ Bacitracin/neomycin/polymyxin B topically applied three times a day<br>  ○ Oral antibiotics such as cephalexin for mastitis or wound infection |
| Grade 4 | • Ulceration<br>• Hemorrhage<br>• Full thickness necrosis | 14–30 days | • Referral to wound care specialist, plastic surgery, and/or dermatology<br>  ○ Full thickness skin graft, surgical debridement, myocutaneous flap, pedicle flap |

NSAIDs, nonsteroidal anti-inflammatory drugs; RT, radiation therapy.

## LATE RADIATION TOXICITY OF THE BREAST

While early skin toxicity is related to slowed repopulation of the epidermis, late toxicity in the skin is caused by damage to the dermal stroma. Effects can occur as early as 2 months after treatment, but can persist for years.

### Telangiectasias

- *Symptoms:* dilation of the capillaries causing affected skin to exhibit spidery red or purple clusters
- *Timing:* 2 to 6+ months
- *Prevention:*

  - Utilization of a breast boost is associated with increased telangiectasias. The local control benefit of a boost should be weighed against the potential long-term complications (31,32).
  - Use of high-energy electron beams (>10 MeV) is associated with increased telangiectasia rates compared to lower energy electrons or photons (33).
  - Forward planned intensity-modulated radiation therapy (IMRT) decreases telangiectasias compared to standard RT (34). The same results may be achieved with advanced 3D planning utilizing control points to increase dose homogeneity.
- *Management:* long pulsed dye laser treatment.

Nymann et al found improved superficial vessel clearance with long pulsed dye laser treatment compared to intense pulsed light laser treatment (90% versus 50%) (35). Lanigan et al found complete clearance of telangiectasias with pulsed dye laser treatment in all patients treated (8 females). Two patients developed hypopigmentation (36).

### Fibrosis/Chest Wall Pain

- *Symptoms:* pain, breast shrinkage and firmness, cutaneous induration, contraction, ulceration, delayed wound healing, arm edema, decreased shoulder range of motion
- *Timing:* 4 to 12+ months
- *Prevention:*

  - Utilization of a breast boost is associated with increased fibrosis. The local control benefit of a boost should be weighed against the potential long-term complications (31,32).
  - Use of high-energy electron beams (>10 MeV) is associated with increased fibrosis rates compared to lower energy electrons or photons (33).
  - Use of 3D-based planning to assess and minimize the amount of breast receiving over 107% of the prescribed dose. If this is not achievable with 3D technique, consider using IMRT.
  - Counsel risk associated with reconstructive options.
  - Consider prophylactic oral pentoxifylline (PTX) 400 mg two to three times a day and oral vitamin E (400–1,000 IU daily) for at least

6 months in patients at high risk for radiation fibrosis (ie, severe acute dermatitis, breast edema, planning to undergo reconstruction).
- Patients should not take PTX while on blood thinners. If patients develop nausea while taking PTX, the dose may be reduced to 200 mg twice a day. PTX and vitamin E should be discontinued 1 week before any planned invasive procedure.

- *Management:* Treatment options in order of recommended use/increasing symptom toxicity
  - Anti-inflammatories
    - Ibuprofen 400 mg two to three times a day
    - Naproxen 250 to 500 mg twice a day
  - Neuropathic pain
    - Duloxetine 60 mg once a day
    - Gabapentin 300 to 1,200 mg three times a day
    - Pregabalin 75 to 150 mg twice a day
  - Oral PTX (400 mg two or three times a day) and oral vitamin E (400–1,000 IU daily) for at least 6 months
  - No evidence to support hyperbaric oxygen therapy.

Breast of chest wall fibrosis can present as early as 4 to 12 months. Prevention predominantly relies on careful utilization of radiation and keeping dose hotspots under 107%. There is some evidence to support use of PTX and vitamin E to prevent or treat radiation fibrosis.

Immediate reconstruction tissue expander placement increases the difficulty of postmastectomy RT planning. Expanders should be maximally expanded prior to RT and not further expanded after RT owing to RT-induced edema and tightening of the skin around the expander (37).

In addition, radiation can cause significant complications with reconstructive surgery. Radiation-related adverse cosmetic outcomes including implant removals and capsular contraction are the highest in patients undergoing immediate implant reconstruction prior to RT (38,39). Autologous tissue flap reconstruction is associated with improved cosmetic rates after RT compared to implant reconstruction due to the transfer of unirradiated tissue into the treatment field. Delaying transverse rectus abdominis musculocutaneous flap reconstruction after RT is associated with decreased complication rates compared to reconstruction prior to RT (9% versus 88%) (40).

Consider prophylactic PTX in women undergoing reconstruction or those with other risk factors for fibrosis. Jacobson et al randomized 53 breast cancer patients to oral PTX 400 mg three times a day with vitamin E 400 IU daily for 6 months after RT or standard follow-up. Objective fibrosis rates were evaluated by differentiating the tissue compliance meter (TCM) measurements in the treated breast compared to the untreated breast. At 18 months, TCM measurements showed less progression in the intervention arm, signaling decreased rates of fibrosis with PTX and vitamin E (41). Magnusson et al randomized 83 patients to PTX (400 mg three times a day) and vitamin E (100 mg) for 12 months starting 1 to 3 months after completion of breast RT and noted a reduction in arm volume compared to vitamin

E plus placebo group. No difference in improvement of passive abduction of shoulder was noted among the groups, which was the primary endpoint of the study (42).

Evidence supporting PTX and vitamin E in the setting of established fibrosis is controversial. A single-arm phase II trial examined PTX (800 mg/d) and vitamin E (1,000 IU/d) for at least 6 months in patients with symptomatic fibrosis after RT and found a reduction in the mean radiation-induced fibrosis (RIF) surface area and subjective, objective management, and analytic (SOMA) injury evaluation score at 6 months compared to baseline (43). An open-label trial evaluated PTX (400 mg three times a day for 8 weeks) on 30 patients with radiation fibrosis. Improvements in active range of motion (20 of 23 patients), passive range of motion (19 of 22 patients), and muscle weakness (11 of 19 patients) were observed. Decreased limb girth was noted in 5 of 7 patients and almost half of patient with pain noted a decrease in their pain scores (9 of 20 patients) (44). However, both of these studies were limited by the lack of a control arm. Gothard et al conducted a randomized trial comparing PTX (400 mg twice a day) and vitamin E (400 mg daily) and did not find a difference in arm volume change or fibrosis compared to placebo (45). Delanian et al randomized 22 patients with RIF to PTX (800 mg/d) + vitamin E (1,000 IU/d); PTX + placebo; vitamin E + placebo; placebo-placebo. The combined PTX-vitamin E arm demonstrated superior RIF surface regression (60% versus 43%, $P$ = .038). Benefit with PTX or vitamin E monotherapy was not seen (46). In a follow-up study, Delanian et al observed a 68% reduction in RIF surface area among 44 patients with PTX (400 mg twice a day) and vitamin E (500 IU twice a day). Thirty-seven patients received treatment for 24 to 48 months and seven patients for 6 to 12 months. Mean time to maximal effect in all patients was 24 months, but was shorter (16 months) in patients who were treated for fibrosis within 6 years of RT. Both the short-term and long-term treatment groups had a 50% reduction in symptom severity as measured by SOMA score. A rebound effect was noted after discontinuation of treatment, but was higher in the short course treatment group compared to the long course group (+40% versus 8.5% increase in RIF surface area). Taken together, prolonged treatment with PTX and vitamin E may decrease the chance of rebound fibrosis after discontinuation (47).

## Lymphedema

- *Symptoms:* increases extremity girth and heaviness and/or pain, and increases the risk of delayed wound healing and cellulitis
- *Timing:* 6+ months
- *Prevention:*
    - In clinically node-negative patients, sentinel node dissection is associated with a four times lower risk of developing lymphedema compared to axillary lymph node dissection (5% vs 20%) (48).
    - In patients with up to 2 positive nodes after sentinel node dissection, axillary radiation is associated with a lower incidence of lymphedema compared to completion nodal dissection (23% vs 11%) (49).

- Addition of a supraclavicular field (9.9%), posterior axillary boost (14.7%), and internal mammary boost (8.3%) are risk factors for developing lymphedema (50).
- Recommended prophylaxis
  - Maintain ideal body weight
  - Aggressively manage localized infections to prevent cellulitis
  - Range of motion and weight-bearing exercise
  - Physiotherapy
- Recommended screening for symptoms
  - Serial arm circumference measurements (compared to unaffected limb)
    - Measure in at least two reproducible points: for instance 10 cm above and 10 cm below the olecranon process
  - Volumetric measurement via water displacement
  - Perometry (uses infrared light to estimate cross-sectional measurements) (51)
- *Management:* Treatment options in order of recommended use/increasing symptom toxicity
  - Exercise
  - Limb elevation (52)
  - Properly fitted compression garments (53)
  - Avoid introducing infectious risks in affected limb
  - Manual lymphatic drainage
  - Complete decongestive therapy
  - Intermittent pneumatic compression
  - Lymphatic bypass procedures
  - Vascularized lymph node transfer

Lymphedema is perhaps the most feared late toxicity of irradiation for breast cancer.

Prevention first relies on appropriate reduction of axillary surgery and nodal irradiation based on disease characteristics.

While not proven to improve lymphedema volume, upper extremity exercise was found to improve symptoms of pain, tenderness, and quality of life (54). Schmitz et al randomized 141 breast cancer survivors with lymphedema to a supervised weight training program or observation. Exercise resulted in a lower incidence of lymphedema exacerbations, reduced severity of symptoms, and improved strength. There was no effect of exercise on limb swelling (55). The Cancer and Leukemia Group B (CALGB) 70305 randomized patients to education alone versus education + exercise. Addition of exercise did not prevent incidence of lymphedema at 18 months (45% versus 42% in the education-only arm), although poor adherence in the exercise arm may have been a confounding factor (56). Compression therapy has been shown to reduce lymphedema compared solely to exercise and self-massage (86% versus 36%) (57). Badger et al demonstrated that multilayered short-stretch bandaging in combination with elastic hosiery reduced lymphedema compared to elastic hosiery alone (31% versus 15.8% reduction at 24 weeks) (53). Casley-Smith et al suggested an increased lymphedema exacerbation risk during air travel due to low cabin pressure (58). This finding was not reproduced in subsequent studies and *there is no compelling evidence to suggest that compression garments especially need to be worn during air travel* (59).

Evidence supporting avoidance of blood pressure measurements on the affected arm is conflicting. Hayes et al conducted a retrospective observational study which found that patients who had blood pressure measurements on the affected arm increased the risk of lymphedema by 3.4 fold (60). In this analysis, 88% of patients underwent axillary lymph node dissection. However, other studies failed to show blood pressure measurements as a risk factor for lymphedema (61–63). Similarly, there is little evidence supporting use of ipsilateral tourniquets as a risk factor for lymphedema formation (59). In the absence of level I evidence, the National Lymphedema Network recommends avoidance of excessive constriction on the affected arm, if possible (64).

Invasive skin procedures, such as lab draws, have been shown in one study by Clark et al to increase the risk of lymphedema by as much as 2.5 fold (65). This study suffered from recall bias as patients who developed lymphedema were more likely to remember that they underwent needle sticks at some point than those who did not. Numerous other studies failed to demonstrate a causative effect of invasive arm procedures on lymphedema (66). It is rather thought that resulting potential infection and cellulitis is the causative factor for lymphedema development (59).

Manual lymphatic drainage is a technique, performed by a specially trained physical therapist, which has been shown to improve limb volume and quality of life compared to self-lymphatic drainage (67). Data demonstrating the benefit of lymphatic drainage have been conflicting. Dayes et al found no improvement in lymphedema with utilization of complete decongestive therapy compared to compression garments. The randomized trial only included 103 women, so the small sample size may have obscured any potential observable difference (68). Intermittent pneumatic compression has shown some effectiveness in small studies, but a meta-analysis of seven randomized trials failed to show a benefit of the pneumatic pump compared to routine lymphedema management (69).

For severe lymphedema that is refractory to nonoperative management, surgical intervention may be considered. Lymphatic bypass procedures include lymphatic-lymphatic transfer (harvests lymphatic vessels from unaffected limbs for direct anastomosis), lymphovenous transfer (uses harvested vein to connect affected lymphatic vessels), lymphaticovenular (microsurgical technique which anastomoses small subdermal lymphatic vessels and corresponding venules), and vascularized lymph node transfer (transfers lymph node from groin or other unaffected area without an anastomosis) (70–73).

Hyperbaric oxygen is not effective. Gothard et al conducted a nonrandomized phase II trial which found no benefit of hyperbaric oxygen in the reduction of lymphedema (74).

## 4. RADIATION THERAPY EFFECTS IN BREAST CANCER

### Brachial Plexopathy

- *Symptoms:* hand/arm paresthesias, pain in affected shoulder or upper arm, weakness, sensory loss typically involving axillary nerve distribution, atrophy, and/or loss of deep tendon reflexes
- *Timing:* 8 to 12+ months
- *Prevention:*
  - Decrease total dose and dose per fraction
- Recommended prophylactic/screening for symptom
  - MRI of the brachial plexus
    - MRI may be helpful in distinguishing neoplastic plexopathy (which will demonstrate a mass) from radiation-induced plexopathy. The former may manifest with T2 hyperintensity in the affected nerve (75).
  - Electromyography (EMG)
    - EMG may reveal fasciculations more pronounced than clinical symptoms but is otherwise of little diagnostic benefit (76). Myokymia (localized quivering of muscles) is present in radiation plexopathy 60% of the time and less often in neoplastic plexopathy (77).
- *Management:* Treatment options in order of recommended use/increasing symptom toxicity
  - Symptomatic treatment and supportive care
    - Gabapentin 300 to 1,200 mg three times a day or pregabalin 75 to 150 mg twice a day for neuropathic pain
    - Benzodiazepines (such as diazepam 2 to 10 mg three to four times a day) for paresthesias
    - Physical therapy for weakness
  - No evidence to support hyperbaric oxygen
  - Nerve transfer (minimal evidence to support)

Brachial plexopathy can be significantly debilitating, but fortunately is not common. Prevention involves care during radiation planning. Incidence of plexopathy was 6% in patients receiving 45 Gy in 15 fractions versus 1% for patients receiving 54 Gy in 30 fractions (78). However, more recent studies found that modest hypofractionation (46 Gy in 20 fractions) to the infraclavicular lymph node region was not associated with brachial plexopathy (79). RT to the supraclavicular lymph nodes and large volume of irradiated brachial plexus ($V_{40Gy} \geq 13.5$ cm$^3$) and max dose to brachial plexus of 55.0 Gy or higher were associated with increased incidence of paresthesias (80).

There is very little evidence supporting any treatment for brachial plexopathy other than supportive care. Pritchard et al conducted a double-blind phase II randomized trial and found that hyperbaric oxygen did not result in improved warm sensory threshold compared to 100% oxygen in patients with radiation-induced brachial plexopathy (81). Tung et al published a case report of microsurgical transfer of median and ulnar nerve fascicles which resulted in a patient with radiation-induced brachial plexopathy regaining elbow flexion after surgery. However, the limited data regarding surgical intervention for plexopathy should be interpreted with caution due to the risk of surgically induced plexopathy exacerbation (82).

## Heart

- *Symptoms:* chronic pericarditis, coronary artery disease, restrictive cardiomyopathy (diastolic dysfunction), congestive heart failure with a preserved ejection fraction, valvular dysfunction, and conduction disorders
- *Timing:* 5 to 30 years
- *Prevention:*
   - Ensure that dose to the heart is as low as possible.
   - Encourage lifestyle modifications (smoking cessation, diabetes control, weight loss, dietary modifications, and exercise) to minimize cardiac risk.
- Recommended prophylactic/screening for symptoms
   - Echocardiogram
- *Management:* treatment options in order of recommended use/increasing symptom toxicity
   - Refer to a cardiologist if heart failure or coronary artery disease is suspected.

Cardiotoxicity is a late toxicity presenting many years after RT. Anthracyclines and anti-Her2/neu antibodies such as trastuzumab increase the risk of cardiomyopathy and display a toxic synergistic effect with RT (83). Risk factors such as a history of ischemic heart disease, diabetes, hypertension, hyperlipidemia, and smoking increase the risk of radiation-induced cardiotoxicity (84,85). Thus, lifestyle modifications are important (smoking cessation, diabetes control, weight loss, dietary modifications, and exercise).

Left-sided breast cancers and irradiation of the internal mammary nodes increase risk for coronary artery disease due to the increased volume of heart irradiated (86). For every 1-Gy increase in mean heart dose, Darby et al demonstrated a 7.4% relative increased risk of a coronary event with no apparent threshold (84). If possible, it is recommended to not let the mean heart dose exceed 5 Gy. Darby et al estimated the risk of death from ischemic heart disease by age 80 years in a 50-year-old woman with no risk factors to be 1.9%. A mean heart dose of 3 Gy would increase that risk to 2.4% (84). Darby et al estimated the risk of cardiac death in a 50-year-old woman with a single coronary risk factor to be 4.5% by age 80 years. A mean heart dose of 3 Gy would increase this risk to 5.4%, while a mean dose of 10 Gy would increase this risk to 7.7% (84).

In left-sided breast cancers, or right-sided breast cancers involving irradiation of the internal mammary nodal chain, consider techniques to displace the heart from the high-dose RT region, such as deep inspiration breath hold or respiratory gating (87). Beam arrangement and energy selection should be optimized to avoid dose to the heart while ensuring appropriate target coverage. Improvement in RT technique explains the decrease in RT-attributed cardiac mortality in patients treated from the mid 1980s or later compared to patients treated prior to the 1980s (88).

Screening echocardiograms are often obtained in patients receiving anti-Her2/neu or anthracycline-based systemic therapy to establish a baseline. Systemic therapy–related dysfunction often presents as dilated cardiomyopathy. Radiation-induced myocardial injury results from endothelial cell damage resulting in ischemia and interstitial fibrosis, which is more often restricted to areas of the myocardium in the high-dose region. This fibrosis results in decreased heart compliance resulting in restrictive cardiomyopathy (89). On echocardiogram, this appears as a decreased left ventricular mass, an increased wall thickness, and a decrease in the left ventricular chamber size. As congestive heart failure advances and myocytes become damaged, systolic failure may occur, which results in a reduced ejection fraction (89).

## Lung

- *Symptoms:* Pneumonitis—cough, shortness of breath, increased oxygen requirements, pleuritic chest pain, and/or pyrexia; fibrosis—dyspnea
- *Timing:* pneumonitis—4 weeks to 12 months; fibrosis 12+ months
- *Prevention:*
    - When treating comprehensive nodal RT, keep ipsilateral lung V20 at less than 35% if possible. When treating standard tangents, keep ipsilateral lung V20 at less than 20% if possible (90).
    - When treating supraclavicular nodes and internal mammary nodes, consider deep inspiration breath hold to decrease lung volume and displace alveoli outside of the irradiated field (91).
- Recommended prophylactic/screening for symptoms
    - Chest x-ray (CXR) or chest CT when symptomatic
- *Management* (see Chapter 3 for more details):
    - Antitussives
    - Prednisone 60 mg per day for 2 weeks following dose reduction by 10 mg per 1 to 2 weeks

Lung toxicity from radiation can occur in two phases: a subacute inflammation known as radiation pneumonitis, and a late fibrotic phase (radiation fibrosis). Radiation pneumonitis occurs within 4 weeks to 1 year after RT, presenting as cough, shortness of breath, increased oxygen requirements, pleuritic chest pain, and/or pyrexia. If treated, radiation pneumonitis typically resolves. Radiation fibrosis is an irreversible effect which can result in reduced lung capacity.

Use of comprehensive nodal RT is associated with a higher rate of grade 2 or higher radiation pneumonitis than standard tangent fields (1.2% versus 0.2%) (92).

## SUMMARY TABLE

| Organ | Ailment | Usual timing | Mild (first step) | Moderate/severe (second steps) | Preventative strategies |
|---|---|---|---|---|---|
| Skin | Telangiectasia | 2–6+ months | Observation | Referral to dermatology for pulsed dye laser treatment | Limit use of high energy (>10 Mev electron beams) |
| | Fibrosis/chest wall pain | 4–12+ months | Anti-inflammatories<br>• Ibuprofen 400 mg two to three times a day<br>• Naproxen 250–500 mg twice a day<br>Duloxetine, gabapentin, pregabalin for neuropathic pain<br>• Duloxetine 60 mg once a day<br>• Gabapentin 300–1,200 mg three times a day<br>• Pregabalin 75–150 mg twice a day | Oral PTX and vitamin E for at least 6 months<br>• PTX (400 mg two or three times a day)<br>• Vitamin E (400–1,000 IU daily) | Limit use of high energy (>10 Mev electron beams) PTX and vitamin E For reconstructed patients, avoid implantation prior to RT |
| Lymphatics | Lymphedema | Immediately after surgery to 6+ months after RT | RT avoid invasive procedures, blood pressure measurements on affected limb<br>Manual lymphatic drainage<br>Complete decongestive therapy<br>Intermittent pneumatic compression | Lymphatic bypass procedures<br>Vascularized lymph node transfer | Sentinel node dissection<br>Maintain ideal body weight<br>Exercise<br>Limb elevation<br>Properly fitted compression garments |

(*continued*)

| Organ | Ailment | Usual timing | Mild (first step) | Moderate/severe (second steps) | Preventative strategies |
|---|---|---|---|---|---|
| Brachial plexus | Brachial plexopathy | 8–12 months | Gabapentin or pregabalin for neuropathic pain<br>Benzodiazepines for paresthesia (ie, diazepam 2–10 mg three or four times a day)<br>Physical therapy | | Decrease dose per fraction |
| Heart | Cardiotoxicity | 5–10 years | Referral to cardiology | Referral to cardiology | Minimize mean dose to the heart<br>Tobacco cessation, diet, exercise, diabetes control |

PTX, pentoxifylline; RT, radiation therapy.

## REFERENCES

1. American Cancer Society. *Cancer Facts & Figures 2016*. Atlanta: American Cancer Society; 2016. http://www.cancer.org/acs/groups/content/@research/documents/document/acspc-047079.pdf
2. Early Breast Cancer Trialists' Collaborative Group. Effect of radiotherapy after breast-conserving surgery on 10-year recurrence and 15-year breast cancer death: meta-analysis of individual patient data for 10 801 women in 17 randomised trials. *Lancet*. 2011;378(9804):1707–1716.
3. van Maaren MC, de Munck L, de Bock GH, et al. 10 year survival after breast-conserving surgery plus radiotherapy compared with mastectomy in early breast cancer in the Netherlands: a population-based study. *Lancet Oncol*. 2016;17(8):1158–1170.
4. Mahmood U, Hanlon AL, Koshy M, et al. Increasing national mastectomy rates for the treatment of early stage breast cancer. *Ann Surg Oncol*. 2013;20(5):1436–1443.
5. Halkett GK, Kristjanson LJ, Lobb EA. 'If we get too close to your bones they'll go brittle': women's initial fears about radiotherapy for early breast cancer. *Psychooncology*. 2008;17(9):877–884.
6. Demirci S, Nam J, Hubbs JL, et al. Radiation-induced cardiac toxicity after therapy for breast cancer: interaction between treatment era and follow-up duration. *Int J Radiat Oncol Biol Phys*. 2009;73(4):980–987.
7. Roy I, Fortin A, Larochelle M. The impact of skin washing with water and soap during breast irradiation: a randomized study. *Radiother Oncol*. 2001;58(3):333–339.
8. McQuestion M. Evidence-based skin care management in radiation therapy: clinical update. *Semin Oncol Nurs*. 2011;27(2):e1–e17.
9. Salvo N, Barnes E, van Draanen J, et al. Prophylaxis and management of acute radiation-induced skin reactions: a systematic review of the literature. *Curr Oncol*. 2010;17(4):94–112.
10. Boström A, Lindman H, Swartling C, et al. Potent corticosteroid cream (mometasone furoate) significantly reduces acute radiation dermatitis: results from a double-blind, randomized study. *Radiother Oncol*. 2001;59(3):257–265.
11. Schmuth M, Wimmer MA, Hofer S, et al. Topical corticosteroid therapy for acute radiation dermatitis: a prospective, randomized, double-blind study. *Br J Dermatol*. 2002;146(6):983–991.
12. Miller RC, Schwartz DJ, Sloan JA, et al. Mometasone furoate effect on acute skin toxicity in breast cancer patients receiving radiotherapy: a phase III double-blind, randomized trial from the North Central Cancer Treatment Group N06C4. *Int J Radiat Oncol Biol Phys*. 2011;79(5):1460–1466.
13. Shukla PN, Gairola M, Mohanti BK, Rath GK. Prophylactic beclomethasone spray to the skin during postoperative radiotherapy of carcinoma breast: a prospective randomized study. *Indian J Cancer*. 2006;43(4):180–184.
14. Olm-Shipman M, Gelblum D, Lacouture ME, et al. Efficacy of mometasone furoate in the reduction of moderate/severe radiation dermatitis in breast cancer patients following mastectomy. *Int J Radiat Oncol Biol Phys*. 2016;96(2S):S5.
15. Théberge V, Harel F, Dagnault A. Use of axillary deodorant and effect on acute skin toxicity during radiotherapy for breast cancer: a prospective randomized noninferiority trial. *Int J Radiat Oncol Biol Phys*. 2009;75(4):1048–1052.

16. Lewis L, Carson S, Bydder S, et al. Evaluating the effects of aluminum-containing and non-aluminum containing deodorants on axillary skin toxicity during radiation therapy for breast cancer: a 3-armed randomized controlled trial. *Int J Radiat Oncol Biol Phys*. 2014;90(4):765–771.

17. Watson LC, Gies D, Thompson E, Thomas B. Randomized control trial: evaluating aluminum-based antiperspirant use, axilla skin toxicity, and reported quality of life in women receiving external beam radiotherapy for treatment of stage 0, I, and II breast cancer. *Int J Radiat Oncol Biol Phys*. 2012;83(1):e29–e34.

18. Morley L, Cashell A, Sperduti A, et al. Evaluating the relevance of dosimetric considerations to patient instructions regarding skin care during radiation therapy. *J Radiother Pract*. 2014;13(3):294–301.

19. Richardson J, Smith JE, McIntyre M, et al. Aloe vera for preventing radiation-induced skin reactions: a systematic literature review. *Clin Oncol (R Coll Radiol)*. 2005;17(6):478–484.

20. Sharp L, Finnilä K, Johansson H, et al. No differences between calendula cream and aqueous cream in the prevention of acute radiation skin reactions–results from a randomised blinded trial. *Eur J Oncol Nurs*. 2013;17(4):429–435.

21. Wells M, Macmillan M, Raab G, et al. Does aqueous or sucralfate cream affect the severity of erythematous radiation skin reactions? A randomised controlled trial. *Radiother Oncol*. 2004;73(2):153–162.

22. Pinnix C, Perkins GH, Strom EA, et al. Topical hyaluronic acid vs. standard of care for the prevention of radiation dermatitis after adjuvant radiotherapy for breast cancer: single-blind randomized phase III clinical trial. *Int J Radiat Oncol Biol Phys*. 2012;83(4):1089–1094.

23. Aquino-Parsons C, Lomas S, Smith K, et al. Phase III study of silver leaf nylon dressing vs standard care for reduction of inframammary moist desquamation in patients undergoing adjuvant whole breast radiation therapy. *J Med Imaging Radiat Sci*. 2010;41(4):215–221.

24. Heggie S, Bryant GP, Tripcony L, et al. A phase III study on the efficacy of topical aloe vera gel on irradiated breast tissue. *Cancer Nurs*. 2002;25(6):442–451.

25. Hoopfer D, Holloway C, Gabos Z, et al. Three-arm randomized phase III trial: quality aloe and placebo cream versus powder as skin treatment during breast cancer radiation therapy. *Clin Breast Cancer*. 2015;15(3):181–190.

26. Hemati S, Asnaashari O, Sarvizadeh M, et al. Topical silver sulfadiazine for the prevention of acute dermatitis during irradiation for breast cancer. *Support Care Cancer*. 2012;20(8):1613–1618.

27. Mak SS, Molassiotis A, Wan WM, et al. The effects of hydrocolloid dressing and gentian violet on radiation-induced moist desquamation wound healing. *Cancer Nurs*. 2000;23(3):220–229.

28. Macmillan MS, Wells M, MacBride S, et al. Randomized comparison of dry dressings versus hydrogel in management of radiation-induced moist desquamation. *Int J Radiat Oncol Biol Phys*. 2007;68(3):864–872.

29. Gollins S, Gaffney C, Slade S, Swindell R. RCT on gentian violet versus a hydrogel dressing for radiotherapyinduced moist skin desquamation. *J Wound Care*. 2008;17(6):268–270.

30. Wong RK, Bensadoun RJ, Boers-Doets CB, et al. Clinical practice guidelines for the prevention and treatment of acute and late radiation reactions from the MASCC Skin Toxicity Study Group. *Support Care Cancer*. 2013;21(10):2933–2948.

31. Romestaing P, Lehingue Y, Carrie C, et al. Role of a 10-Gy boost in the conservative treatment of early breast cancer: results of a randomized clinical trial in Lyon, France. *J Clin Oncol.* 1997;15(3):963–968.
32. Bartelink H, Horiot JC, Poortmans PM, et al. Impact of a higher radiation dose on local control and survival in breast-conserving therapy of early breast cancer: 10-year results of the randomized boost versus no boost EORTC 22881-10882 trial. *J Clin Oncol.* 2007;25(22):3259–3265.
33. Murphy C, Anderson PR, Li T, et al. Impact of the radiation boost on outcomes after breast-conserving surgery and radiation. *Int J Radiat Oncol Biol Phys.* 2011;81(1):69–76.
34. Barnett GC, Wilkinson JS, Moody AM, et al. Randomized controlled trial of forward-planned intensity modulated radiotherapy for early breast cancer: interim results at 2 years. *Int J Radiat Oncol Biol Phys.* 2012;82(2):715–723.
35. Nymann P, Hedelund L, Hædersdal M. Intense pulsed light vs. long-pulsed dye laser treatment of telangiectasia after radiotherapy for breast cancer: a randomized split-lesion trial of two different treatments. *Br J Dermatol.* 2009;160(6):1237–1241.
36. Lanigan SW, Joannides T. Pulsed dye laser treatment of telangiectasia after radiotherapy for carcinoma of the breast. *Br J Dermatol.* 2003;148(1):77–79.
37. Schechter NR, Strom EA, Perkins GH, et al. Immediate breast reconstruction can impact postmastectomy irradiation. *Am J Clin Oncol.* 2005;28(5):485–494.
38. Anker CJ, Hymas RV, Ahluwalia R, et al. The effect of radiation on complication rates and patient satisfaction in breast reconstruction using temporary tissue expanders and permanent implants. *Breast J.* 2015;21(3):233–240.
39. Adesiyun TA, Lee BT, Yueh JH, et al. Impact of sequencing of postmastectomy radiotherapy and breast reconstruction on timing and rate of complications and patient satisfaction. *Int J Radiat Oncol Biol Phys.* 2011;80(2):392–397.
40. Rogers NE, Allen RJ. Radiation effects on breast reconstruction with the deep inferior epigastric perforator flap. *Plast Reconstr Surg.* 2002;109(6):1919–1924.
41. Jacobson G, Bhatia S, Smith BJ, et al. Randomized trial of pentoxifylline and vitamin E vs standard follow-up after breast irradiation to prevent breast fibrosis, evaluated by tissue compliance meter. *Int J Radiat Oncol Biol Phys.* 2013;85(3):604–608.
42. Magnusson M, Höglund P, Johansson K, et al. Pentoxifylline and vitamin E treatment for prevention of radiation-induced side-effects in women with breast cancer: a phase two, double-blind, placebo-controlled randomised clinical trial (Ptx-5). *Eur J Cancer.* 2009;45(14):2488–2495.
43. Delanian S, Balla-Mekias S, Lefaix JL. Striking regression of chronic radiotherapy damage in a clinical trial of combined pentoxifylline and tocopherol. *J Clin Oncol.* 1999;17(10):3283–3290.
44. Okunieff P, Augustine E, Hicks JE, et al. Pentoxifylline in the treatment of radiation-induced fibrosis. *J Clin Oncol.* 2004;22(11):2207–2213.
45. Gothard L, Cornes P, Earl J, et al. Double-blind placebo-controlled randomised trial of vitamin E and pentoxifylline in patients with chronic arm lymphoedema and fibrosis after surgery and radiotherapy for breast cancer. *Radiother Oncol.* 2004;73(2):133–139.
46. Delanian S, Porcher R, Balla-Mekias S, Lefaix JL. Randomized, placebo-controlled trial of combined pentoxifylline and tocopherol for regression of superficial radiation-induced fibrosis. *J Clin Oncol.* 2003;21(13):2545–2550.

47. Delanian S, Porcher R, Rudant J, Lefaix JL. Kinetics of response to long-term treatment combining pentoxifylline and tocopherol in patients with superficial radiation-induced fibrosis. *J Clin Oncol*. 2005;23(34):8570–8579.
48. DiSipio T, Rye S, Newman B, Hayes S. Incidence of unilateral arm lymphoedema after breast cancer: a systematic review and meta-analysis. *Lancet Oncol*. 2013;14(6):500–515.
49. Donker M, van Tienhoven G, Straver ME, et al. Radiotherapy or surgery of the axilla after a positive sentinel node in breast cancer (EORTC 10981-22023 AMAROS): a randomised, multicentre, open-label, phase 3 non-inferiority trial. *Lancet Oncol*. 2014;15(12):1303–1310.
50. Shah C, Wilkinson JB, Baschnagel A, et al. Factors associated with the development of breast cancer–related lymphedema after whole-breast irradiation. *Int J Radiat Oncol Biol Phys*. 2012;83(4):1095–1100.
51. Stanton AW, Northfield JW, Holroyd B, et al. Validation of an optoelectronic limb volumeter (Perometer®). *Lymphology*. 1997;30(2):77–97.
52. Swedborg I, Norrefalk JR, Piller NB, Asard C. Lymphoedema post-mastectomy: is elevation alone an effective treatment? *Scand J Rehabil Med*. 1993;25(2):79–82.
53. Badger CM, Peacock JL, Mortimer PS. A randomized, controlled, parallel-group clinical trial comparing multilayer bandaging followed by hosiery versus hosiery alone in the treatment of patients with lymphedema of the limb. *Cancer*. 2000;88(12):2832–2837.
54. McNeely ML, Peddle CJ, Yurick JL, et al. Conservative and dietary interventions for cancer-related lymphedema. *Cancer*. 2011;117(6):1136–1148.
55. Schmitz KH, Ahmed RL, Troxel A, et al. Weight lifting in women with breast-cancer–related lymphedema. *N Engl J Med*. 2009;361(7):664–673.
56. Paskett, Electra, Le-Rademacher J, Oliveri J, et al. *Prevention of lymphedema in women with breast cancer (BC): results of CALGB (Alliance) 70305*. Presentation at ASCO 2017 Cancer Survivorship Program; 2017. http://meetinglibrary.asco.org/content/177040-196
57. Hornsby, R. The use of compression to treat lymphoedema. *Prof Nurse*. 1995;11(2):127–128.
58. Casley-Smith JR, Casley-Smith JR. Lymphedema initiated by aircraft flights. *Aviat Space Environ Med*. 1996;67(1):52–56.
59. Asdourian MS, Skolny MN, Brunelle C, et al. Precautions for breast cancer-related lymphoedema: risk from air travel, ipsilateral arm blood pressure measurements, skin puncture, extreme temperatures, and cellulitis. *Lancet Oncol*. 2016;17(9):e392–e405.
60. Hayes S, Cornish B, Newman B. Comparison of methods to diagnose lymphoedema among breast cancer survivors: 6-month follow-up. *Breast Cancer Res Treat*. 2005;89(3):221–226.
61. Showalter SL, Brown JC, Cheville AL, et al. Lifestyle risk factors associated with arm swelling among women with breast cancer. *Ann Surg Oncol*. 2013;20(3):842–849.
62. Ferguson CM, Swaroop MN, Horick N, et al. Impact of ipsilateral blood draws, injections, blood pressure measurements, and air travel on the risk of lymphedema for patients treated for breast cancer. *J Clin Oncol*. 2016;34(7):691–698.
63. Chan, E. Risk factors for the initiation and aggravation of lymphoedema after axillary lymph node dissection for breast cancer. *Hong Kong Med J*. 2009;15(3, Suppl 4):8–12.

64. NLN Medical Advisory Committee. Position statement of the National Lymphedema Network. http://www.lymphnet.org/pdfDocs/nlnriskreduction.pdf. Revised May 2012.
65. Clark B, Sitzia J, Harlow W. Incidence and risk of arm oedema following treatment for breast cancer: a three-year follow-up study. *QJM*. 2005;98(5):343–348.
66. Cole, T. Risks and benefits of needle use in patients after axillary node surgery. *Br J Nurs*. 2006;15(18):969–974, 976–979.
67. Williams AF, Vadgama A, Franks PJ, Mortimer PS. A randomized controlled crossover study of manual lymphatic drainage therapy in women with breast cancer-related lymphoedema. *Eur J Cancer Care (Engl)*. 2002;11(4):254–261.
68. Dayes IS, Whelan TJ, Julian JA, et al. Randomized trial of decongestive lymphatic therapy for the treatment of lymphedema in women with breast cancer. *J Clin Oncol*. 2013;31(30):3758–3763.
69. Shao Y, Qi K, Zhou QH, Zhong DS. Intermittent pneumatic compression pump for breast cancer-related lymphedema: a systematic review and meta-analysis of randomized controlled trials. *Oncol Res Treat*. 2014;37(4):170–174.
70. Baumeister RG, Siuda S. Treatment of lymphedemas by microsurgical lymphatic grafting: what is proved? *Plast Reconstr Surg*. 1990;85(1):64–74.
71. Campisi C, Boccardo F. Lymphedema and microsurgery. *Microsurgery*. 2002;22(2):74–80.
72. Chang DW. Lymphaticovenular bypass for lymphedema management in breast cancer patients: a prospective study. *Plast Reconstr Surg*. 2010;126(3):752–758.
73. Lin C-H, Ali R, Chen SC, et al. Vascularized groin lymph node transfer using the wrist as a recipient site for management of postmastectomy upper extremity lymphedema. *Plast Reconstr Surg*. 2009;123(4):1265–1275.
74. Gothard L, Haviland J, Bryson P, et al. Randomised phase II trial of hyperbaric oxygen therapy in patients with chronic arm lymphoedema after radiotherapy for cancer. *Radiother Oncol*. 2010;97(1):101–107.
75. Wouter van Es H, Engelen AM, Witkamp TD, et al. Radiation-induced brachial plexopathy: MR imaging. *Skeletal Radiol*. 1997;26(5):284–288.
76. Jaeckle KA. Neurologic manifestations of neoplastic and radiation-induced plexopathies. *Semin Neurol*. 2010;30(3):254–262.
77. Roth G, Magistris MR, Le Fort D, et al. Post-radiation brachial plexopathy. Persistent conduction block. Myokymic discharges and cramps. *Rev Neurol (Paris)*. 1988;144(3):173–180.
78. Powell S, Cooke J, Parsons C. Radiation-induced brachial plexus injury: follow-up of two different fractionation schedules. *Radiother Oncol*. 1990;18(3):213–220.
79. Guenzi M, Blandino G, Vidili MG, et al. Hypofractionated irradiation of infrasupraclavicular lymph nodes after axillary dissection in patients with breast cancer post-conservative surgery: impact on late toxicity. *Radiat Oncol*. 2015;10(1):177. doi:10.1186/s13014-015-0480-y
80. Olsen NK, Pfeiffer P, Johannsen L, et al. Radiation-induced brachial plexopathy: neurological follow-up in 161 recurrence-free breast cancer patients. *Int J Radiat Oncol Biol Phys*. 1993;26(1):43–49.
81. Pritchard J, Anand P, Broome J, et al. Double-blind randomized phase II study of hyperbaric oxygen in patients with radiation-induced brachial plexopathy. *Radiother Oncol*. 2001;58(3):279–286.
82. Tung TH, Liu DZ, Mackinnon SE. Nerve transfer for elbow flexion in radiation-induced brachial plexopathy: a case report. *Hand*. 2009;4(2):123–128.

83. Carver JR, Shapiro CL, Ng A, et al. American Society of Clinical Oncology clinical evidence review on the ongoing care of adult cancer survivors: cardiac and pulmonary late effects. *J Clin Oncol*. 2007;25(25):3991–4008.
84. Darby SC, Ewertz M, McGale P, et al. Risk of ischemic heart disease in women after radiotherapy for breast cancer. *N Engl J Med*. 2013;368(11):987–998.
85. Hooning MJ, Botma A, Aleman BM, et al. Long-term risk of cardiovascular disease in 10-year survivors of breast cancer. *J Natl Cancer Inst*. 2007;99(5):365–375.
86. Gagliardi G, Constine LS, Moiseenko V, et al. Radiation dose–volume effects in the heart. *Int J Radiat Oncol Biol Phys*. 2010;76(3, Suppl):S77–S85.
87. Nissen HD, Appelt AL. Improved heart, lung and target dose with deep inspiration breath hold in a large clinical series of breast cancer patients. *Radiother Oncol*. 2013;106(1):28–32.
88. Darby SC, McGale P, Taylor CW, Peto R. Long-term mortality from heart disease and lung cancer after radiotherapy for early breast cancer: prospective cohort study of about 300 000 women in US SEER cancer registries. *Lancet Oncol*. 2005;6(8):557–565.
89. Adams MJ, Lipshultz SE. Lipshultz. Pathophysiology of anthracycline-and radiation-associated cardiomyopathies: Implications for screening and prevention. *Pediatr Blood Cancer*. 2005;44(7):600–606.
90. Goldman, U. Blom, et al. Radiation pneumonitis and pulmonary function with lung dose–volume constraints in breast cancer irradiation. *J Radiother Pract*. 2014;13(2):211–217.
91. Nissen HD, Appelt AL. Improved heart, lung and target dose with deep inspiration breath hold in a large clinical series of breast cancer patients. *Radiother Oncol*. 2013;106(1):28–32.
92. Whelan TJ, Olivotto IA, Parulekar WR, et al. Regional nodal irradiation in early-stage breast cancer. *N Engl J Med*. 2015;373(4):307–316.

# 5

# Radiation Therapy Effects on the Abdomen

*John Cuaron and Abraham Wu*

## OVERVIEW

- Radiation therapy (RT) is a commonly used neoadjuvant and adjuvant therapy to prevent locoregional recurrence for esophageal, gastric, pancreatic, and hepatobiliary tumors.
- Acute toxicities are related to bowel mucositis and can cause systemic effects such as nausea and fatigue.
- Late toxicities are related to vascular and fibrotic effects, which can result in stricture and scarring.

As a group, gastrointestinal malignancies make up the largest percentage of new cases of cancer in the United States (1). Although many of these tumors occur in the colon, rectum, and anus, more than half of gastrointestinal cancers occur in the abdomen, including the esophagus, gastroesophageal junction, stomach, liver (including both metastases and primary liver tumors), pancreas, gallbladder, and small bowel. RT plays a crucial role in the neoadjuvant treatment of esophageal and gastroesophageal junction tumors, prevents locoregional recurrence for patients with resected gastric, pancreatic, and hepatobiliary tumors with high-risk features, and provides definitive treatment for hepatobiliary and pancreatic cancers that are unresectable owing to vascular involvement or patient comorbidities. Stereotactic body radiation therapy (SBRT) using high doses per fraction may provide a higher chance of tumor response and local control in many of these typically radioresistant histologies, and is a safe and effective treatment for oligometastatic disease to the liver. Finally, radiation therapy can provide effective and durable palliation of dysphagia, pain, bleeding, or obstruction in patients with incurable disease with symptomatic primary tumors. This chapter summarizes the major toxicities to the organs at risk when treating these malignancies and discusses their pathophysiology, timing, presentation, management, and prevention.

## ACUTE TOXICITY (Table 5.1)

### Esophagus

*Esophagitis*

- *Symptoms:* dysphagia, globus sensation, odynophagia
- *Timing:* presents ~2 weeks into radiation treatment
- *Prevention:* H2 blocker or proton pump inhibitor (PPI)

**Table 5.1 Acute Toxicities: Timing, Management, and Prevention**

| Organ | Ailment | Usual timing | Mild (first step) | Moderate/severe (second steps) | Preventative strategies |
|---|---|---|---|---|---|
| Esophagus | Esophagitis | Two weeks after initiation of RT until 2 weeks after RT | • Soften diet<br>• Nutritional supplements as needed | • Sucralfate (Carafate)<br>• Topical analgesics (lidocaine)<br>• Narcotic medication<br>• PEG tube | • PPI (omeprazole)<br>• Histamine H2 antagonists (cimetidine, famotidine, ranitidine) |
| Stomach | Anorexia, nausea, vomiting | Shortly after delivery of each fraction until a few hours afterward | • Ondansetron (Zofran)<br>• Metoclopramide (Reglan)<br>• Prochlorperazine (Compazine) | • Lorazepam (Ativan)<br>• Dexamethasone | • Prophylactic antiemetic prior to therapy<br>• Small dose per fraction<br>• Small frequent meals |
|  | Gastritis | Variable. Start of radiation up to 12 months following | • Antiemetics<br>• PPIs<br>• Histamine H2 antagonists | • Non-NSAID analgesics<br>• Narcotic analgesics | None |
|  | Abdominal cramping | Variable. Start of radiation to several months following | • Metoclopramide (Reglan)<br>• Hyoscyamine (Levsin) | • Endoscopy<br>• Resection/gastrectomy for severe ulceration or stenosis | None |

*(continued)*

**Table 5.1** Acute Toxicities: Timing, Management, and Prevention (*continued*)

| Organ | Ailment | Usual timing | Mild (first step) | Moderate/severe (second steps) | Preventative strategies |
|---|---|---|---|---|---|
| Liver/Biliary System | RILD | Anicteric ascites 2–4 weeks after radiation therapy | • Diuretics | • Paracentesis<br>• Prednisone or dexamethasone | • Limit mean dose to liver 28.5 Gy<br>• Limit D33% 93 Gy and D67% 54 Gy<br>• V15 <700 mL with SBRT |
| | Liver enzyme increase | Variable. Start of radiation up to 6 months following | • Observation<br>• Serial repeat LFTs | • Referral to hepatologist | None |
| Pancreas | Pancreatitis | Extremely rare | • Intravenous hydration<br>• Analgesic medication | • Aggressive intravenous fluid replacement<br>• Bowel rest | None |
| Small Bowel | Diarrhea | Second to third week of radiation therapy | • Dietary modifications (low-fat, low-fiber diet)<br>• Limiting use of exacerbating medications (magnesium, Maalox, Mylanta, Colace, Senna, Prilosec)<br>• Loperamide (maximum 16 mg per day) | • Rule out infectious etiology<br>• Lomotil (maximum 8 tablets per day)<br>• Tincture of opium<br>• Discontinuation of concurrent chemotherapy<br>• Radiation therapy treatment break | • Minimize the amount of small bowel in treatment field when possible |

(*continued*)

**Table 5.1** Acute Toxicities: Timing, Management, and Prevention (*continued*)

| Organ | Ailment | Usual timing | Mild (first step) | Moderate/severe (second steps) | Preventative strategies |
|---|---|---|---|---|---|
| | Duodenitis | Second to third week of radiation therapy | • Antiemetics<br>• Antisecretory medications (PPIs, H2 antagonists)<br>• Non-NSAID analgesics | • Narcotic analgesics<br>• Endoscopic evaluation | • Limit amount of duodenum receiving 50 Gy <45 mL<br>• For SBRT, V33 ≤1 mL, V20 ≤3 mL, V15 ≤9 mL |
| | Increased bowel gas/bloating | First to third week of radiation therapy | • Beano<br>• Simethicone (ie, Gas-X, Maalox) | | • Low residue/antigas diet |

LFTs, liver function tests; PEG, percutaneous endoscopic gastrostomy; PPI, proton pump inhibitor; RT, radiation therapy; SBRT, stereotactic body radiation therapy.

- *Management:*
  - Grade 1: diet change (soft solids, liquid supplements)
  - Grade 2: barrier agents (ie, sucralfate) and analgesics (2% viscous lidocaine, PO opioids)
  - Grade 3+: IV hydration, percutaneous endoscopic gastronomy tube

The esophageal mucosa has an inherently high rate of cellular turnover and is considered to be a radiation-sensitive organ. Most patients receiving definitive RT to the esophagus or mediastinum (such as for lung cancer) will develop at least grade 1 esophagitis.

Esophagitis presents as subtle dysphagia or globus sensation ("lump in the throat") approximately 2 weeks after the initiation of radiation therapy (2). This can progress to moderate to severe odynophagia to both solids and liquids, especially pronounced for hard, spicy, fatty, or acidic foods and beverages.

Management of mild esophagitis is typically conservative, with interventions aimed at decreasing discomfort and ensuring adequate nutrition. For grade 1 esophagitis, softening the diet and adding nutritional supplements is warranted. For grade 2 esophagitis, sucralfate can be used to provide an acid buffer and protective barrier on the mucosal surface. For progressive discomfort, topical analgesics or systemic opioid medication is used. During therapy, patients' weight and nutritional status is monitored. With continued significant esophagitis and compromised ability to nourish and hydrate, patients should be considered for intravenous rehydration, or in severe cases, evaluated for hospitalization and temporary percutaneous endoscopic gastronomy tube placement.

## Stomach

### Anorexia, Nausea, and Vomiting

- *Timing*: at any time during radiation treatment
- *Prevention*: H2 blocker or PPI
- *Management*:
  - Antiemetics (ie, ondansetron, prochlorperazine, and metoclopramide)
  - Benzodiazepines (ie, lorazepam)
  - Dexamethasone

Nausea and vomiting is a well-known sequela of radiation therapy to the abdomen and can present at any point during a course of RT, often shortly after the delivery of each fraction. The pathophysiology is related to acute radiation-induced edema of both the epithelial and stromal tissue. It is typically transient in nature, often lasting a few hours after treatment and resolving 1 to 2 weeks after the end of the course of radiation therapy.

Prior to the initiation of therapy, patients should be considered for either PPI or H2 blocker therapy to prevent acid-induced gastritis, which can exacerbate nausea and vomiting. Antiemetics used for radiation-induced nausea include ondansetron, prochlorperazine, and metoclopramide. Benzodiazepines such as lorazepam can also be substituted or added in refractory cases. For patients treated to an area with high emetic risk, such as the stomach, a short course of dexamethasone to curtail the effects of the edema can also be used (3).

For patients with significant nausea associated with their radiation treatment, prophylactic antiemetic premedication prior to treatment administration can be considered (3). Other preventative measures include using a smaller dose per fraction, if possible, and advising the patient to eat small frequent meals rather than large meals prior to treatment.

### *Gastritis*

- *Symptoms:* nausea, vomiting, abdominal pain
- *Timing:* 3+ weeks into treatment
- *Prevention:* H2 blocker, PPI
- *Management:* H2 blocker, PPI
  - Antiemetics
  - Analgesics (avoid nonsteroidal anti-inflammatory drugs [NSAIDs])

The timing of radiation-induced gastritis is variable and can present between the start of radiation to 12 months after the end of treatment (2). There is a correlation between the development of gastritis and increased dose of radiation therapy delivered to the stomach, increased dose rate and size per fraction, and the use of concurrent chemotherapy. Symptoms include nausea, vomiting, and abdominal pain. Endoscopic findings include mucosal erosions, ulceration, and mucosal atrophy. Treatment is mainly aimed at symptom management, including antiemetics, antisecretory medications (PPIs or H2 blockers), non-NSAID analgesics, and narcotic analgesics.

### *Abdominal Cramping*

- *Symptoms:* abdominal cramping, pain, bloating
- *Timing:* 3+ weeks into treatment
- *Prevention:* diet changes (low residue)
- *Management:*
  - Promotility agents (metoclopramide or hyoscyamine)
  - Endoscopic evaluation

Abdominal cramping can result from acute inflammation of the stomach and intestinal mucosa during the acute stages of treatment. It presents as a paroxysmal sharp pain and bloating that is often relieved by eructation, flatus, or bowel movements. In later periods after therapy, it can be the presenting symptom of chronic complications such as gastric outlet obstruction, antral stenosis, late ulceration, or fistula.

Initial management should include a trial of motility agents, including metoclopramide or hyoscyamine. Refractory cases can be considered for workup with upper endoscopy in order to determine etiology. For uncomplicated dysmotility or mild ulceration, conservative management with reassurance is reasonable. For severe ulceration or stenosis, therapeutic interventions include cessation of RT and consideration of endoscopic interventions, such as stenting (for obstruction).

## Liver/Bile Duct System
### Radiation-Induced Liver Disease

- *Symptoms:* anicteric ascites with fatigue, bloating, and weight gain
- *Timing:* presents 2 to 4 weeks into radiation treatment
- *Prevention:* careful radiation dose planning with consideration of baseline liver function
- *Management:* supportive (diuretics, paracentesis, steroids, treatment of coagulopathies)

Radiation-induced liver disease (RILD) is a serious and potentially fatal complication of radiation treatment to the abdomen. The current model of pathogenesis suggests that this form of injury is caused by radiation-induced fibrin deposition into the central veins, resulting in veno-occlusive disease and retrograde congestion. The disease presents 2 to 4 weeks after radiation treatment as anicteric ascites with fatigue, bloating, and weight gain. Pathognomonic laboratory values show a marked increase in alkaline phosphatase, mild to moderate elevations in aspartate transaminase (AST)/alanine transaminase (ALT), and little to no increase in bilirubin.

The risk of RILD is related to radiation dose–volume parameters, as well as underlying hepatic conditions (including cirrhosis). The TD5/5, the radiation dose that would result in a 5% risk of severe complications 5 years after radiation therapy, to the entire liver is 30 Gy in 2-Gy fractions (4,5). Partial volume tolerances are 93 Gy to one-third of the liver and 54 Gy to two-thirds of the liver (6). Extrapolation of these constraints to the hypofractionated setting suggests that no more than 700 mL of the liver (which represents 25% of a typical liver volume and the minimum volume that must be spared during liver resection) can receive more than 15 Gy when using SBRT (7). At our institution, we typically constrain the mean liver dose to 28.5 Gy when using conventional fractionation, and for hypofractionated cases, we spare at least 700 mL of the normal liver to 15 Gy or lesser.

The only known treatment for RILD is supportive. Interventions include diuretics, paracentesis, and steroids to relieve the discomfort of ascites, and correction of coagulopathy. The majority of patients will recover within 6 months. A minority of patients, especially those with underlying liver conditions, will experience fibrosis, cirrhosis, and fulminant hepatic failure. RILD is associated with a 10% to 20% mortality rate.

### Liver Enzyme Increase

In the absence of the clinical presentation of RILD, transient elevation in liver transaminases or alkaline phosphatase is typically mild and self-limiting. If elevation in liver enzymes persists for more than 6 months after the end of radiation, referral to a hepatologist for further workup and management should be considered.

## Pancreas
### Pancreatitis

Acute radiation-induced pancreatic toxicity is exceedingly rare. Management is similar to acute pancreatitis of other etiologies and includes supportive care with intravenous fluid replacement and pain management in mild cases. Severe or refractory cases require intensive fluid status monitoring, pain control, and bowel rest.

## Small Bowel

### Diarrhea

- *Timing:* presents 2 to 3 weeks into radiation treatment
- *Prevention:* low-fat low-fiber diet
- *Management:*
  - Grade 1: loperamide
  - Grade 2: diphenoxylate/atropine (Lomotil) or tincture of opium
  - Grade 3+: IV hydration, cessation of chemotherapy or radiation

Diarrhea (increased, loose, watery bowel movements with our without bleeding) typically presents in the second to third week of conventionally fractionated radiation when at least some portion of the small bowel is being irradiated. The pathophysiology is multifactorial and due to a combination of malabsorption of lactose and bile salts owing to radiation-induced epithelial denudation, altered intestinal motility, and bacterial floral disturbance (8).

Initial management includes dietary and lifestyle modifications. Having patients adopt a low-fat, low-fiber diet can significantly improve symptoms. Limiting the use of medications that exacerbate diarrhea (including aluminum/magnesium/simethicone, docusate sodium, senna, magnesium supplements, and omeprazole) can also provide relief. If conservative measures are insufficient, over-the-counter (OTC) antidiarrheals, such as loperamide, can be used as needed after loose bowel movements, up to eight times per day.

If diarrhea remains refractory to OTC agents, consideration should be made regarding other etiologies, including infectious enteritis or colitis. Stool cultures should be considered. If an infectious cause is ruled out, pharmacological therapy can be escalated to include diphenoxylate/atropine (Lomotil) or tincture of opium. Concurrent chemotherapy may also contribute to refractory diarrhea and may need to be discontinued.

Weight and volume status should be closely monitored and intravenous fluid replacement should be used as needed while diarrhea persists.

### Duodenitis

The duodenum's close proximity to the pancreas and hepatobiliary structures puts this organ at unique risk for radiation-induced toxicity during and after the treatment of pancreatic, liver, and gallbladder tumors. Duodenitis presents with anorexia, nausea, vomiting, cramping, and diarrhea. Significant ulceration and hemorrhage can present as dark, tarry stools, hematemesis, and decreasing hemoglobin.

Acute management is similar to that of gastritis and includes conservative trials of antiemetics, antisecretory medications (PPIs or H2 blockers), non-NSAID analgesics, and narcotic analgesics. Refractory cases or significant hemorrhage should be managed with endoscopic evaluation for possible local therapies.

Duodenal inflammation and enteritis is rare with conventional doses less than 40 Gy, whereas the incidence increases when a substantial portion of the duodenum is irradiated beyond 50 Gy. Our institutional constraints include limiting the duodenal volume receiving 50 Gy to 45 mL or lesser and limiting the maximum point dose to 58 Gy.

Duodenal toxicity is of particular concern when using SBRT. High doses per fraction can cause severe mucositis, ulceration, and perforation. When using SBRT at our institution for pancreas SBRT, we prefer to constrain the duodenal V33, V20, and V15 to 1, 3, and 9 mL respectively.

## LATE TOXICITY (Table 5.2)

### Esophagus

*Stricture*

- *Symptoms:* dysphagia, odynophagia, pain
- *Timing:* 1 to 6+ months
- *Prevention*: not defined
- *Management:* endoscopic dilation

Late radiation toxicity of the esophagus can include stricture and dysmotility. This manifests predominantly as dysphagia, although odynophagia and spastic pain can also occur. The presentation is as early as 4 to 6 weeks following therapy with a median time to presentation of 6 months (9).

Workup includes upper endoscopy and barium swallow. The latter imaging modality is important in evaluating locations of strictures and peristaltic functionality.

The mainstay of treatment for radiation-induced strictures is manual endoscopic dilation. This results in a favorable initial success rate of 83% to 85% but is associated with a high long-term recurrence rate of 33% (10,11). For patients with significant weight loss and malnutrition, tube feedings may be required.

When portions of the esophagus are treated with 56 to 60 Gy, the incidence of stricture is 12% to 30% (2,9). Specific dose-limit recommendations are difficult to generate because of the large range of dose volume parameters that have been associated with esophageal toxicity (12). The most widely used dose-volume constraint (including at our institution) is to limit the mean dose to the entire esophagus to no more than 34 Gy, but this may not be entirely relevant when small volumes of the esophagus are treated to very high doses (as high as 74 Gy), which anecdotal experience and randomized evidence suggest to be safe. A practical approach is to limit the amount of the organ that is electively treated to a high dose. The use of image guidance with smaller treatment margins and intensity-modulated radiation therapy (IMRT) can be useful in achieving this goal.

*Fistula*

- *Timing:* months to years after end of RT
- *Prevention:* not defined
- *Management:* surgical repair

**Table 5.2 Late Toxicities: Timing, Management and Prevention**

| Organ | Ailment | Usual timing | Mild (first step) | Moderate/severe (second steps) | Preventative strategies |
|---|---|---|---|---|---|
| **Esophagus** | Stricture | Six months | • Endoscopic dilation | • PEG tube | • Limit volume receiving high dose<br>• Mean dose <34 Gy<br>• Image guidance for smaller margins<br>• IMRT when appropriate |
| | Fistula | Variable | • N/A | • Intubation<br>• Bypass<br>• Excision | • For SBRT, limit max point dose <22 Gy, V14 <2.5 mL |
| **Stomach** | Gastric outlet obstruction | Variable | • Endoscopic dilation | • PEG tube | • Limit volume receiving high dose<br>• Image guidance for smaller margins<br>• IMRT when appropriate |
| | Ulceration, bleeding, perforation | Latency period of 5 months | • Antiemetics<br>• PPI<br>• Histamine H2 antagonists<br>• Non-NSAID analgesics<br>• Narcotic analgesics | • Surgery for severe ulceration or perforation | • Antisecretory medication (PPIs, H2 blockers) during and after therapy<br>• Limit the full stomach dose <45 Gy |

*(continued)*

Table 5.2 Late Toxicities: Timing, Management, and Prevention (continued)

| Organ | Ailment | Usual timing | Mild (first step) | Moderate/severe (second steps) | Preventative strategies |
|---|---|---|---|---|---|
| Liver/Biliary System | Biliary stricture | Many years after radiation therapy | • N/A | • Surgical bypass<br>• Stenting | • Limit max point dose to 40Gy or less in 5 fractions<br>• Limit V40 <21 mL and V37.7 <24 mL for 5 fraction regimens<br>• Limit V33.8 <21 mL and V32 <24 mL for 3 fraction regimens |
| Pancreas | Chronic pancreatitis/exocrine insufficiency | Extremely rare | • Analgesic medication<br>• Enzyme supplementation<br>• Dietary modification | • Celiac nerve block<br>• Lipase supplementation | None |
| Small Bowel | Ulceration, obstruction, fistula | Eight— to twelve months post radiation therapy | • Dietary modifications (low-fat, low-fiber diet)<br>• Imodium<br>• Cholestyramine | • Severe bleeding: endoscopic cautery or laser treatment<br>• Partial bowel obstruction: bowel rest and decompression<br>• Fistula, perforation, complete obstruction: Surgical intervention | • Limit small bowel in field when possible<br>• For SBRT, limit the max point dose to 30 Gy, V12.5 Gy <30 mL, or V33, V20, and V15 to be 1, 3, and 9 mL |

IMRT, intensity-modulated radiation therapy; PEG, percutaneous endoscopic gastrostomy; PPI, proton pump inhibitor; SBRT, stereotactic body radiation therapy.

Esophageal fistula is a rare but potentially devastating late complication of high-dose radiation. The time to development is variable but is generally months to years after the end of RT. It typically presents as a persistent cough that is exacerbated by eating or drinking. Management includes efforts to prevent further fistulization and protection of the airway, either by intubation, bypass, or surgical excision (13).

Precise risk factors and preventative strategies have not been well defined. However, a number of recent reports have provided more recognition of the scope of this issue and suggested dose-volume constraints to minimize this risk in the context of SBRT (14,15).

## Stomach

### Gastric Outlet Obstruction

With a mechanism and presentation similar to esophageal stricture, gastric outlet obstruction can occur secondary to radiation-induced antral dysmotility and stenosis. The acute inflammation of gastritis eventually gives way to mucosal atrophy and fibrosis of the submucosal tissues.

Similar to esophageal stricture, radiation-induced antral stenosis is typically treated with serial endoscopic dilation.

### Ulceration, Bleeding, and Perforation

- *Timing:* 5+ months after end of RT
- *Prevention:* PPIs, H2 blockers
- *Management:*
  - Grade 1: PPIs or H2 blockers, non-NSAID analgesics
  - Grade 2: narcotic analgesics
  - Grade 3: severe ulceration, fistula, or perforations require surgical intervention

Late ulceration and bleeding of the gastric mucosa has a median latency period of 5 months (2), after which time patients present with epigastric pain, hematemesis, and dark tarry stools. Endoscopy demonstrates mucosal erosion and atrophy along with ulcerations indistinguishable from non–radiation-induced ulcerations. The pathogenesis of late ulceration is radiation-induced necrosis of acid-secreting cells with resultant chronic inflammation, mucosal thinning, and ulceration. Ulcerations can later form aberrant gastric-involved fistulous tracts or perforations.

The risk of late gastric ulceration is related to the dose delivered, with risk estimates extrapolated from historical clinical series. These include a reported risk of 4% ulceration for doses less than 50 Gy and 16% for doses equal to or greater than 50 Gy among men treated for testicular cancer (16). Among 516 patients treated with 40 Gy for Hodgkin disease with the stomach in the field, the rates of ulceration, perforation, and gastritis were acceptably low at 4.8%, 1.7%, and 0.38% (17). Limiting the full stomach dose to 45 Gy results in a late ulceration risk of approximately 5% to 7% (18).

Prevention efforts should include the use of antisecretory medication (PPIs, H2 blockers) during and after therapy. Acute management of mild bleeding includes conservative trials of antisecretory medications (PPIs or H2 blockers), non-NSAID analgesics, and narcotic analgesics. Severe ulceration, fistula, or perforations require surgical intervention.

## Liver/Bile Duct System
### Biliary Stricture

- *Timing:* years after end of RT
- *Prevention:* constraining dose to the central hepatobiliary tract
- *Management:* surgical bypass or stent

The most significant late toxicity after treatment to the liver and biliary system is radiation-associated stricture of the bile duct. It typically presents years after radiation treatment of the abdomen with obstructive jaundice with or without pruritus. Laboratory values indicate conjugated hyperbilirubinemia and imaging with ultrasound, CT, and magnetic resonance cholangiopancreatography (MRCP) show thickening of the bile duct. Endoscopic retrograde cholangiopancreatography and cholangioscopy can be used to confirm luminal narrowing or obstruction. Histologic hallmarks are collagen deposition, fibrosis, and vasculitis (19).

Untreated biliary obstruction can put patients at risk for ascending cholangitis, sepsis, and liver failure. Management of biliary stricture aims to relieve obstruction and is accomplished either by surgical bypass or stenting.

Biliary stenosis is rare after conventional radiation therapy. There is a higher incidence of 4% to 15% among patients treated with SBRT (15,20). Prevention hinges on constraining dose to the central hepatobiliary tract. Published suggested dose constraints include limiting the max point dose to 40 Gy or less in 5 fractions (21) and limiting V40 to less than 21 mL and V37.7 to less than 24 mL for 5 fraction regimens, and V33.8 to less than 21 mL and V32 to less than 24 mL for 3 fraction regimens (20).

## Pancreas
### Chronic Pancreatitis and Exocrine Insufficiency

- *Timing:* 5+ months
- *Prevention:* PPIs, H2 blockers
- *Management:*
  - Grade 1: low-fat diet, lipase supplementation, OTC analgesics, nutrition counseling
  - Grade 2+: analgesics, celiac nerve block

Compared to luminal gastrointestinal organs, pancreatic parenchymal cells have a low turnover rate and are considered more resistant to radiation therapy. Although the incidence of pancreatitis and exocrine insufficiency among patients with pancreatic cancer is substantial (22), direct injury from radiation therapy is rare and appears only as isolated case reports in the literature (16,23,24). Presentation and duration of symptoms is variable but most commonly presents as paroxysmal severe postprandial pain and symptoms of malabsorption, including weight loss, vitamin deficiency, and steatorrhea.

Pancreatitis due to radiation injury is managed similarly to pancreatitis from other causes. Principles of treatment include pain management with enzyme supplementation, analgesics, and consideration of celiac nerve block if refractory. Patients should be advised to restrict fat intake, both to prevent hyperstimulation and to mitigate the effects of steatorrhea. Lipase supplementation may be indicated to prevent malabsorption. Patients should also be monitored for glucose intolerance, as diabetes mellitus can develop as a late complication.

## Small Bowel

### *Ulceration, Obstruction, and Fistula*

Chronic injury to the small bowel presents a median of 8 to 12 months after radiation treatment (2). Symptoms include frequent, urgent stools with blood or mucous, fecal urgency, and abdominal cramping. The pathophysiology of the condition is driven by fibrosis within the bowel wall with resultant ischemia, ulceration, and mucosal smoothing with impaired reabsorption. Severe fibrosis can cause luminal narrowing or adhesions that may precipitate obstruction. Ulcerations can cause fistula formation.

Mild cases of late small-bowel toxicity should be managed with conservative measures including a low-fat, low-fiber diet and antidiarrheal medication as needed. Cholestyramine can alleviate diarrhea from malabsorption by reducing intraluminal bile salts. Severe bleeding should be evaluated for endoscopic management, including cautery or laser ablation. Partial small-bowel obstructions should be managed with bowel rest and decompression initially, with consideration of surgery if refractory to conservative management. Severe ulceration, fistula, perforations, or complete bowel obstruction require surgical intervention.

The risk of small-bowel complications appears to have a threshold dose, with the incidence sharply increasing to 15% to 25% if a substantial portion of small bowel is treated to doses of approximately 50 to 55 Gy of conventionally fractionated RT (2). With the increasing use of SBRT for hepatobiliary and pancreatic tumors, dosimetric consideration of the duodenum and small bowel is crucial. Reported dose constraints are heterogenous and evolving as groups and institutions report experience with different SBRT regimens (15). Quantitative Analyses of Normal Tissue Effects in the Clinic (QUANTEC) recommendations are to limit V12.5 Gy to less than 30 mL and to limit the maximum point dose to 30 Gy (18). At our institution, we use identical constraints as when treating pancreas tumors with SBRT, and limit the small bowel V33, V20, and V15 to be 1, 3, and 9 mL respectively.

## REFERENCES

1. Siegel RL, Miller KD, Jemal A. Cancer statistics, 2016. *CA Cancer J Clin*. 2016;66: 7–30.
2. Coia LR, Myerson RJ, Tepper JE. Late effects of radiation therapy on the gastrointestinal tract. *Int J Radiat Oncol Biol Phys*. 1995;31:1213–1236.

3. Basch E, Prestrud AA, Hesketh PJ, et al. Antiemetics: American Society of Clinical Oncology clinical practice guideline update. *J Clin Oncol*. 2011;29:4189–4198.
4. Emami B, Lyman J, Brown A, et al. Tolerance of normal tissue to therapeutic irradiation. *Int J Radiat Oncol Biol Phys*. 1991;21:109–122.
5. Lawrence TS, Robertson JM, Anscher MS, et al. Hepatic toxicity resulting from cancer treatment. *Int J Radiat Oncol Biol Phys*. 1995;31:1237–1248.
6. Dawson LA, Ten Haken RK. Partial volume tolerance of the liver to radiation. *Semin Radiat Oncol*. 2005;15:279–283.
7. Rusthoven KE, Kavanagh BD, Cardenes H, et al. Multi-institutional phase i/ii trial of stereotactic body radiation therapy for liver metastases. *J Clin Oncol*. 2009;27:1572–1578.
8. Classen J, Belka C, Paulsen F, et al. Radiation-induced gastrointestinal toxicity. Pathophysiology, approaches to treatment and prophylaxis. *Strahlenther Onkol* 1998;174(Suppl 3):82–84.
9. O'Rourke IC, Tiver K, Bull C, et al. Swallowing performance after radiation therapy for carcinoma of the esophagus. *Cancer*. 1988;61:2022–2026.
10. Choi GB, Shin JH, Song HY, et al. Fluoroscopically guided balloon dilation for patients with esophageal stricture after radiation treatment. *J Vasc Interv Radiol*. 2005;16:1705–1710.
11. Agarwalla A, Small AJ, Mendelson AH, et al. Risk of recurrent or refractory strictures and outcome of endoscopic dilation for radiation-induced esophageal strictures. *Surg Endosc*. 2015;29:1903–1912.
12. Werner-Wasik M, Yorke E, Deasy J, et al. Radiation dose-volume effects in the esophagus. *Int J Radiat Oncol Biol Phys*. 2010;76:S86–S93.
13. Little AG, Ferguson MK, DeMeester TR, et al. Esophageal carcinoma with respiratory tract fistula. *Cancer*. 1984;53:1322–1328.
14. Cox BW, Jackson A, Hunt M, et al. Esophageal toxicity from high-dose, single-fraction paraspinal stereotactic radiosurgery. *Int J Radiat Oncol Biol Phys*. 2012;83:e661–e667.
15. Thomas TO, Hasan S, Small W Jr, et al. The tolerance of gastrointestinal organs to stereotactic body radiation therapy: what do we know so far? *J Gastrointest Oncol*. 2014;5:236–246.
16. Brick IB. Effects of million volt irradiation on the gastrointestinal tract. *AMA Arch Intern Med*. 1955;96:26–31.
17. Cosset JM, Henry-Amar M, Burgers JM, et al. Late radiation injuries of the gastrointestinal tract in the h2 and h5 eortc hodgkin's disease trials: emphasis on the role of exploratory laparotomy and fractionation. *Radiother Oncol*. 1988;13:61–68.
18. Kavanagh BD, Pan CC, Dawson LA, et al. Radiation dose-volume effects in the stomach and small bowel. *Int J Radiat Oncol Biol Phys*. 2010;76:S101–S107.
19. Fajardo LF, Berthrong M. Radiation injury in surgical pathology. Part I. *Am J Surg Pathol*. 1978;2:159–199.
20. Osmundson EC, Wu Y, Luxton G, et al. Predictors of toxicity associated with stereotactic body radiation therapy to the central hepatobiliary tract. *Int J Radiat Oncol Biol Phys*. 2015;91:986–994.
21. Eriguchi T, Takeda A, Sanuki N, et al. Acceptable toxicity after stereotactic body radiation therapy for liver tumors adjacent to the central biliary system. *Int J Radiat Oncol Biol Phys*. 2013;85:1006–1011.
22. Tseng DS, Molenaar IQ, Besselink MG, et al. Pancreatic exocrine insufficiency in patients with pancreatic or periampullary cancer: a systematic review. *Pancreas*. 2016;45:325–330.

23. Strole WE Jr, Castleman B. Case 32-1969 — Abdominal irradiation followed by diarrhea and twenty-five years later by malabsorption, diabetes, headaches and diplopia. *N Engl J Med*. 1969;281:314–323.
24. Fajardo LF, Berthrong M. Radiation injury in surgical pathology. Part III. Salivary glands, pancreas and skin. *Am J Surg Pathol*. 1981;5:279–296.

# 6
# Radiation Therapy Effects on the Pelvis

*Elizabeth B. Jeans and Peter J. Rossi*

## INTRODUCTION

- Radiation therapy (RT) is a common and effective treatment for anorectal cancer, bladder and prostate cancer, and gynecologic cancers.
- Advanced radiation planning technology can reduce, but not prevent, pelvic toxicity.
- The pelvis is a common site for brachytherapy as a strategy to deliver high doses to a tumor while minimizing doses to the pelvic organs.
- To date, prospective data comparing proton therapy with photon external beam therapy shows similar side effect profiles.
- Patient-reported outcomes through validated questionnaires are commonly used to understand patient experience and provide another facet of radiotoxicity.

RT has proven to be an effective treatment modality for various cancers of the male and female pelvis. The success of definitive RT has been well established as a primary treatment in anorectal cancer. More recently, concurrent chemotherapy and RT has been used for bladder conservation in patients with bladder cancer. While level I evidence of bladder preservation versus radical cystectomy is lacking, recent studies have demonstrated satisfactory quality of life (QOL) and bladder function after concurrent chemoradiation (1). In males, RT remains a predominant treatment modality for prostate carcinoma and an option for penile preservation in patients with penile carcinoma. RT can also be used for ureteral and testicular cancer to improve local control in certain cases. In females, RT has been utilized in treating vulvar, vaginal, cervical, and uterine cancer, with demonstrated efficacy postoperatively or definitely for nonsurgical candidates.

Current pelvic therapy can utilize various treatment techniques such as brachytherapy, three-dimensional conformal radiation therapy (3DCRT), intensity-modulated radiation therapy (IMRT) (with or without advanced image guidance), proton therapy, and utilization of concurrent chemotherapy, which increases frequency and severity of toxicity. The treatment choice is based upon the patient's clinical presentation, burden of disease, the physician's training and experience with differing techniques, as well as the available treatment machines at the facility coupled with the expertise of the staff. Therefore, given the differing methods of treatment for patients who receive RT to the pelvis, the incidence of radiotoxicity to nearby structures can be vastly different. Regardless, understanding the array of toxicities that can occur in these anatomical areas, as well as the evidence behind prophylactic and treatment measures for various toxicities is imperative to improved success in overall patient satisfaction, patient QOL, and patient compliance with treatment plans.

## PATIENT-REPORTED OUTCOMES VERSUS PHYSICIAN-REPORTED TOXICITY

- Both physician-reported toxicity and patient-reported outcomes through validated questionnaires offer insight into the pelvic cancer patient's experience of treatment-related toxicity.
- Recognize that patient-reported outcomes offer snapshots in time, but may be more sensitive than physician-reported toxicity, which can describe cumulative risk over time.

An additional component of discussing radiotoxicity to the pelvis comes with the subjective, as well as objective, differences in patient-reported versus physician-reported outcomes. Across numerous different RT sites, demonstrated discrepancies in patient-related outcomes versus physician-related outcomes has been established. Rosati et al (2) analyzed 42 patients treated to 25 to 33 Gy in 5 fractions with stereotactic body radiation therapy (SBRT). In this subset, discrepancies from patient to physician were noted in toxicities such as constipation and diarrhea, as well as a discrepancy among physician-reported outcomes and patient-reported overall health or QOL.

## USE OF RADIATION TECHNOLOGY

### Image Guidance and IMRT

Despite the great efficacy of RT on the female and male pelvis, the proximity of these tumors to nearby critical organs creates an environment that can easily be subjected to radiotoxicity. Over the past decade, the advancements in RT have allowed for firmer target delineation and decreased dosage to surrounding organs. 3DCRT was introduced in the 1980s, which allowed for CT-based three-dimensional volume planning of internal anatomy. Subsequently, in the late 1990s, IMRT became a more commercialized and standardized method of RT delivery. This, along with improvements of image guidance (IG) through placement of fiducial/gold markers and placement of cone beam CT on machines, allowed for reduction in margins on planning volumes. Conceptually, this reduction in planning volume and improvement in daily setup should lead to improved acute and late toxicities with suspected equivalent, if not improved, disease outcomes as compared to older external beam radiation therapy (EBRT) techniques.

- Wortel et al (3) compared the toxicity profile of 3DCRT ($n$ = 189) to IG-IMRT ($n$ = 242) using 78 Gy in 39 fractions in patients with localized prostate cancer. At 5 years, patients treated with IG-IMRT were noted to have a 24.9% incidence of grade 2 or greater gastrointestinal toxicity, as compared to 37.6% with 3D-CRT. Genitourinary toxicity of grade 2 or higher with IG-IMRT was 46.2% as compared to 36.4% with 3D-CRT.

Significant reductions in proctitis (hazard ratio [HR]: 0.37, $P = .047$) and increased stool frequency (HR: 0.23, $P \leq .001$) were noted.

- Because of increased cost of IMRT, 3DCRT remains the primary treatment modality for many cancers while awaiting trial data due to limited data supporting benefit with other advanced technologies.

### Brachytherapy and Proton Therapy

Brachytherapy, either as seed implantation or interstitial radiation therapy (RT), is a common well-established treatment option for patients with specific criteria of disease state for prostate, cervical, and endometrial cancer. Brachytherapy, due to rapid dose falloff, often reduces the dose delivered to large volumes of organs at risk (OARs), and decreases treatment time and equivalent retrospective disease outcomes compared to EBRT. Proton therapy has gained recognition over the past decade for its potentially better dose distribution owing to depth-dose characteristics with equivalent tissue response per unit dose (as compared to photons). However, patient-reported outcomes comparing 3DCRT, IMRT, and proton beam therapy have failed to demonstrate superiority in toxicity profile with photon treatment. No prospective randomized trial for demonstrating superiority of proton therapy in pelvic tumors yet exists.

- Gray et al (4) analyzed prospectively collected patient-reported outcomes of toxicities in patients with prostate cancer. Patients were treated with 3DCRT ($n = 123$), IMRT ($n = 153$), or proton therapy ($n = 95$) and followed up at 2 to 3 months, 12 months, and 24 months. While short-term QOL was decreased with protons (bowel) or IMRT (urinary), these detriments recovered by 12 or 24 months.

## USE OF DOSE-VOLUME CONSTRAINTS TO REDUCE TOXICITY RISK

Predicting a patient's likelihood for toxicity has long been studied in a quantitative fashion through dose-volume effects on OARs. With the increased use of IMRT, a greater push exists to quantify the dose-volume effects of RT on OARs to detail dose-volume constraints that can be readily incorporated into the radiation oncologist's practice. The majority of studies detailing toxicities of the pelvis are focused within the use of IMRT for prostate cancer. Of greatest interest has been the toxicity of the rectum. However, regardless of the vast amount of published literature quantifying dose-volume toxicities, predicting radiotoxicity remains imprecise. Physician predictions should be based on historical observation of radiation-induced changes, dosimetric analysis of treatment plan, as well as patient's personal and genetic risk factors.

## TOXICITY BY PELVIC ORGAN

### Rectum

#### Acute Proctitis

- *Symptoms:* diarrhea, urgency, mucus discharge, and tenesmus
- *Timing:* during RT to within 6 months after treatment

- *Prevention:* minimizing bowel/rectum receiving high dose
- *Management:* hydration, antidiarrheal agents (Table 6.1)

### Chronic Proctitis (ie, Pelvic Radiation Disease)

- *Symptoms:* diarrhea and tenesmus, rectal bleeding, excessive flatulence, incontinence, fistula formation, and intestinal stricture
- *Timing:* 3 months to years after RT
- *Prevention:* hyaluronic acid gel spacers, advanced radiation techniques
- *Management:*
  - Grade 1: antidiarrheal agents, hydrocortisone suppositories
  - Grade 2: sucralfate enemas
  - Grade 3+: endoscopic procedures (ie, formalin, argon plasma coagulation [APC] laser), hyperbaric oxygen therapy, surgical fistula repair

Note increased risk of fistula with invasive procedures, particularly formalin or rectal biopsies.

Acute radiation proctitis occurs during RT or within six months of the end of RT. Symptoms include diarrhea, urgency, and tenesmus. Acute toxicity stems from local tissue ischemia caused by radiation injury to the colonic and rectal wall leading to connective tissue fibrosis and obliterative endarteritis. Most often, acute radiation proctitis is self-limiting, but can have a severe impact on QOL and therefore often demands physician intervention.

Chronic radiation proctitis is a misnomer as inflammation of the bowel wall is typically minimal and observation of the colon is noted for fibrosis and vascular sclerosis. Better-suited terms for chronic radiation proctitis include chronic radiation proctopathy or pelvic radiation disease. Chronic radiation proctopathy, by definition, occurs beyond 3 months after the end of RT; however, occasionally symptoms can begin several years following the end of treatment. Symptoms can include diarrhea and tenesmus, as well as rectal bleeding, incontinence, excessive flatulence, fistula formation, and intestinal stricture leading to narrowing of the bowel and potential intestinal blockage. Chronic symptoms often prelude to physician intervention, given increased impact to patient QOL and risk of complications.

Incidence and Prevention

- IG-IMRT in prostate RT has shown significantly lower grade 2 or greater proctitis compared to 3DCRT of equal dose.
- The use of endorectal balloons or perirectal injected "spacers" in decreasing dose to the rectum may be helpful to prevent radiation-related morbidities.
- Both oral and enema sucralfate and misoprostol have failed to provide prophylaxis for radiation-induced rectal symptoms.

Many studies have attempted to predict the incidence of acute rectal proctitis; however, given the inconsistency of reporting among physicians, the

*(text continues on page 125)*

## Table 6.1 Radiation-Induced Rectal Symptom Treatment

| Symptom | Intervention | Evidence for treatment | Rationalization |
|---|---|---|---|
| Diarrhea | Supportive management: hydration, antidiarrheals (ie, loperamide, Lomotil) | None | Help control symptoms and allow for natural healing process to occur |
| Rectal bleeding, tenesmus | Sucralfate enemas | RCT ($n = 37$) randomized to sulfasalazine (3g/day) plus prednisolone enemas (20 mg twice a day) or sucralfate enemas (2 mg twice a day) noted clinical improvement with no difference between groups; however, clinical response and tolerance were greater with sucralfate enemas (5). Has also demonstrated efficacy in rectal bleeding. Kochhar et al (6) prospectively studied 26 patients with severe radiation proctosigmoiditis. Each patient was treated with sucralfate enemas (20 mL of 10% suspension twice a day), 77% demonstrated reduction in bleed by 4 weeks and 92% by 16 weeks. At 46-months (median follow-up), 71% had no further bleeding. | May have positive healing effects on epithelial microvascular injury by stimulating mucosal glutathione and angiogenesis (7) |

*(continued)*

**Table 6.1 Radiation-Induced Rectal Symptom Treatment** *(continued)*

| Symptom | Intervention | Evidence for treatment | Rationalization |
|---|---|---|---|
| Rectal bleeding, tenesmus | Glucocorticoid suppositories or enemas: Hydrocortisone 2% PR hydrocortisone enema 100 mg twice a day | Reduces blood loss, mucus production, endoscopy appearance, but one RCT was significantly less effective when compared to sucralfate-like suppositories (8). | Improve inflammatory mechanism of acute proctitis leading to symptomatic improvement |
| Diarrhea | Selenium | RCT with cervical cancer ($n = 11$) and uterine cancer ($n = 70$) patients with initial selenium concentrations of less than 84 mcg/L. Randomized to 500 mcg of selenium on days of RT and 300 mcg selenium on non-RT days versus placebo. Demonstrated reduced grade 2+ toxicity of diarrhea (20.5% versus 44.5%) (9). | |
| Diarrhea Rectal bleeding | Metronidazole | RCT ($n = 60$) with rectal bleeding and diarrhea randomized to mesalamine plus betamethasone enemas with or without metronidazole (400 mg three times a day). At 4 weeks, 3 months, and 12 months, rectal bleeding, diarrhea, edema, and mucosal ulcers were reduced (10). Demonstrating potential role for synergistic effect with topical steroids. | Unclear mechanism how it reduces bleeding |

*(continued)*

**Table 6.1** Radiation-Induced Rectal Symptom Treatment (*continued*)

| Symptom | Intervention | Evidence for treatment | Rationalization |
|---|---|---|---|
| | Bile acid sequestrants: Cholestyramine (4–8 g twice a day) Colesevelam (625 mg, up to 6 times/day) (11) | None | Beneficial if etiology is secondary to bile acid malabsorption |
| | Opioids (11) | None | If taken 30–60 min prior to meals, delay transit time allowing for increased absorption of food contents and decreased osmotic effect in the gut |
| | Minimally absorbed antibiotics: rifaximin (200 mg two or three times a day) Or Broad-spectrum oral antibiotics: ciprofloxacin/doxycycline for 7–10 days (11) | None | If etiology is related to small-intestinal bacterial overgrowth, treatment could allow for resolution of bacterial cultivation decreasing clinical symptoms |

(*continued*)

**Table 6.1 Radiation-Induced Rectal Symptom Treatment** *(continued)*

| Symptom | Intervention | Evidence for treatment | Rationalization |
|---|---|---|---|
| | **NOT RECOMMENDED—NEGATIVE TRIALS** | | |
| | Supportive management: octreotide | None<br>RTOG 0315 ($n = 215$) with rectal or anal cancer. Randomized to 30 mg long-acting octreotide 4–7 days prior to RT and on day 22 versus placebo. Demonstrated **no difference** in grade 2+ diarrhea | Octreotide is inhibitor of GI motility, as well as intestinal fluid and electrolyte transport |
| | Short-chain fatty acid enemas | None<br>Treatment in patients with chronic proctitis in multiple RCTs demonstrated no superiority to placebo (12–14) | May help to accelerate healing. Specifically SCFA enemas may quicken the process due to preferred energy source for epithelium of the colon in regeneration |

Adapted from UpToDate: Clinical manifestations, diagnosis, and treatment of radiation proctitis.
GI, gastrointestinal; RCT, randomized controlled trial; RT, radiation therapy; SCFA, short-chain fatty acid enemas.

true estimated amount of acute proctitis is unclear. One study, Lesperance et al (15), predicted acute proctitis among prostate cancer patients treated with EBRT to be as high as around 43% ($n = 183$), indicating quite a large proportion of treated patients, especially when compared to brachytherapy at 6% ($n = 50$). Chronic proctitis is likely to be lower, with IMRT series noting a 10% to 20% risk of grade 2+ proctitis (16). Lesperance et al (15) determined chronic proctitis incidence to be higher with EBRT compared to patients receiving brachytherapy. In Radiation Therapy Oncology Group (RTOG) 9513, incidence of late gastrointestinal (GI) toxicity (grade 3 or worse) in the absence of hormonal treatment was dependent upon treatment field: whole pelvis RT patients had late GI toxicity of 5% as compared to prostate-only RT, 1% (17). These studies demonstrate that incidence is truly dependent upon individual treatment plan.

The most significant factor that can prevent radiation-induced proctitis, at this point, includes dose-volume constraints, localized RT techniques, especially the use of IG, and advanced planning and treatment methods, such as IMRT, coupled with decreasing patient risk factors for radiation-related morbidities. Ali et al (18) compared patients treated with IMRT plans from CT alone ($n = 53$) versus CT-MRI (n = 28). CT-MRI demonstrated significantly less contoured prostate volumes (43.0 cm$^3$ versus 55.7 cm$^3$, $n = 15$), as well as decreased bladder and rectal V20, V30, and V70. While genitourinary (GU) grade 2 toxicity rates were similar, CT-MRI demonstrated significantly less rates of GI grade 2 toxicity: 50% versus 72%, respectively.

Quantifying chronic proctitis in relation to treatment strategy has been more difficult as the current studies and the duration of follow-up is limited. Those with long-term follow-up show that 10% to 20% of patients develop chronic GI toxicities during a 10-year period. One study (16) analyzed 1,571 patients between 1988 and 2000 treated for T1 to T3 prostate cancer. Patients were treated with 3DCRT to prescription doses between 66 and 81 Gy or IMRT to a dose of 81 Gy. Median follow-up time was 8 years, and 10-year actuarial rates demonstrated the likelihood of developing a grade 2 or greater GI toxicity was 9%. Of the patients who experienced acute GI symptoms, the 10-year likelihood of late toxicity was 42% as compared to 9% for those who did not experience acute toxicities ($P < .001$). Analysis of patients with IMRT versus 3DCRT once again demonstrated that while those treated with IMRT had higher prescription dose than 3DCRT, the patients had lesser amounts of chronic proctitis denoting less dose delivered to adjacent structures.

Recent investigations into further techniques to reduce rectal toxicity in the planning part of RT have yielded interesting results. Smeenk et al (19) investigated the use of an endorectal balloon to spare the anal wall during 3DCRT or IMRT in localized prostate carcinoma. Two planning CTs were performed, with and without the endorectal balloon. Endorectal balloon was identified to significantly reduce the mean and max dose to the anorectal wall. Perirectal fat injections have also been investigated in the setting of brachytherapy and EBRT. Prada et al (20) randomized 69 patients with low- and intermediate- risk prostate cancer to brachytherapy alone versus brachytherapy and protection of the rectal wall with hyaluronic acid (6–8 mL into perirectal fat). Patients with hyaluronic acid injections had less mucosal damage on proctoscopic examination

(5% versus 36%, respectively, $P = .002$) as well as no macroscopic rectal bleeding (0% versus 12% respectively, $P = .047$) at median follow-up of 18 months. Newer methods, such as Hydrogel Spacer, have been studied in randomized clinical trials. Mariados et al (21) and Hamstra et al (22) reported on 222 men with T1 or T2 prostate cancer undergoing IMRT who were randomized 2:1 to spacer injection versus control. In addition to dosimetric advantages during treatment planning, the use of spacer injection with more than 3 years follow-up showed decreased bowel toxicity (grade 2+ 6% versus 0%, $P = .012$) compared to control. Additionally, fewer declines in urinary and bowel QOL were reported when the spacer agent was used versus the control group. Further, there was no significant late toxicity in the spacer group. As well, 15 month follow-up demonstrated a significantly less percentage of patients having 10-point decline in bowel QOL in the spacer group (11.6% versus 21.4%, respectively). Continued clinical trials and long-term follow-up are necessary to further analyze the role of these interventions in preventing RT-induced toxicity by advanced planning.

Due to the uncertainty with which patients could be dealing with symptoms incurred during treatment, prophylactic medical interventions for radiation-induced proctitis have been investigated. Most investigated is prophylactic sucralfate. While sucralfate has demonstrated efficacy in treatment, it has failed to provide prophylaxis for patients undergoing therapy. Prophylactic misoprostol suppositories yielded similar results. As of date, no prophylactic medical interventions have proven to decrease the incidence of radiation-induced proctitis.

- Kreebone et al (23) administered 3 g of oral sucralfate suspension or placebo twice a day to 338 patients with localized prostate cancer undergoing RT. There was no difference in the two groups regarding symptom burden from RT: stool frequency ($P = .41$), consistency ($P = .20$), flatus ($P = .25$), mucus ($P = .54$), and pain ($P = .73$). Of note, the sucralfate group had more rectal bleeding (64% versus 47%, $P = .001$).
- An additional study randomized 86 patients with localized prostate cancer undergoing RT to a daily enema of 3 g sucralfate versus placebo (24). At 5-year follow-up, grade 2 toxicity was noted at 12% for placebo versus 5% for sucralfate ($P = .26$). Late rectal bleeding was 59% versus 54%, respectively.
- One hundred patients undergoing therapy for prostate cancer were randomized to daily misoprostol or placebo suppositories. Grade 2 toxicity was reported in 36% of the misoprostol patients versus 26% in the placebo group. In addition, more patients with misoprostol experienced rectal bleeding (25).

Important patient factors predisposing to proctitis include smoking history, obesity, diabetes mellitus, and irritable bowel disorder, and previous pelvic or abdominal surgery, history of collagen vascular diseases, such as scleroderma or systemic lupus erythematosus, and immunodeficiency states. The role of hypertension in relationship to development of proctitis is still uncertain. Some studies have demonstrated a direct correlation while others have suggested a protective effect of hypertension on development of radiation-induced proctitis.

More recent studies have focused on genetic predisposition to developing proctitis after RT. Valdagni et al (26) looked at patients' genetic predispositions toward late rectal bleeding by analyzing 30 patients, at a minimum follow-up of 48 months, who underwent 3DCRT to prescription doses higher than 70 Gy for prostate cancer. Patients were stratified into low-risk and high-risk groups based on dosimetric parameters. All patients received gene analysis of 35 different genes responsible for DNA repair. Overall, there were nine genes downregulated in low-risk bleeders versus high-risk bleeders. As well, there were four genes that were significantly upregulated in high-risk nonbleeders as compared to both other cohorts. Given these results, the role of genetics in predicting one's likelihood of toxicity to RT is becoming an area that could provide clinical practices with a better understanding of preventative and treatment strategies for higher risk patients.

## Management: Acute Proctitis

Regardless of strategies to minimize rectal dose for pelvic RT patients who are at highest likelihood of developing radiation proctitis, a physician must have an understanding of how to manage toxicity if and when it does occur. There are a multitude of therapies available, some demonstrating strong therapeutic evidence in literature while others are unproven. Very few large randomized clinical trials have been studied in patients with radiation-induced proctitis. Therefore, management paradigms are concentrated from small clinical trials, case reports, and physician experience.

Diarrhea is the most common GI-associated radiotoxicity complaint to the physician in the acute setting. Determining the etiology of radiation-induced diarrhea can help the physician determine appropriate treatment if primary empiric treatments fail. There are numerous possible etiologies for radiation-induced diarrhea. Fuccio et al (11) give an elaborate explanation of such etiologies including small intestinal bacterial overgrowth, bile acid malabsorption, carbohydrate malabsorption, or any change in GI transit time. Table 6.1 lists empirical treatment and dosages that can be used when radiation-induced rectal symptoms occur. Other symptoms of acute radiation proctitis include rectal urgency, rectal pain, and tenesmus. These symptoms are often also improved with the previously listed treatment options. Based on the current evidence, recommendations include supportive treatment with consideration of utilizing butyrate or sucralfate and glucocorticoid enemas.

Patient improvement should be closely followed for indications that further treatment is required. If no improvement is seen after 3 to 4 weeks of treatment, alternative treatment options or testing, specifically endoscopy, should be considered. If patients are unable to tolerate treatment side effects, RT breaks should be considered to allow for symptomatic improvement to prevent compromising further treatments or disease outcomes. Despite high likelihood that symptoms are related to pelvic RT, alternative diagnoses should always be considered if patient fails to improve. Differential diagnosis should include inflammatory bowel disease, infectious colitis, diverticulitis/diverticulosis, medication-induced symptoms, and ischemic colitis, specifically in the elderly.

## Management: Chronic Proctitis

Symptoms of chronic radiation proctitis include symptoms similar to acute radiation proctitis, but patients are more likely to have bleeding (especially that which is clinically significant). Symptom management, including previously mentioned interventions, is warranted if symptoms are minimal. Specifically, sucralfate enemas (20 mL in 10% sucralfate suspension twice a day), which we prefer to hydrocortisone suppositories, have shown to significantly decrease bleeding in patients with chronic radiation proctitis. When patients have bleeding that fails to respond to sucralfate therapy, other treatments including endoscopic therapy with argon plasma coagulation is warranted.

Before endoscopic intervention, a trial of formalin therapy can be considered in specific patient populations. Formalin is known to cause coagulative tissue necrosis, therefore if symptomatic bleeding is present, use of formalin to induce necrosis of bleeding tissue should be considered. However, formalin is also associated with fistula formation. Therefore, this therapy should be avoided in patients with rectal cancer or those who are more prone to fistula formation (inflammatory bowel patients or patients with a significant history of infectious colitis or diverticulitis). Given the severity of side effects and the high tolerability of endoscopic intervention, argon plasma coagulation is usually preferred.

- Ma et al (27) studied 24 patients with medical treatment–resistant grade 2 or 3 rectal bleeding post RT (mean time from end of treatment: 11.1 ± 9.0 months). Of the 24 patients, 19 required one course of formalin irrigation and 5 required a second course. One month post topical irrigation treatment, complete blood cessation was noted in 5 patients and decreased bleeding was noted in 14 patients. On long-term follow-up, 5 of 16 had bleeding at 1 year, 1 of 9 at 2 years, and 0 of 6 at 5 years. No acute side effects of treatment were noted, but three rectovaginal fistulas were found at 1 month, 3 months, and 2 years postformalin treatment. In other case reports, serious complications of fistula formation required a colostomy and also bowel resection.

- Formation of strictures and worsening of fecal incontinence have been noted in case reports of formalin application, specifically in patients postradiotherapy for anal cancer (28). The largest study, 100 patients, treated with 10% buffered formalin solution by proctoscope navigation of bleeding vessel, noted 93% had bleeding cessation after an average of 3.5 applications within 2 to 4 weeks (29).

Argon plasma coagulation (APC) is a well-studied therapy for chronic radiation proctitis. APC use in postradiation bleeding has been reported in case studies dating back to the early 1990s. On average, patients required two to four treatments in order to stop rectal bleeding. Case reports noting its effectiveness in refractory hemorrhagic radiation proctitis is also noted. Side effect profile of APC includes rectal ulceration, of which glucocorticoid and mesalamine suppositories can provide benefit. Morbidity with bowel explosion has been noted (30) and complete bowel lavage is now recommended prior to APC. Due to the high risk of fistula formation in the postradiation setting, current recommendations include combined consultation with a urology and radiation oncologist before APC administration in order to predict likelihood of such a morbidity.

Other interventions for rectal bleeding have included argon lasers, cryoablation, bipolar electrocoagulation and heater probe, and radiofrequency ablation. While some have proven efficacy in case reports, large studies as well as long-term follow-up are warranted to assess their efficacy, as well as long-term morbidity. In addition, due to the expense of many of these technologies, randomized clinical trials with APC are warranted to assess the necessity of such treatments with current practice.

Obstructive symptoms such as constipation, rectal pain and urgency, and occasionally fecal incontinence are other common symptoms associated with chronic radiation proctitis. Obstructive symptoms are often a sign of stricture formation and endoscopic evaluation is warranted. Stool softeners provide symptomatic relief for patients with obstructive symptoms and balloon or Savary-Gilliard dilation should be considered for patients who do not get relief with stool softeners. However, the correlation of colonic rupture increases with length of stricture, and colorectal surgical evaluation should be considered based on imaging findings.

Fecal incontinence is a morbid complication following RT. Once fecal incontinence has occurred, medical therapy is very limited. Fiber supplementation can help in bulking the stool and improving continence; however, comorbidity with other radiation-induced side effects may limit use of fiber. Rather, fecal incontinence is ideally prevented by limiting dose to the anal sphincter muscles and iliococcygeal muscle.

- Schaake et al (31) analyzed 262 patients with localized or advanced prostate cancer (T1–T3 stage) to analyze side effects with dosimetric variables. Fecal incontinence was associated with V15 to the external sphincter and V55 to the iliococcygeal muscle. Also of note in the study was increase in stool frequency with V45 to iliococcygeal muscle and V40 to levator ani, as well as increase in rectal bleeding with V70 to anorectum and anticoagulation use.

Anti-inflammatories have long been investigated as therapy for acute and chronic radiation proctitis; 5-ASA drugs such as sulfasalazine and aminosalicylates have demonstrated efficacy in case reports. In Table 6.1, the efficacy in sulfasalazine (3g/day) plus prednisolone enemas (20 mg twice a day) was demonstrated in a randomized clinical trial (32). However, the role of other oral 5-ASA drugs such as mesalamine, balsalazide, olsalazine, as well as 5-ASA enemas and foams remains unclear. The need for randomized controlled trials (RCTs) demonstrating the efficacy of these drugs for radiation-induced proctitis is necessary.

Pentosan polysulfate (PPS) demonstrated in a study of 13 patients with chronic radiation-induced proctitis to alleviate clinical symptoms completely in 82% and partially in 9%. Nine percent of patients failed to respond (33). A subsequent phase III randomized clinical trial of PPS (100 mg three times a day or 200 mg three times a day) versus placebo was planned in 168 patients. This failed to demonstrate improvement of radiation-induced proctitis (34). Further investigation has not occurred.

Given the free radical damage of RT, antioxidants have been investigated as methods of treatment and prophylaxis for RT-induced proctitis. One study, involving 10 patients, administered vitamin E (400 IU three times a day) and vitamin C (500 mg three times a day) to patients with improvement in diarrhea and urgency (35). In another trial, patients ($n = 18$) with radiation proctitis were randomized to vitamin A or placebo for 90 days. Significant improvement in symptoms were correlated with vitamin A: 77% versus 22%, respectively. Similarly, a small randomized controlled study ($n = 40$) of 6 months of pentoxifylline has failed to duplicate case reports of improvement in radiation-induced proctitis (36). Regardless of historical case reports and these aforementioned small clinical trials, large randomized clinical trials with internal and external validity are necessary to validate any correlation between antioxidants or anti-inflammatories and improvement in symptoms.

Much research has been allocated toward hyperbaric oxygen therapy (HBOT) for chronic radiation proctitis. Radiation-induced injury is known to occur by oxidative stress and hypoxia to tissue. Animal studies have shown increased tissue regeneration, decreased oxidative damage by free radicals, decreased tissue fibrosis, and increased activity of antioxidant enzymes (11). Therefore, hypothetically, in humans, HBOT should cause quickened regeneration and prevent further radiation-induced injury of normal tissue, allowing for symptomatic improvement. Controlled trials have attempted to demonstrate the beneficial results of HBOT across many tumor sites and radiation side effects. However, if a patient is refractory to medical therapy, is a nonsurgical candidate, and/or prefers to avoid surgery, HBOT should be utilized. Patients demonstrated improvement in symptoms and QOL.

- In an RCT of patients with refractory radiation proctitis ($n = 120$) randomized to 2.0 atm HBOT or 1.1 atm HBOT (control), HBOT was noted to improve healing responses with an absolute risk reduction of 32% and number needed to treat of 3 (37). However, limitations in this study included a large dropout percentage, as well as unclear blinding.

For some patients with severe chronic rectal injury, surgical intervention may deem necessary. These patients include those with perforation, stricture formation unamenable to dilation, fistula formation, or uncontrollable pain or bleeding. Due to the likelihood of numerous adhesions from RT, surgical intervention comes with a large chance of complications and patients should be educated that such risks are more likely. Surgical options for patients include diversion, as well as construction of ileocecal reservoir for select patients.

## Bladder

### Radiation Cystitis

- *Symptoms:* frequency, dysuria, hematuria, obstruction
- *Timing:* Acute: within 2 to 3 weeks of RT; Chronic: 6 months+ (mean 3 years)
- *Prevention:* respect dose constraints during planning
- *Acute management:* test for urinary tract infection (UTI)
    - Grade 1, 2: phenazopyridine, alpha blockers, anticholinergics (use with caution in elderly)

- *Chronic management:*
  - Grade 1: anticoagulation reversal (when appropriate), transfusion, bladder irrigation
  - Grade 2: sodium PPS or conjugated estrogens, botulinum A
  - Grade 3: cystoscopy with fulguration, HBOT
  - Grade 4: surgical excision/repair/cystectomy

Radiation cystitis, much like radiation proctitis, is a collective term that includes irritative bladder symptoms, such as frequency, dysuria, nocturia, or of most clinical concern, hematuria. Radiation cystitis can occur during RT or soon following treatment completion, commonly called acute radiation cystitis. Acute radiation cystitis is commonly marked by symptoms of frequency and dysuria, which are often self-limiting. Late radiation cystitis has been noted in case reports to begin anywhere from 6 months to 20 years after treatment with a mean latent period of 35 months (38). Symptoms of late radiation cystitis include frequency and dysuria, but often includes hematuria lending to the term hemorrhagic radiation cystitis (HRC).

The diagnosis of radiation cystitis should be highly scrutinized in the clinical setting. Many patients may be receiving chemotherapy for their pelvic tumors and chemotherapeutic drugs, such as ifosfamide, cyclophosphamide, busulfan, doxorubicin, fludarabine, and cabazitaxel are known to cause nonhemorrhagic and hemorrhagic cystitis. Although important to recognize, it may be nearly impossible to discern the origin of cystitis if patients are receiving concurrent chemoradiotherapy. Also, given the immunodeficient state of the average cancer patient, as well as the commonality of infections of the urinary tract, dipstick urinalysis and urine culture should always be performed to exclude infection. Although uncommon, secondary malignancy should always be considered. Therefore, radiation-induced cystitis should be considered as a diagnosis of exclusion to ensure for proper follow-up.

Radiation toxicity to the bladder is noted by damage to the bladder mucosa leading to an inflammatory state with marked tissue edema (39). The pathophysiology of the bladder during acute toxicity leads to patient symptoms of dysuria, frequency, and less likely hematuria. With late radiation cystitis, obliterative endarteritis causes a hypoxic environment leading to atrophy and fibrosis of the bladder mucosa causing tissue breakdown and sloughing of the necrotic tissue (38). The pathophysiology of late radiation-induced changes explains the greater likelihood for patients with late radiation-induced cystitis to develop hematuria. The slow replicative nature of vascular and connective tissue discerns the delayed presentation of late radiation-induced cystitis (39).

## Incidence and Prevention

Similar to acute radiation proctitis, the incidence of acute radiation cystitis is difficult to predict, given the gaps in reporting these symptoms on both the patient and physician part. It is estimated that up to half of patients treated with pelvic RT will experience some version of acute cystitis (clinically significant or not) during treatment. This incidence is highly dependent on the pelvic site of RT and the inclusion of the bladder in the treatment plan: those treated with RT for bladder cancer are almost certain to develop some symptoms of acute radiation cystitis, while those treated for prostate cancer with newer treatment techniques are less likely.

Late radiation cystitis incidence is more accurate to predict given increased severity and chronicity of symptoms and the high likelihood that patients and physicians will report such symptoms. Late radiation cystitis has an incidence of 5% to 10% (38). In a questionnaire collected from 192 prostate cancer patients treated with standard four-field box technique RT of 60 to 66 Gy over 6.5 weeks, 4% of patients claimed significant bladder symptoms impacting QOL at a median follow-up of 33 months after RT (40), while 83% noted no changes or improvement in urinary stream post-treatment. Seventy percent noted improvement or stable nocturia. Only 2% noted needing some form of protection for urinary incontinence following treatment, while 0.5% described frequent hematuria and 2% moderate or severe dysuria.

Radiotoxicity to the bladder can result in urinary incontinence. Although highly unlikely given modern methods of delivery-focused treatment, a recent retrospective review of 29 patients (41) who underwent cystectomy for treatment-refractory disease secondary to RT demonstrated 41.4% was due to refractory fistulas, 41.4% due to radiation cystitis, 13.8% due to pelvic pain, and 3.4% due to incontinence. While any of the afore-mentioned symptoms of acute and late radiation-induced cystitis can result in incontinence, prolonged incontinence severely impacts QOL for patients. Al Awamlh et al (41) demonstrated through patient surveys that although surgical risk exists with cystectomy and urinary diversion in this subgroup, significant improvement in patient's physical and mental QOL is noted. Therefore, patients should be promptly referred to a urologist when QOL due to prolonged incontinence is noted on behalf of the radiation oncologist.

Other toxicities of radiation to the bladder can include urethral strictures and fistula formation. Urethral strictures, of varying degrees, following RT are predicted to occur in 1% to 12% of patients (42). The incidence is highly dependent on treatment type and dose delivery. Diez et al (43) analyzed the rate of urethral strictures in 213 patients treated with high dose rate (HDR) brachytherapy (34 Gy in 4 fractions, 36 Gy in 4 fractions, 31.5 Gy in 3 fractions, or 26 Gy in 2 fractions). The rate of strictures was 3%, 4%, 6%, and 4%, respectively. Overall incidence was 4.7%, demonstrating an infrequent incidence (43). Obliterative strictures have become less common given modern RT techniques. When these strictures do occur, however, they require immediate intervention, typically urethroplasty, as bladder distention can lead to bladder rupture. Brachytherapy is more likely to cause obliterative strictures as compared to EBRT (42).

Similar to other toxicities within the pelvis, the likelihood of developing acute and late radiation cystitis is proportional to the volume of the bladder irradiated, as well as the dose it receives. It is also highly dependent on mode of delivery (brachytherapy versus 3DCRT versus IMRT). Similar to discussion of radiation proctitis, patient factors and comorbidities play a large role in the likelihood of developing radiation cystitis, specifically hemorrhagic radiation cystitis. Such patient factors include diabetes, hypertension, tobacco abuse, and previous abdominal surgery.

Management: Acute Cystitis

While acute radiation-induced cystitis is often self-limiting, the physician should be prepared to aid the patient in symptom management when symptoms are causing deterioration in patient QOL. For patients with symptomatic urgency and urinary frequency, anticholinergic drugs can help to decrease urinary burden and stress (see Table 6.2). While anticholinergic drugs can provide significant relief, prescription of these drugs on behalf of the physician should urge a review of other medications to prevent polypharmacy leading to anticholinergic toxicity, specifically within the elderly. In addition, treatment options have included phenazopyridine hydrochloride (anesthetic) and flavoxate hydrochloride (antispasmodic, nonanticholinergic) with improvement in symptoms (44). However, of these two drugs, flavoxate has been noted to have decreased side effects with equivalent efficacy in symptomatic relief (45).

In acute radiation-induced cystitis, patients can have mild hematuria; however, it is usually clinically insignificant and warrants observation for resolution. The majority of patients will have resolution of their symptoms within 4 to 6 weeks.

Management: Chronic Cystitis

Chronic radiation cystitis is estimated to occur between 5% and 10% of patients who receive pelvic RT (46). Patients with chronic radiation cystitis are more likely to experience hematuria of clinical significance, warranting further treatment options. Table 6.3 lists pharmaceutical interventions used in symptomatic hemorrhagic cystitis, as well as the evidence that supports and/or discredits their use.

The potential for hematuria ranging from mildly symptomatic to life threatening warrants an array of interventions. Although the aforementioned incidence of late radiation-induced cystitis is between 5% and 10%, in a retrospective study analyzing women with the Federation of Gynecology and Obstetrics (FIGO) stage IB cervical carcinoma treated with RT, HRC occurred and was severe in less than 5% (57).

For the patient with minimal symptoms, conservative measures may include intervention with fluid and blood product replacement. Other

**Table 6.2** Anticholinergic Drugs

| Drug | Dosing |
| --- | --- |
| Propantheline bromide | 15–30 mg every 4–6 h |
| Oxybutynin chloride | 5 mg three times a day |
| Imipramine hydrochloride | 25 mg four times a day |

*Source:* From Ref. (44). Rubin P, Constine LS, Marks LB. *ALERT - adverse late effects of cancer treatment. Vol. 2: normal tissue specific sites and systems.* Heidelberg: Springer-Verlag; 2014:488.

**Table 6.3** Pharmaceutical Agents Used in Symptomatic HRC

| Intervention | Administration | Evidence |
|---|---|---|
| Sodium pentosan polysulfate (SPPS) | Sublingual, also available in IV | Hampson and Woodhouse (47): 14 patients (8 requiring no transfusions, 2 requiring <6U without other intervention, 4 requiring >6U with other intervention [formalin or more]) received 100 mg SPPS three times a day. Seventy-one percent CR by maximum of 2 years, 3% PR, 1% no response. No adverse side effects.<br>Sandhu et al (48): 60 patients treated with SPP (53 cases secondary to RT) received 100 mg three times a day. Twenty-one patients achieved dose deescalation to 100 mg daily and 10 patients discontinued therapy all together due to cessation of hematuria. Response rate 58%. |
| Conjugated estrogen | Oral/IV | Liu et al (49): 5 patients with radiation-induced or cyclophosphamide treated with IV (1 mg/kg) conjugated estrogen twice a day for 2 days followed by 5 mg PO ($n = 2$) or 5 mg conjugated oral estrogen once daily ($n = 3$). For IV/oral patients, hematuria decreased by 6–8 hours and urine appeared normal at 1–3 days. For oral only patients, urine appeared normal by 4–7 days. Four patients (80%) received daily conjugated estrogen at 1.25 mg daily and did not have recurrence during 12–22 months. One patient had persistent mild hematuria at 10 mg/day dose. No toxicity. |
| WF10 (Tetrachlorodecaoxygen [TCDO]) | IV | RCT (50): Cervical cancer patients with grade 2 or 4 late HRC randomized to WF10 0.5 mL/kg diluted in 250 mL saline or 5% dextrose in water (D5W) for two cycles ($n = 50$) (given over 5 days with 3-week break) or standard treatment ($n = 50$). At 7 weeks, 74% WF10 patients and 64% standard treatment had CR (NS). However, 47% WF10 patients as compared to 77% standard therapy patients had recurrent hematuria ($P = .01$). At 1 year follow-up, overall general improvement between two groups with no differences. |

*(continued)*

## Table 6.3 Pharmaceutical Agents Used in Symptomatic HRC (continued)

| Intervention | Administration | Evidence |
|---|---|---|
| | | Phase II study (51): 30 symptomatic patients with grade 2 and 3 late hemorrhagic cystitis ($n = 16$) and proctitis ($n = 14$) treated with IV WF10 (0.5 mL/kg BW in 250 mL 5% D/W), given over 2 h on 5 consecutive days, every 3 weeks, for 2–4 cycles. Eighty-eight percent of cystitis patients and 100% patients improved to grade 0–1 hematuria and rectal bleeding, respectively, within 3 month; 28% cystitis patients had recurrent bleeding and 14% proctitis patients had recurrent rectal bleeding (grade 2–3). No toxicity. |
| Formalin | Topical | Retrospective review—Dewen et al (52): 35 patients with HRC from RT for cervical cancer. All had failed conservative management. Treated with 1% ($n = 22$), 2% ($n = 10$), 4% ($n = 4$) topical formalin irrigation for 20–30 min and continuous saline irrigation for 12–48 h. Eighty-nine percent CR, 8% PR. Recurrence of hematuria in 23% of CR at mean of 8 months; 54% mild complications including mild fever, frequency, dysuria, suprapubic pain, temporary incontinence, unilateral hydronephrosis, grade 2 ureterovesical reflux and decreased bladder capacity; 31% major complications including bilateral hydronephrosis due to ureteral stenosis, vesicovaginal fistula, and decreased bladder capacity; 14% required diversion and 1 patient death due to bleeding and formalin toxicity; 1% formalin demonstrated CR with less morbidity. |
| | | Retrospective review—Lojanapiwat et al (53): 19 women with HRC from RT to the cervix for cervical cancer. Group 1: 4% formalin for half of the bladder volume (15 min) followed by saline irrigation (12–14 h) ($n = 11$). Group 2: 10% formalin soaked pledgets (1×1cm) on bleeding points (15 min) ($n = 8$). Median pledges was 5.5. Group 1 had 82% CR. Group 2 had 75% CR. Four major complications in group 1 versus none in group 2. These included anuria, bilateral hydronephrosis, two vesiculovaginal fistula, and one septic death. Eleven minor complications occurred in group 1 vs three in group 2. Average follow-up was 25 months. |

*(continued)*

## Table 6.3 Pharmaceutical Agents Used in Symptomatic HRC (continued)

| Intervention | Administration | Evidence |
| --- | --- | --- |
| Hyaluronic acid | Topical | RCT—Shao et al (54): Randomized to 40 mg HA in bladder by Foley catheter for 20 min weekly for 1 month, then monthly for following 2 months ($n = 16$) versus HBOT of 2.5 atm for 60 min, 7 days a week, for 1 month ($n = 20$). Complications included increased UTI in HA group. HA group at 6 months had CR of 88% versus 75% HBOT patients. CR at 12 months: 75% vs 50%. CR at 18 months: 50% vs 45%. |
| Aluminous salts | Topical | Arrizabalaga et al (55): 15 patients with hematuria (13 tumor related, 1 HRC, 1 transurethral resection) treated with 1% aluminum potassium sulfate solution in sterile distilled water using catheter for intravesical lavage. Sixty-six percent CR, 15% PR, 20% failure. No toxicity. Mild symptoms of vesical tenesmus/spasms and suprapubic pain. |
| Prostaglandins | Topical | Hemal et al (56) reports a case of one female with stage IIB uterine cervical cancer post-RT with persistent radiation cystitis. Received 15 (S)-15-methyl prostaglandin F2-alpha (1 mg in 100 mL normal saline) daily for 2 days. Bleeding decreased with return on day 21. Subsequent 15 (S) 15-Me PGF2 alpha mixed with hydroxyethyl cellulose gel to 10 mL instilled with no recurrence on 5-month follow-up. |
| Silver nitrate | Topical | |

CR, complete response; HBOT, hyperbaric oxygen therapy; HRC, hemorrhagic radiation cystitis; PR, partial response; RCT, randomized controlled trial; RT, radiation therapy.

conservative measures should include stopping all anticoagulation and antiplatelet therapies, unless comorbidities are severe enough to allot for current use. If symptoms do not resolve with conservative measures, initial management can also include bladder irrigation and clot evacuation. For patients with HRC, attempting repeat trials of cystoscopy for bladder irrigation and clot evaluation is worthwhile. However, the physician must analyze the patient's clinical status and response to cystoscopy to determine if more aggressive measures are needed to control hematuria.

- Kaplan and Wolf (58) evaluated records of 33 patients with cyclophosphamide or radiation-induced hemorrhagic cystitis who underwent cystoscopy and clot evacuation. Sixty-one percent ($n = 20$) had resolution of hematuria with one cystoscopy; however, none of these patients were found to have hematuria of HRC etiology. Only 4 of 11 (36%) had resolution with two or more cystoscopies and these 4 patients were all of HRC etiology. Nine patients were refractory to cystoscopy. This study identified that patients who fail to respond to initial cystoscopy are less likely to respond to subsequent cystoscopies. However, of those who will respond on future cystoscopies, they are most likely to have HRC as compared to chemotherapy-induced cystitis.

If bladder irrigation and clot evacuation fails to control HRC, oral, parenteral, or IV agents can be considered. Although no randomized clinical trials exist for the use of radiation-induced refractory cystitis, single arm studies demonstrate significant improvement in mean frequency, pain, and nocturia at 6 months after botulinum A injection for some patients with refractory interstitial cystitis (59). Extrapolating beyond the evidence in interstitial cystitis, a trial of botulinum toxin A for anticholinergic refractory radiation-induced cystitis is reasonable and should be considered for patients without evidence of hematuria.

- In a case report, Chuang et al (60) investigated the use of botulinum toxin A for six patients with radiation cystitis refractory to anticholinergics. They were treated with 200 U botulinum toxin A injection into 20 different submucosal sites in the trigone and the floor of the bladder via cystoscope guidance. Of these six patients, five noted moderate to significant clinical improvement. Bladder capacity increased from an average of 105 to 250 mL, while urinary frequency decreased from an average of 14 to 11 episodes per day.

Of the aforementioned interventions, all could be considered treatment options for patients who have failed conservative management. However, an analysis of the side effects, timeliness, and expense of application of treatment juxtaposed to the evidence-based response rate and applicability and strength of evidence should be analyzed for each specific patient and case (see Table 6.4).

If bleeding does not cease by using any of the aforementioned methods, other interventions such as cystoscopy with fulguration or HBOT can be considered. HBOT for HRC is a highly researched area as its potential to cure refractory disease with minimal side effects is imperative. Numerous studies have looked at the necessary length of treatment session, number of treatment sessions, as well as ideal atmospheric pressure of treatments.

**Table 6.4** Summary of Response Rate for Pharmaceutical Intervention

| Intervention | Complete response rate (%) | Follow-up (months) | Number of studies | Number of patients treated |
|---|---|---|---|---|
| PPS | 58–69 | NR | 2 | 65 |
| Conjugated estrogens | 80 | 15 | 1 | 5 |
| WF10 | 74–88 | 12–51 | 2 | 66 |
| Soaked pledgets: formalin | 75 | | 1 | 8 |
| 1% formalin | 83–89 | | 2 | 43 |
| 2% formalin | 89 | NR | 1 | 10 |
| 4% formalin | ~ 82 | | 2 | 15 |
| 5% formalin | 78 | | 1 | 91 |
| 10% formalin | 83–93 | | 3 | 143 |
| Hyaluronic acid | 88 | 6 | 1 | 16 |
| 1% aluminum | 50–100 | NR | 4 | 43 |
| Prostaglandins | 100% (case reports) | NR | 3 | 2 |

NR, not reported; PPS, sodium pentosane polysulfate.
Adapted from Ref. (38). Smit SG, Heyns CF. Management of radiation cystitis. *Nat Rev Urol.* 2010;7(4):206–214. doi:10.1038/nrurol.2010.23

There is generally no consensus on these measures as well as the overall effectiveness of this therapy.

- Smit et al (38) compared seven of the most recent studies using HBOT for patients with radiation cystitis. They noted a 62% to 92% response rate with a median follow-up time ranging from 2 to 61 months. The length of each session was fairly uniform at 90 minutes, with one study using 120-minute sessions, and the number of treatment sessions ranging from 14 to 60. There were no trends in regard to response rate and the number of treatment sessions or median follow-up time.
- An upcoming study called Hyperbaric Oxygen Radiation Tissue Injury Study (HORTIS) III (study III of VIII) is on the horizon and gives hope to clarifying the role of HBOT in late radiation-induced toxicity. It will be a multicenter, randomized controlled trial specifically in refractory cystitis.

Various methods of cystoscopy with fulguration or intravesical endoscopic procedures have proven effective. They include electrocoagulation, diathermy, argon laser, and neodymium-doped yttrium-aluminum-garnet (Nd:YAG) laser. Various studies analyzed these techniques in refractory HRC patients with various outcomes (see Table 6.5). Despite the relative success of these interventions, the chance for severe morbidity with these procedures means they should be used for refractory cases or for those whose side effects to pharmaceutical treatments would be too large.

When all of the aforementioned interventions fail, surgical interventions should be considered. Atheroembolic procedures can include embolization of vesicular artery or embolization/ligation of the iliac arteries. Other options include urinary diversion (via percutaneous nephrostomy, cutaneous ureterostomy, or intestinal conduit) with or without cystectomy. Given the history of pelvic radiation in these patients, the morbidity of the procedure is increased and patients have a high risk of fistula formation and increased likelihood of bowel obstructions in the future. Given this risk, alternatives should be sought and if in the end surgical intervention

**Table 6.5** Intravesical Endoscopic Procedures

| Study | Number of patients | Treatment | Outcomes | Morbidity |
|---|---|---|---|---|
| Ravi et al (61) | 42 | Nd:YAG laser, laser power ≤30 W and pulse duration ≤3 seconds | CR: 98% 93% (after one treatment) 5% (after two treatment) | One patient with severe hematuria (requiring blood transfusion) failed to respond |
| Wines, Lynch (62) | 7 | Argon plasma coagulation at 40–60W power with gas flow rate of 1.5 L/min | CR: 100% 86% (after one treatment) 14% (after two treatments) | None |
| Zhu et al (63) | 10 | Transurethral greenlight KTP laser | CR: 100% 100% (after one session) | One patient with recurrent hematuria after 7 months and underwent second laser procedure |
| Kushik et al (64) | 4 | Standard cystoscopic electrocautery with laser fulguration (980 nm diode laser) | CR: 100% 100% (after one treatment) | None |

CR, complete response; KTP, potassium titanyl phosphate; Nd:YAG, neodymium-doped yttrium aluminium garnet.
*Source:* From Ref. (65). Mendenhall WM, Henderson RH, Costa JA, et al. Hemorrhagic radiation cystitis. *Am J Clin Oncol*. 2015;38:331–336. http://journals.lww.com/amjclinicaloncology/Abstract/2015/06000/Hemorrhagic_Radiation_Cystitis.18.aspx

is deemed necessary, these procedures should be undertaken by an experienced surgeon.

For patients who have symptomatic strictures (difficulty with urination or suprapubic pain/discomfort), regardless of severity, referral to a surgeon should be given. This will allow for evaluation of urethral stenting with a likelihood to improve patient's QOL. When stenting fails or stricture worsens, patients should be considered for urethroplasty, urinary diversion, or nephrectomy.

Fistula formation is also a rare occurrence for pelvic RT patients. Fistula formation can occur between the bladder and the rectum, vagina in women, or bowel. When fistula formation does occur, surgical intervention should be considered due to the morbidity of the fistula tract. However, surgery in itself should be weighed against conservative measures, as the irradiated pelvis increases the morbidity of any surgery.

Overall, the toxicities from radiation to the bladder are vast and a systematic approach should be taken to treat these toxicities. Supportive care followed by pharmaceutical measures should be employed prior to endoscopic or surgical interventions. Regardless of the systematic approach, each patient should be evaluated on an individual basis and if the patient fails conservative treatment or warrants immediate intervention, the clinician should use a team-based approach to correlate the literature to the specific case and discern next treatment options. Much like radiation-induced proctitis, the severity of radiation-induced cystitis has decreased with newer treatment modalities, allowing for more focused and targeted treatment. However, for some patients, especially those receiving RT to the bladder, acute toxicity and potentially late toxicities are inevitable and the radiation oncologist should be knowledgeable with the treatment paradigm.

## Female Reproductive Organs

### Female Sexual Dysfunction

- *Symptoms:* vaginal atrophy (dryness, thinning), stenosis/fibrosis (dyspareunia)
- *Timing:* acute 2 to 3+ weeks into RT; chronic: 6+ months after RT
- *Prevention:* tobacco cessation, dilute hydrogen peroxide douches for cleansing
- *Acute management:*
  - Vaginal mucositis: vulvar cleansing with mild soap or sitz, topical or oral antifungal
- *Chronic symptom management:*
  - Vaginal atrophy: topical lubricants, topical estrogen, or benzydamine
  - Stenosis: vaginal dilator, topical mitomycin C
  - Necrosis: pentoxifylline or hyperbaric oxygen

While the majority of research regarding sexual dysfunction involves erectile dysfunction (ED) following prostate RT, RT can also have significant impact on women and their sexual function. Female sexual dysfunction (FSD) is an inclusive term that marks all side effects following RT and/or surgery that make sexual intercourse more difficult, including physical and psychological factors. Physicians are still very hesitant to address this comorbidity with their patients. For this reason, similar to other mentioned radiotoxicities of the pelvis, incidence cannot be accurately estimated. This, coupled with the difference in symptoms and severity of symptoms with differing treatment sites and modalities, makes predicting FSD for the radiation oncologist very difficult.

Incidence and Prevention

Vaginal stenosis is the most commonly noted side effect after RT to the pelvis, regardless of EBRT versus brachytherapy. A study by Fossa et al (66) noted that physician-assessed vaginal morbidity was 23%, while patient-reported outcomes were much higher at 58%. Pelvic examination often shows mucosal pallor and telangiectasias. Vaginal fibrosis and stenosis can significantly impact a woman's ability to have vaginal intercourse. The highest incidence rate of FSD is in definitive therapy for locally advanced cervical cancer, in which over half of patients report sexual dysfunction (67).

- Bergmark et al (68) analyzed 256 women with early-stage cervical cancer (as compared to 350 controls), 26% of women with cancer (as compared to 11% of controls), and reporting insufficient vaginal lubrication for intercourse. Twenty-six percent of cancer patients (as compared to 3% of controls) reported a short vagina, and 23% (as compared to 4%, respectively) reported an insufficient elastic vagina. Twenty-three percent of cancer patients were concerned with their vaginal symptoms as compared to 8% controls. There was no noted difference in sexual orgasms or orgasmic pleasure; however, dyspareunia was more commonly mentioned among previous cervical cancer patients. Of the cancer patients treated, 36% received surgery alone, 22% received intracavitary RT, 9% received EBRT, and 21% received intracavitary and EBRT. Notably, there was no significant difference on specific therapy type related to patient-reported vaginal changes.
- In a more recent study, Jensen et al (69) noted that FSD as a patient-reported outcome is noted within the literature of endometrial and rectal cancers, but very little literature about FSD is noted within bladder, vulva, or anal cancers. Of note, they recognized very limited data on FDS within modern RT modalities.

The factors impacting sexual dysfunction noted within these patients included a physical nature (vaginal shortening, dyspareunia, or bleeding) and psychological factors (concern of bleeding and/or concerned about risk of recurrence). FSD is more common with RT and surgery combined, as compared to surgery alone (67).

Overall dose also matters. Significant (more than grade 2) vaginal toxicity is more common with high-dose definitive treatment as compared to adjuvant treatment. As well, modern day techniques, such as HDR vaginal brachytherapy (VB) have been noted to have significantly less toxicity.

- In one study of 414 patients with stage IA to stage II endometrial adenocarcinoma treated with HDR VB alone (24 Gy in 6 fractions), no grade 2 or higher vaginal toxicities were seen (70).

To date, there are essentially no large-scale randomized controlled clinical studies that have evaluated treatment or prophylactic strategy for FSD from RT. The strongest evidence (grade IC) surrounds topical estrogen and benzydamine douches (not available in the United States) coupled with supportive measures for acute radiation changes. Primary intervention should include conservative measures, such as risk factor management, dilute hydrogen peroxide douches for cleansing, as well as antibiotics, if acute infection is of concern. Given the lack of true knowledge surrounding prevention and treatment around FSD, the physician should make treatment options based on the clinical presentation, as well as the patient's response to acute intervention. The physician should keep in mind that FSD is also highlighted by psychological changes on behalf of the patient, and discussion regarding potential physical and psychological changes that can occur with the patient during and after therapy is warranted prior to initiating treatment. As well, the physician should always consider psychological or psychiatric referral if the patient eludes to psychological distress and is interested in or would benefit from such an intervention.

## Management: Acute Toxicity

Patients undergoing RT to the pelvis can develop acute vaginal mucositis, vaginal ulcerations, and necrosis. Mucosal tissues are subjugated to RT changes and can range from erythema to superficial ulceration, predisposing to infection (71). Current approach to vaginal mucositis includes supportive measures: vulvar cleansing with mild soap or sitz baths (71). This prevents the accumulation of irritants in the area of therapy, preventing further skin breakdown, leading to necrosis. Denton et al (72) reviewed the evidence for alternative treatment options of acute mucositis. Results included grade IC evidence for topical estrogen and benzydamine (commonly used in a douche preparation, acts as an anti-inflammatory and local anesthetic). Although level I evidence was present, the studies were not recent, as well as the studies were convoluted by poor design (unclear allocation concealment and variable level of assessment of response to treatment). Therefore, a prospective randomized clinical trial involving the use of topical estrogen, as well as benzydamine and hydrogen peroxide douches, should be completed in order to know its true efficacy in treatment. However, despite the lack of level I evidence in these treatment options, the known side effect of these treatments are minimal, and therapy with them can be considered if a patient fails to respond to conservative measures.

## Management: Chronic Toxicity

Vaginal stenosis can have a significant impact on FSD as it can cause shortening of the vagina, vaginismus, and dyspareunia. Additionally, stenosis can impact patient follow-up, as pelvic exams can become very uncomfortable. Vaginal stenosis typically begins 3 to 6 months following RT, and has greatest incidence in those undergoing pelvic RT plus VB. The primary method for vaginal stenosis is application of a vaginal dilator. While lack of level I evidence exists, vaginal dilators are often recommended to patients as both a prophylactic and treatment option. Caution should be used as some studies have shown that dilator use can cause psychological and physical damage.

- Miles and Johnson (73) reviewed the limited literature available on the efficacy of vaginal dilator therapy, noting that two studies (74,75) were the only studies examining sexual function in women randomized to more dilation therapy as compared to less. These trials noted no support of dilation therapy during RT.

More recent studies have suggested that the use of dilation after acute inflammation postradiotherapy has ceased can perhaps prevent vaginal stenosis. These studies are noted to have bias as gauging true outcomes is difficult owing to poor compliance and intrinsic reporting bias on behalf of the patient (73). Given there is grade IIC evidence supporting vaginal dilator use posttreatment, this can be recommended to patients (particularly those who are not having routine intercourse).

Recent research regarding the application of local mitomycin C to prevent or treat vaginal stenosis has been studied in a small RCT. Sobotkowski et al (76) used local mitomycin C in 31 patients after brachytherapy and EBRT for locally advanced cervical cancer. In the mitomycin C group ($n = 16$), vaginal shortening still occurred, but complete vaginal occlusion and fibrotic vault changes were less frequent. Given the small study size, as well as the potential bias in observation of findings, the use of mitomycin C has yet to be used on a larger scale.

While vaginal atrophy and fibrosis are common, vaginal and cervical necrosis, as well as full thickness ulceration, are uncommon toxicities. Etiology is proposed as loss of progenitor cells from the mucosal basal layer (71), preventing regeneration of the mucosa and impairing wound healing, lasting beyond 3 months.

- Fawaz et al (77) demonstrated five case reports of women presenting with cervical necrosis following chemoradiation for cervical cancer. Mean time to presentation was 9.3 months. All patients were managed conservatively with tobacco cessation, antibiotics (metronidazole), hydrogen peroxide vaginal douches, and use of opioids for pain relief. All patients had clinical improvement within 1 to 4 months with no recurrence at median follow-up of 19 months.

Studies involving the use of pentoxifylline or hyperbaric oxygen for persistent nonhealing necrosis (Table 6.6) have demonstrated high rates of resolution; however, there is a lack of level I evidence surrounding the true efficacy of these interventions.

Rectovaginal and vesiculovaginal fistulas are extremely rare. The physician should be suspicious for fistulae formation if the patient is receiving high-dose RT, interstitial brachytherapy, necrosis develops, or tumor is noted to have invasion of the bladder or rectum (81). Treatment for fistulae formation warrants consideration of the patient's comorbidities. The potential for further fistula formation with surgery should be weighed against the potential benefit from surgical intervention. Conservative management should be considered if the patient has other comorbidities that warrant against acute intervention.

**Table 6.6** Studies of Alternative Therapies for Unresolved Vaginal/Cervical Necrosis

| Study | Methods | Findings |
|---|---|---|
| Williams et al (78): Prospective observational study | Fourteen patients with necrotic wounds failing to heal after 3 months undergoing 15 courses of HBOT | All had treatment resolution with one treatment failure |
| Dion et al (79): Prospective observational study | Twelve patients with 15 sites of late radiation necrosis of soft tissue treated with pentoxifylline: four were of female genitalia | 87% response among all patients |
| Safra et al (80): Prospective observational study | Thirteen women treated with HBOT. Five had long-standing vaginal ulcers and fistulas. Twenty-seven median session at 2 atm. | NCI CTC decreased from 3.3 +/−0.75 prior to therapy to 0.3 +/−0.63 after treatment |

HBOT, hyperbaric oxygen therapy; NCI CTC, National Cancer Institute Common Toxicity Criteria.

*Fertility and Early Menopause*

- The threshold dose to the two ovaries and uterus is approximately 4 Gy.
- Prevention primarily through awareness and avoidance of ovaries/uterus when possible.
- For those who require RT in that region, consider embryo and oocyte cryopreservation or laparoscopic ovarian transposition.
- New experimental techniques with promise include in vitro maturation or harvested immature eggs and ovarian tissue cryopreservation.
- Hormone replacement therapy for patients with premature ovarian failure is key (for those in whom estrogen replacement is not contraindicated because of a hormonally driven tumor).

Pelvic RT dosed to the ovaries can lead to infertility and premature ovarian failure (POF), resulting in early menopause. Unlike many of the other organs in the pelvis, the ovaries are extremely sensitive to radiation, and damage can be expected at lower radiation doses than other pelvic organs. The effective sterilizing dose (ESD) to expect POF is dependent on age: ESD is lower with increasing age (82). At birth, ESD is predicted to be 20.3 Gy, 10 years 18.4 Gy, 20 years 16.5 Gy, and 30 years 14.3 Gy (82). Safely, the threshold dose to the two ovaries and uterus is approximately 4 Gy (83). Therefore, patients who receive lower doses from ESD can potentially see recovery of estrogen levels within 6 to 18 months (71). RT has a direct gonadotoxic effect on primordial follicles, resulting in a decrease in oocyte number. As well, RT has been shown to have a direct effect on uterine tissue, resulting in decreased volume, elasticity, and vascularity, which can impact future pregnancies (83).

### Prevention

Primary intervention in female patients includes plan-based prevention. The goal of newer RT techniques is to limit dose to the ovaries in order to prevent infertility and POF. However, in some cases, some dose may be delivered and next step intervention should include discussion with the patient regarding the risk of infertility and POF. Some patients' treatment decisions may be altered by fertility issues. Physicians should discuss early with the patient their interest in having children after radiation treatment and fertility preservation techniques.

While all patients should be offered referral to a fertility specialist if it coincides with their future wishes, it should be made known to the patient that the rate of treatment-related infertility is based on numerous other factors. These can include age, comorbidities, history of previous infertility with or without previous infertility treatment, chemotherapy as part of treatment plan, or use of adjuvant endocrine therapy (84). Lee et al (85) demonstrated that from a RT perspective, women with the highest risk of future infertility (>80% permanent amenorrhea) are those receiving EBRT (with a field including the ovaries). Therefore, fertility counselling should be personalized to the patient and their treatment plan.

Primary fertility-sparing methods include embryo and oocyte cryopreservation, as well as laparoscopic ovarian transposition. Laparoscopic ovarian transposition is an option for patients who are premenopausal and have a low likelihood of metastases to the ovaries. These patients can undergo transposition of the ovary with an 80% to 88% rate of ovary preservation. Analysis of the RT plan should be considered prior to consideration of surgical transposition, as ovaries should be relocated to a safe margin (often quoted as 3 cm) from the RT treatment field. Dependent on the treatment modality chosen by the radiation oncologist, this may not be a possibility, but should be thoroughly investigated, especially in younger children.

Embryo and oocyte cryopreservation encompass hormonal stimulation of the ovaries and collection of oocytes. In oocyte cryopreservation, oocytes remain unfertilized for future fertilization via in vitro fertilization (IVF) immediately prior to implantation. With new techniques on cryopreservation, this technique has similar efficacy to embryo cryopreservation (83). In embryo cryopreservation, oocytes and partner/donor sperm are used to create embryos in real time via IVF for future implantation.

Newer experimental techniques include in vitro maturation (IVM). IVM is a technique in which oocytes are matured in vitro and subsequently used for cryopreservation for oocytes and embryos (83). This has been an important discovery when considering infertility issues in women who cannot receive hormonal stimulation (such as estrogen receptor [ER]/progesterone receptor [PR]+ breast cancer). Ovarian tissue cryopreservation is also a newer experimental technique in which the goal is to collect ovarian tissue (the ovarian cortex) to preserve eggs within the primordial follicles. This is a technique of interest in prepubertal adolescents in whom future fertility is of grave concern with pediatric cancer therapy. The cortical tissue is extracted via laparoscopic ovarian cortical biopsy or oophorectomy. This tissue is frozen and after treatment retransplanted into the patient. Approximately 20 live births have been successful with this method. It has proven to be more successful when reimplanted into its native site (83).

A new intriguing area of research is focused around finding radioprotective agents for the ovaries, so as to ensure ovarian function following RT. In Mahran et al (86), female rats were exposed to whole body irradiation (3.2 Gy) and/or treated with growth hormone (GH). Those rats treated with GH regained fertility that was lost following irradiation. The mechanism of action of GH on ovarian follicles is suspected to be by increasing insulin-like growth factor (IGF)-1 levels (known to stimulate and sustain granulosa cells) and counteracting oxidative stress and apoptosis caused by RT (86). In other body areas, GH has demonstrated similar radioprotective effects.

Women who have premature ovarian failure will suffer from premature menopause secondary to estrogen deficiency. Similar to primary ovarian failure, these women can expect symptoms of vaginal dryness, hot sweats, flushing, fatigue, and mood changes. Patients are also at greater risk of decreased libido, osteopenia and osteoporosis, as well as cardiovascular morbidity and mortality. Treatment for menopause-induced symptoms includes symptomatic management. Symptoms can be controlled predominantly by hormonal replacement therapy, usually estradiol, unless contraindicated.

## Male Reproductive Organs

### Erectile Dysfunction

- *Symptoms:* incomplete or lack of erection, anejaculation
- *Timing:* 12+ months after RT
- *Prevention:* treatment of co-morbidities, review of concurrent medications, radiation-treatment planning for avoidance of penile bulb
- *Management:* phosphodiesterase-5 inhibitor (PDE-5) inhibitors, vacuum erection device, intraurethral or intracavernosal prostaglandins, penile implant

For men receiving RT to the pelvis, ED is a potential side effect that has a dire effect on QOL. Similar to other pelvic toxicities, difficulty in predicting the likelihood of impotence after treatment comes from the discrepancies that exist in reporting symptoms in an objective manner. In one study, ED was reported by physicians and patients who were potent prior to brachytherapy (87). At 2 years, 66% of patients reported ED as compared to 48% by physicians. This discrepancy between physician- and patient-reported incidence of ED post-RT is presumed to be due to underreporting/lack of ascertainment during follow-up visits. Therefore, ED is being commonly measured using validated patient-reported survey measures such as the Mount Sinai Erectile Function Score (MSEFS) for physicians and Sexual Health Inventory for Men (SHIM), International Index of Erectile Function (IIEF), and Extended Prostate Cancer Index Composite (EPIC) (88).

The rate of ED is dependent on prefunction assessment, treatment selection, and time from treatment. Other studies have noted similar findings (see Table 6.7), thus concluding that a significant factor in determining patient likelihood of impotence is preradiotherapy function.

- Talcott et al (92) reported symptoms before therapy, as well as 3 and 12 months following therapy for early prostate cancer (surgery versus RT). Pretreatment, 32% of surgical patients and 45% of RT patients claimed either or both of these symptoms. The discrepancy in the two groups was easily rationalized by the difference in average age: surgical patients tended to be younger. At 3 months, 85% of those undergoing radical prostatectomy reported complete impotence and 96% reported incomplete erections. At 12 months, sexual dysfunction among radical prostatectomy patients was 75% and 93%, respectively. This 12-month mark, as compared to RT patients, showed a decreased rate of complete impotence among patients at 33% and incomplete erections at 67%. While notably sexual dysfunction was lower in RT patients as compared to surgical patients, RT patients still noted worsening sexual dysfunction as compared to baseline.

Other factors that predict the likelihood of becoming impotent include numerous patient comorbidities (especially vascular disease, such as smoking and hypertension, and diabetes [89]), as well as patient's age, which tends to lead to impotence independent of treatment. A recent model by

**Table 6.7** Studies of Sexual Dysfunction for EBRT for Localized Prostate Cancer

| Study | Methods | Findings |
|---|---|---|
| Mantz et al (89): Retrospective study | 114 patients receiving EBRT for stage A–C prostate cancer. Median follow-up time was 18.5 months | At 1, 12, 24, and 36 months: potency rates were 98%, 92%, 75%, 66%. Median time to impotence was 14 months<br><br>Risk factors predicting post-EBRT impotence: pre-EBRT partial potency ($P < .001$), vascular disease ($P < .001$), and diabetes ($P = .003$)<br><br>EBRT patient potency was 76.1%, as compared to historical data of prostatectomy patients, which was 66.2% |
| Potosky et al (90): Retrospective study | Patients receiving radical prostatectomy ($n = 1156$) vs EBRT ($n = 435$) for localized prostate cancer. Two-year follow-up | Impotence among radical prostatectomy 79.6% as compared to EBRT, 61.5% ($P < .001$) |
| Hamilton et al (91): Retrospective study | 497 patients with localized prostate cancer treated with EBRT. Followed up at 6, 12, 24 months | At 24 months, decline of sexual function to 28.9%. Forty-three percent of men who were potent before diagnosis became impotent after treatment |

EBRT, external beam radiation therapy.

Alemozaffar et al (93) was designed to help predict the likelihood of functional erections suitable for intercourse 2 years following treatment. This model, entitled the PROSTQA (Prostate Cancer Outcomes and Satisfaction With Treatment Quality Assessment) model, was designed by analyzing pretreatment patient characteristics, sexual health–related QOL (using a scored assessment), and treatment details, as compared to erectile function after treatment, in 1,027 patients. Patient therapy included prostatectomy ($n = 524$), EBRT (n = 241), or brachytherapy ($n = 262$). At 2-year follow up, 35% of patients with prostatectomy had functional erections. This is compared to 37% treated with EBRT and 43% treated with brachytherapy. For patients receiving EBRT, multivariable analysis indicated that a lower prostate-specific antigen (PSA) level, better pretreatment sexual functioning score, and no use of neoadjuvant hormone therapy were associated with increased log-odds of functional erection after treatment. Using the PROSTQA model, the physician can predict that for a patient without planned neoadjuvant hormonal therapy, with a pretreatment sexual health–related QOL score of 83, a predicted functional erection after treatment of 83% is predicted, if the patient had a pretreatment PSA level of less than 4 ng/mL as compared to a predicted 60% functional erection after treatment with a pretreatment PSA level of greater than or equal to 4 ng/mL. For this same patient, if neoadjuvant hormonal therapy is planned, the model predicts that functional erection after treatment remains at 60%, if pretreatment PSA level is less than 4 ng/mL, and drops to 31% if pretreatment PSA level is greater than 4 ng/mL. Similarly, the PROSTQA model demonstrates an increased log-odds of better erectile function following brachytherapy with better pretreatment sexual function, younger age, African American race, and lower body-mass index (BMI) (93). These models were validated by application among the Cancer of the Prostate Strategic Urologic Research Endeavor (CaPSURE) cohort group demonstrating a 0.77, 0.87, and 0.90 correlation for predicting erections in prostatectomy, EBRT, and brachytherapy, respectively.

Another questioned component in order to predict the likelihood of developing impotence after RT is an analysis of the treatment plan. Specifically with prostate cancer, the shift from 3DCRT and IMRT has allowed for decreased dose to nearby structures, including penile bulb (94). Recent studies have focused on dose constraints surrounding the penile bulb and corporal bodies in an effort to avoid dose delivery to the erectile tissue to decipher its effect on ED. Numerous studies have attempted to highlight the importance of dose constraints to the penile bulb with some incongruence potentially related to either contouring inaccuracy or incorrect biologic explanation for radiation-induced ED. Unfortunately, other studies have failed to demonstrate the relationship of ED to penile bulb or corporal bulb dose altogether, and numerous studies could be limited by compounding factors (particularly the arrival of hormonal therapy use). Therefore, the ability to predict the role the plan and dose have on developing ED remains limited. Other etiologies have included damage to the vascular supply such as neurovascular bundles or internal pudendal arteries. However, this has yet to be proven as well. Therefore, in the future, limiting dose to these structures could be considered as well. However, in the meantime, limiting the dose to the erectile tissue without compromising outcomes could perhaps be of some benefit.

- Roach et al (95) analyzed 10 studies looking at dose constraints to the penile bulb and percentage of patients developing ED after treatment. This data demonstrated that ED was limited with V95 to the penile bulb being less than 50 Gy. As well, this meta-analysis suggests that limiting the penile bulb V70 to 70 Gy and V90 to 50 Gy may also decrease the risk of ED.

Erectile dysfunction remains a very common complication of RT to the pelvis. It has been noted to be more common in men receiving EBRT, as compared to brachytherapy. There has been no proven benefit in proton therapy to decrease ED, as compared to IMRT. Due to the unknown etiology of ED following RT, dose constraints on erectile tissues have had noncongruent results in yielding decreased ED; however, limiting this dose to the erectile tissue with modern therapy does not seem unreasonable. Other factors likely impacting the onset of ED posttherapy include age, pretreatment function, comorbidities, and the use of androgen deprivation therapy (ADT).

Of recent interest has been the role in transforming growth factor (TGF)-B1 B1 single nucleotide polymorphisms and RT complications. TGF-B1 is a cytokine produced by numerous cells implicated in the normal healing response after RT (88). TGF-B1 single nucleotide polymorphisms (small DNA variants of a single base pair) became of interest owing to the correlation at the −509 T/T and 869 position with developing clinically significant fibrosis in breast cancer patients postradiation treatment. In the pelvis, Peters et al (96) studied 141 patients with prostate cancer treated with RT at a median follow up time of 51.3 months. Results noted a direct correlation with decline in erectile function for patients who had the −509 T/T genotype, the 869 C/C genotype, or the 915 G/C genotype: 56% versus 24%, respectively (96). Although not yet clinically significant for predicting incidence, the study shows the variation in patient factors that contribute to the development of radiation ED.

## Management

Regardless of the ability to predict the likelihood of developing ED after therapy, it is important for physicians to know any treatment studies that exist. Phosphodiesterase type 5 inhibitors have been the pharmaceutical drug of exploration, given their known mechanism of action of promoting degradation of cyclic guanosine monophosphate, which indirectly increases blood flow to the penis allowing for erection. RTOG 0215 randomized patients with known ED after RT and ADT to 12 weeks of sildenafil or placebo followed by 1 week of no therapy and subsequent cross-over treatment. Of 115 patients enrolled in the study, 55% of them completed all three of the IIEF assessments. Results showed sildenafil had an overall significant benefit on the probability of erectile response (0.17) ($P = .009$), and a higher overall probability (0.21) for patients who received less than 120 days of ADT (97). Overall, this study indicated that patients could benefit from therapy with sildenafil (especially those on no or shorter ADT), but overall, the response to treatment is unpredictable and the low response rate warrants investigation into preventative measures (98).

A subsequent trial, RTOG 0831, randomized patients to tadalafil 5 mg ($n = 121$) or placebo ($n = 121$) for 24 weeks while completing EBRT (63%)

or brachytherapy (37%). All patients had intact erectile function prior to the start of RT. Patients completed IIEF responses before RT, at 2 weeks and 4 weeks, between 20 and 24 weeks, between 28 and 30 weeks, and 1 year after treatment. Between 28 and 30 weeks, there was no significant difference between maintained erectile function on tadalafil versus placebo (79% versus 74%, $P = .49$) (99). Also, no significant difference was noted at 1 year: 72% versus 71%, $P = .93$ (99). Partners of the men taking tadalafil did not notice significant effects on sexual satisfaction or an improvement in marital adjustment, as compared to placebo (99). Therefore, RTOG 0831 demonstrated that prophylactic tadalafil 5 mg use during therapy does not improve overall erectile function.

In an institutional study, Zelefsky et al (100) studied 279 potent men with localized prostate cancer treated with RT who were randomized 2:1 to sildenafil citrate (50 mg daily) or placebo concurrent with RT, and continued daily for 6 months. Patients completed the IIEF questionnaire before therapy, and at 3, 6, 9, 12, 18, and 24 months after RT. Results showed that at 12 months, those treated with sildenafil citrate had no or minimal ED (73% versus 50%, respectively, $P = .024$). Those treated with sildenafil were also noted to have superior overall satisfaction and IIEF total scores ($P = .027$ and $0.043$, respectively). At 24 months, erectile function and IIEF scores were no longer significantly different between the groups ($P = .172$ and $.09$, respectively), but overall satisfaction was higher in the sildenafil group as compared to placebo ($P = .033$). Zelefsky et al (100) also separated out men on ADT (~10%), and noted that these men tend to have worse erectile function than those not on ADT regardless of the use of sildenafil citrate or placebo. As well, the variation in scores among time points for the men on ADT suggested a potential mitigation effect of ADT on the perhaps beneficial effect of prophylactic sildenafil.

If PDE-5 inhibitors are unsuccessful or contraindicated, referral to a urologist who can manage ED is beneficial—other therapies such as vacuum erection device, which mechanically increases flow into the penis and through the use of a penile ring obstructs venous outflow, and prostaglandin injections are highly successful. These therapies do require a more motivated patient. Penile implant surgery is uncommon but results in high satisfaction scores for those who proceed with such treatment.

### *Anejaculation*

This late effect is very common after prostate irradiation, whether for prostate cancer or as a nearby organ for other therapy. The prostate is a gland producing much of the seminal fluid. Radiation dose as low as 15 to 20 Gy can result in reduced or absent seminal fluid.

While patients are still able to orgasm, they can describe that the sensation has changed. Some men note significant distress with this symptom, and while there is no effective management, education of the risk of this effect during the consultation and reassurance when it occurs can greatly alleviate concern.

### *Fertility*

- Doses less than 0.8 Gy can cause oligospermia, 0.8 to 2 Gy transient azoospermia, and 2 to 3 Gy irreversible azoospermia.

- Best prevention is avoidance.
- When testes will be irradiated, fertility preservation options include sperm cryopreservation or surgical sperm extraction.

Men, like women, are at risk of infertility with the toxic effects of radiation on both the testicular somatic cells (Sertoli and Leydig cells) and germ cells. Etiology is believed to be related to the depletion of the proliferating germ cell pool (83). The damage to the generation of sperm cell can lead to oligospermia (defined as sperm density less than $20 \times 10^6$ sperm/mL measured in an ejaculate sample) or azoospermia. Like the ovaries, the testes are extremely sensitive to radiation. It has been suspected that doses less than 0.8 Gy can cause oligospermia, 0.8 to 2 Gy transient azoospermia, and 2 to 3 Gy irreversible azoospermia (101,102). Given the high likelihood of developing infertility with testicular irradiation, preventative measures in planning should be taken and patient conversations should be held early on likelihood of infertility based on individual patient treatment plan.

While not all men will choose fertility preservation prior to treatment, evaluation by sperm analysis may be warranted to determine those most at risk. For men deciding to undergo fertility preservation, options include sperm cryopreservation or surgical sperm extraction. Sperm cryopreservation consists of collecting and freezing sperm. Sperm frozen for up to 28 years has been successfully used in IVF resulting in live birth (103). Another fertility preservation method is surgical sperm extraction, in which sperm are obtained via differing surgical techniques (testicular sperm extraction, testicular sperm aspiration, and microsurgical epididymal sperm aspiration) (83). This technique can be used for patients who cannot ejaculate. Much less common methods of cryopreservation included urine collection and processing for sperm after retrograde ejaculation or electroejaculation (83). These methods can be considered for patients who are less likely to be successful ejaculating.

Intracytoplasmic sperm injection (ICSI) is a new technique for men with severe oligospermia. Sperm are retrieved from the testes typically by testicular sperm extraction (TESE). ICSI typically follows IVF retrieval of female oocytes with subsequent reimplantation of an embryo or embryos. One study showed a 37% successful sperm retrieval in 73 patients with suspected postchemotherapy azoospermia (104).

While all of the aforementioned preservation techniques are focused on the postpubertal man, new experimental methods help to allow for future fertility for prepubertal boys as well. Similar to women, testicular tissue cryopreservation is an emerging fertility treatment option, although still considered experimental at this time. It involves surgically removing a portion of the testicular tissue and cryopreserving it. Tissue thawing and transplantation can occur post treatment with a viability of up to 95% (83). Spermatogonial stem cells (SSCs) have been frozen and transplanted posttreatment with a lower viability of 66% (83).

Overall, there are various fertility-preserving techniques for men and women, and correct physician-patient interaction includes early conversation regarding the patient's individualized risk and next step in treatment planning.

## Lymphatic System

- *Symptoms:* swelling, edema
- *Timing:* 12+ months after RT
- *Prevention:* weight control, exercise, and avoidance of skin injury due to risk of infection
- *Management:* limb elevation, compression bandaging, physiotherapy

RT can be associated with lymphedema. The most well-studied area of increased risk for lymphedema is in breast cancer patients. However, lower limb lymphedema (LLL) following whole pelvic RT is also common and potentially debilitating. Risk of lymphedema increases with combined surgery and radiation or chemoradiation.

- Dunberger et al (105): 616 patients received RT alone or combined treatment (surgery and RT) for gynecological cancer. Thirty-six percent ($n$ = 218) reported LLL with negative impact on physical activity, housework, and social activities.
- Pieterse et al (106) studied 229 women, 94 (41%) of whom received RT for cervical cancer. At 12 months, lymphedema in RT group was 26% as compared to 12% (RR = 2.75 [1.24–6.10]). At 24 months, 29% as compared to 13%, respectively (RR = 2.81 [1.23–6.40]).
- In one study of 802 patients with gynecological cancer, 76.2% ($n$ = 611) had no lower leg swelling, 13.7% ($n$ = 110) undiagnosed lower limb swelling, and 10.1% ($n$ = 81) diagnosed lymphedema (107). Authors calculated through multivariate analysis that cervical cancer survivors have a 3.5-fold higher odds of LLL with RT as part of their treatment plan.

Regardless, these studies demonstrate the correlated effects of RT to the pelvis on the lymph system marked by increased risk of lymphedema that can cause a considerable QOL change. It is imperative to assess patients for LLL in order to appropriately refer them for lymphedema management.

Lymphedema is a chronic condition that is extremely difficult to resolve, but can generally be managed. General management includes self-monitoring, limb elevation, diet and exercise, and avoidance of skin injury due to risk of infection. Compression bandaging, as well as compression garments and pneumatic compression devices can provide relief. Physiotherapy consists of manual lymphatic drainage or complete decongestive therapy, which is reserved for more severe lymphedema. Lymphedema specialists can help to clinically stage patient's severity and provide appropriate recommendations.

## Bone

- *Symptoms:* pelvic insufficiency fractures
- *Timing:* years after RT
- *Prevention:* minimize dose, calcium/vitamin D supplementation, weight-bearing exercise
- *Management:* immobilization/bed rest, analgesics

Radiation can have a long-term side effect on mature bone exhibiting after several years. Patients who undergo EBRT with significant bone dose are at risk to develop pelvic or sacral insufficiency fractures. The etiology of this risk is due to the formation of intimal fibrosis and endothelial damage by RT. This reduces blood flow to allow for healthy regeneration posttreatment. Furthermore, RT affects osteoblast proliferation (71). Collectively, diminished regeneration leads to focal osteopenia that is susceptible to fractures, particularly at the weight-bearing areas. These are commonly pelvic insufficiency fractures, a subtype of stress fracture caused by weakened bone. The incidence of pelvic insufficiency fractures is related to treatment site, treatment modality, which determines radiation dose to site, as well as age, comorbidities, and other general osteoporosis risk factors. Pelvic insufficiency fractures (PIF) most commonly occur at the sacroiliac joint and present with low back or pelvic pain. MRI has increased detection of these fractures and should be considered if a patient has received higher than 50 Gy to the site of symptoms and normal x-ray is nondiagnostic.

- Baxter et al (108) analyzed 6,428 women diagnosed with pelvic malignancies who underwent RT ($n$ = 2,855) versus no RT ($n$ = 3,573). Ninety percent of fractures in both groups collectively occurred at the hip. The 5-year fracture rates were higher in each site of disease for the women who underwent RT: 14.0% versus 7.5% in anal cancer patients, 8.2% versus 5.9% in cervical cancer patients, and 11.2% versus 8.7% in rectal cancer patients. No difference in rate of spine or arm fractures was noted.
- A subsequent study by Ikushima et al (109) investigated 158 gynecological cancer patients who underwent EBRT. Insufficiency fractures were developed by 11.4% ($n$ = 158) in the irradiated field with a mean timeline of 6 months. All women were treated with bed rest and analgesics with symptoms ranging from 3 to 20 months.

The main method to prevent PIF is to limit the dose delivered to the pelvic bone, as well as other bones of the area. Oh et al (110) determined that radiation dose of 50.4 Gy or higher was a significant risk factor for developing PIF ($P$ = .005). As well, patients undergoing EBRT to the pelvis should be placed on calcium and vitamin D supplementation, as well as subscribe to a regular weight-bearing exercise program to further reduce risk of osteopenia. Also, further ways to decrease risk of osteoporosis should be implemented: decreased alcohol intake and smoking cessation. Patients should discuss with their primary care physician when they should begin dual energy x-ray absorptiometry (DEXA) scans. If PIF does occur, treatment includes immobilization and rest coupled with symptoms relief.

## Bone Marrow

- *Symptoms:* fatigue, easy bruising/bleeding, increased risk of infection
- *Timing:* 1+ week into RT
- *Prevention:* keep pelvic bone marrow V 40 Gy less than or equal to 25% and V 20 Gy less than or equal to 90%
- *Management:* attention to symptoms, transfusion, infection prophylaxis, antibiotics as necessary

Up to 25% of the bone marrow is located in the bones of the pelvis (71), and hematopoietic stem cells are quite sensitive to radiation dose; therefore, hematologic toxicities can be of concern. In addition, the treatment of multiple pelvic malignancies utilizes concurrent chemotherapy, further affecting this risk. RTOG 0418 patients ($n$ = 83) were treated with postoperative IMRT of 50.4 Gy to the pelvic lymphatics and vagina. Of those treated with V40 to the pelvic bone of more than 37%, 75% had grade 2 or higher hematologic toxicity when on concurrent cisplatin (111). Similarly, Rose et al (112) studied hematologic outcomes during chemotherapy and volume of bone marrow receiving greater than 10 and 20 Gy. Patients with a higher bone marrow V10 or greater were more likely to experience grade 3 or greater leukopenia (68.8% versus 24.6% and 57.7% versus 21.8%, respectively). Both of these studies demonstrate that the dose of radiation delivered to the bone marrow is significantly correlated with hematologic toxicity, specifically when patients are treated with concurrent chemotherapy. Therefore, in order to reduce the incidence of toxicity to the pelvic bone marrow, dose should be limited to the pelvic bone marrow. While many differing theories exist as to the exact parameters of these dose constraints, recent studies have suggested that a V40 Gy less than or equal to 25% and V20 Gy of less than or equal to 90% can significantly decrease hematologic toxicity to the bone marrow (113). With the modern use of IMRT for many malignancies of the pelvis, delivering low doses to the pelvic marrow is straightforward for most cases. Fortunately, marrow suppression usually recovers quickly as stem cells repopulate from other nonirradiated areas.

### Skin

- *Symptoms:* erythema, pain, dry and moist desquamation
- *Timing:* 2 to 3+ weeks into radiation
- *Prevention:* IMRT, loose fitting clothing, moisturizers, good hygiene
- *Management:* moisturizers, loose fitting clothing, topical steroids/analgesics, antifungal treatment as needed

Skin reactions are common with treatment to the pelvis, although advances with radiation delivery via IMRT have dramatically decreased the rate of grade 2 and grade 3 dermatitis. Treatment is most likely for cancers which involve or come close to the skin, such as anal, vulvar, and low rectal cancers. Acutely, patients may notice erythema and moist or dry desquamation. Rarely does ulceration occur. For photon therapy, skin reaction is proportional to treatment time and dose delivered.

The treatment for acute dermatitis has been studied for numerous years, with little convincing evidence. It is recommended that patients should begin treatment for skin reactions with conservative measures: hygienic measures with mild unscented soap, avoid sun exposure, wear loose-fitted clothing, avoid irritants, and use lanolin-free water-based creams and ointments (114). These are also suggested to patients as preventative measures. While these suggestions are not rooted in evidence, they do not pose any harm to the patient and have been interpreted by many physicians, based on previous clinical experience, to be of sufficient aid. More specific additional interventions have been more thoroughly discussed in literature and are analyzed in Table 6.8.

As noted in Table 6.8, there is a tremendous lack of clarity on the benefit of various treatments. Apart from the evidence in using IMRT, there is no level I evidence for prophylactic measures for radiodermatitis in pelvic RT patients. Strong data by Pommier et al (118) supports the use of calendula for prevention of grade 2 or higher acute dermatitis in breast cancer patients. Kassab et al's (122) review of literature demonstrated support of the efficacy of topical calendula: one study demonstrated use of topical calendula over trolamine to prevent radiodermatitis. These studies should be discussed with pelvic RT patients prior to treatment; however, prophylactic measure for radiodermatitis demands more investigation and search for level I evidence.

**Table 6.8** Evidence-Based Interventions for Acute Skin Toxicity During RT

| Intervention | Study | Findings |
|---|---|---|
| Aquaphor, Biafine, RadiaCare | Gosselin et al (115): RCT | Patients randomized to placebo ($n = 49$), Aquaphor ($n = 53$), Biafine ($n = 53$), RadiaCare ($n = 53$). No difference noticed between products in reducing grade 2–4 skin reaction |
| Aloe vera | Heggie et al (116): RCT | Randomized to aloe vera ($n = 107$) versus aqueous cream ($n = 101$). Higher prevalence of dry desquamation in aloe group |
| Biafine (trolamine) | Fenig et al (117): RCT | Randomized to Biafine ($n = 25$), Lipiderm ($n = 24$), no treatment ($n = 25$). No difference in groups |
| Calendula cream | Pommier et al (118): RCT | Randomized to calendula ($n = 126$) versus trolamine ($n = 128$). Calendula group with significant reduced pain and reduced grade 2 or greater skin reactions |
| Steroids | Omidvari et al (119): RCT | Randomized to betamethasone ($n = 19$) versus petrolatum ($n = 17$) versus control ($n = 15$). No benefit of steroids |
| Sucralfate | Wells et al (120): RCT | Randomized to aqueous cream ($n = 120$) versus sucralfate cream ($n = 122$) versus no cream ($n = 124$). No difference in groups |

RCT, randomized controlled trial; RT, radiation therapy.
*Source:* From Ref. (121). McQuestion M. Evidence-based skin care management in radiation therapy: clinical update. *Semin Oncol Nurs.* 2011;27(2):e1–e17.

Management

If desquamation occurs, low to mild potency topical steroids can be tried (114). Moist desquamation could respond to calendula cream, as well as formulations of hyaluronic acid (121). Specific to the pelvis, use of sitz baths or frequent baths/showers are helpful to keep the perineal area clean after bowel movements. Use of moist towelettes (ie, baby wipes) are gentler on skin than toilet paper. After cleansing, circulating air through loose clothing, fan, or hair dryer set on cool can help to dry the area or reduce residual moisture, which can promote chafing/yeast infection. Mild acute dermatitis symptoms can be watched and usually resolve in 1 to 3 weeks. Moist desquamation of clinical significance warrants wound care consult for dressing changes, as well as a consideration of treatment break to prevent further skin breakdown.

Late radiation effects predominantly include chronic radiation dermatitis, hyperpigmentation, and radiation-induced fibrosis. Patients with chronic dermatitis (ulcers and erosions) should see a wound care specialist for specific guidelines, as well as be considered for debridement, if applicable, or surgical interventions for nonhealing ulcers, if necessary (114).

## SECONDARY MALIGNANCY OF THE PELVIS

A recent meta-analysis (123) has attempted to quantify the risk of second primary cancer (SPC) from RT. In this analysis, 19 publications, 21 institutional series, and 7 other studies were used. Conclusively, the analysis suggested that the risk of radiation-induced SPC appears small: 1 in 220 to 1 in 290. For patients receiving older radiation techniques, the incidence may be increased to as little as 1 in 70 (123). There is not enough information at this time to understand the risk of SPC with IMRT and brachytherapy, although more conformal dose delivery suspects less incidence of SPC. While significant to predict and acknowledge the risk of SPC, this study was marked by heterogeneity and therefore limited to its applicability.

## CONCLUSION

The content presented attempts to quantify and summarize the collective evidence-based data available on the incidence, effect, prophylactic measures, interventions, and outcomes of common and uncommon toxicities associated with RT to the pelvis by organ and event: damage to the rectum, bladder, bone, bone marrow, skin, and lymphatic organs, and event of sexual function, fertility, and secondary malignancies. The authors hope that this can serve as a guide to better inform patients for potential side effects of RT, and also to effectively treat patients if a side effect occurs. Furthermore, the authors hope this may serve as a guide to the treatment team, to best predict and prevent toxicities for our patients' survivorship and well-being. Finally, continuing education by the treatment team, participating in QOL trials, and utilizing the most advanced treatment techniques and imaging for various pelvic tumors (brachytherapy, 3DCRT, protons and IMRT/volumetric arc therapy (VMAT)/SBRT with or without advanced IG) will help best mitigate these issues for our patients in our current and future practices.

## REFERENCES

1. Lagrange JL, Bascoul-Mollevi C, Geoffrois L, et al.; Study Group on Genito-Urinary Tumors. Quality of life assessment after concurrent chemoradiation for invasive bladder cancer: results of a multicenter prospective study. *Int J Radiat Oncol Biol Phys*. 2007;79(1):172–178.

2. Rosati LM.. Patient- versus physician-reported outcomes in patients enrolled in a prospective study involving stereotactic body radiation therapy in unresectable or recurrent pancreatic cancer. *J Clin Oncol*. 2015;33(29 Suppl):84.

3. Wortel RC, Incrocci L, Pos FJ, et al. Late side effects after image guided intensity modulated radiation therapy compared to 3D-conformal radiation therapy for prostate cancer: results from 2 prospective cohorts. *Int J Radiat Oncol Biol Phys*. 2016;95(2):680–689.

4. Gray PJ, Paly JJ, Yeap BY, et al. Patient-reported outcomes after 3-dimensional conformal, intensity-modulated, or proton beam radiotherapy for localized prostate cancer. *Cancer*. 2013;119(9):1729–1735. doi:10.1002/cncr.27956

5. Kochhar R, Patel F, Dhar A, et al. Radiation-induced proctosigmoiditis. prospective, randomized, double-blind controlled trial of oral sulfasalazine plus rectal steroids versus rectal sucralfate. *Dig Dis Sci*. 1991;36(1):103–107.

6. Kochhar R, Sriram PV, Sharma SC, et al. Natural history of late radiation proctosigmoiditis treated with topical sucralfate suspension. *Dig Dis Sci*. 1999;44(5):973–978.

7. Sandor Z, Nagata M, Kusstatscher S, et al. Stimulation of mucosal glutathione and angiogenesis: new mechanisms of gastroprotection and ulcer healing by sucralfate. *Scand J Gastroenterol*. 1995;30:19–21.

8. Lucidarme D, Marteau P, Foucault M, et al. Efficacy and tolerance of mesalazine suppositories vs. hydrocortisone foam in proctitis. *Aliment Pharmacol Ther*. 1997;11(2):335–340.

9. Muecke R, Schomburg L, Glatzel M, et al. Multicenter, phase 3 trial comparing selenium supplementation with observation in gynecologic radiation oncology. *Int J Radiat Oncol Biol Phys*. 2010;78:828–835.

10. Cavcić J, Turcić J, Martinac P, et al. Metronidazole in the treatment of chronic radiation proctitis: clinical trial. *Croat Med J*. 2000;41(3):314–318.

11. Fuccio L, Guido A, Andreyev HJ. Management of intestinal complications in patients with pelvic radiation disease. *Clin Gastroenterol Hepatol*. 2012;10(12):1326.e4–1334.e4.

12. Talley NA, Chen F, King D, et al. Short-chain fatty acids in the treatment of radiation proctitis: a randomized, double-blind, placebo-controlled, cross-over pilot trial. *Dis Colon Rectum*. 1997;40(9):1046–1050.

13. Hanson B, Macdonald R, Shaukat A. Endoscopic and medical therapy for chronic radiation proctopathy: a systematic review. *Dis Colon Rectum*. 2012;55(10):1081–1095.

14. Al-Sabbagh R, Sinicrope FA, Sellin JH, et al. Evaluation of short-chain fatty acid enemas: treatment of radiation proctitis. *Am J Gastroenterol*. 1996;91(9):1814–1816.

15. Lesperance RN, Kjorstadt RJ, Halligan JB, et al. Colorectal complications of external beam radiation versus brachytherapy for prostate cancer. *Am J Surg*. 2008;195(5):616–620.

16. Zelefsky MJ, Levin EJ, Hunt M, et al. Incidence of late rectal and urinary toxicities after three-dimensional conformal radiotherapy and intensity-modulated radiotherapy for localized prostate cancer. *Int J Radiat Oncol Biol Phys*. 2008;70(4):1124–1129.

17. Lawton CA, Desilvio M, Roach M, et al. An update of the phase III trial comparing whole pelvic to prostate only radiotherapy and neoadjuvant to adjuvant total androgen suppression: updated analysis of RTOG 94-13, with emphasis on unexpected hormone/radiation Interactions. *Int J Radiat Oncol Biol Phys.* 2007;69(3):646–655.

18. Ali AN, Rossi PJ, Godette KD, et al. Impact of magnetic resonance imaging on computed tomography-based treatment planning and acute toxicity for prostate cancer patients treated with intensity modulated radiation therapy. *Pract Radiat Oncol.* 2013;3(1):e1–e9. doi:10.1016/j.prro.2012.04.005

19. Smeenk RJ, van Lin EN, van Kollenburg P, et al. Anal wall sparing effect of an endorectal balloon in 3D conformal and intensity-modulated prostate radiotherapy. *Radiother Oncol.* 2009;93(1):131–136.

20. Prada PJ, Gonzalez H, Menéndez C, et al. Transperineal injection of hyaluronic acid in the anterior perirectal fat to decrease rectal toxicity from radiation delivered with low-dose-rate brachytherapy for prostate cancer patients. *Brachytherapy.* 2009;8(2):210–217.

21. Mariados N, Sylvester J, Shah D, et al. Hydrogel spacer prospective multicenter randomized controlled pivotal trial: dosimetric and clinical effects of perirectal spacer application in men undergoing prostate image guided intensity modulated radiation therapy. *Int J Radiat Oncol Biol Phys.* 2015;92(5):971–977.

22. Hamstra DA, Mariados N, Sylvester J, et al. Continued benefit to rectal separation for prostate radiation therapy: final results of a phase III trial. *Int J Radiat Oncol Biol Phys.* 2017;97(5):976–985. doi:10.1016/j.ijrobp.2016.12.024

23. Kneebone A, Mameghan H, Bolin T, et al. The effect of oral sucralfate on the acute proctitis associated with prostate radiotherapy: a double-blind, randomized trial. *Int J Radiat Oncol Biol Phys.* 2001;51(3):628–635.

24. O'Brien PC, Franklin CI, Poulsen MG, et al. Acute symptoms, not rectally administered sucralfate, predict for late radiation proctitis: longer term follow-up of a phase III trial—trans-Tasman radiation oncology group. *Int J Radiat Oncol Biol Phys.* 2002;54(2):442–449.

25. Hille A, Schmidberger H, Hermann RM, et al. A phase III randomized, placebo-controlled, double-blind study of misoprostol rectal suppositories to prevent acute radiation proctitis in patients with prostate cancer. *Int J Radiat Oncol Biol Phys.* 2005;63(5):1488–1493.

26. Valdagni R, Rancati T, Ghilotti M, et al. To bleed or not to bleed. A prediction based on individual gene profiling combined with dose-volume histogram shapes in prostate cancer patients undergoing three-dimensional conformal radiation therapy. *Int J Radiat Oncol Biol Phys.* 2009;74(5):1431–1440.

27. Ma TH, Yuan ZX, Zhong QH, et al. Formalin irrigation for hemorrhagic chronic radiation proctitis. *World J Gastroenterol.* 2015;21(12):3593–3598.

28. de Parades V, Etienney I, Bauer P, et al. Formalin application in the treatment of chronic radiation-induced hemorrhagic proctitis—an effective but not risk-free procedure: a prospective study of 33 patients. *Dis Colon Rectum.* 2005;48(8):1535–1541.

29. Haas EM, Bailey HR, Faragher I. Application of 10 percent formalin for the treatment of radiation-induced hemorrhagic proctitis. *Dis Colon Rectum.* 2007;50(2):213–217.

30. Ben Soussan E, Mathieu N, Roque I, et al. Bowel explosion with colonic perforation during argon plasma coagulation for hemorrhagic radiation-induced proctitis. *Gastrointest Endosc.* 2003;57(3):412–413.

31. Schaake W, van der Schaaf A, van Dijk LV, et al. Normal tissue complication probability (NTCP) models for late rectal bleeding, stool frequency and fecal incontinence after radiotherapy in prostate cancer patients. *Radiother Oncol.* 2016;119(3):381–387.
32. Vernia P, Fracasso PL, Casale V, et al. Topical butyrate for acute radiation proctitis: randomised, crossover trial. *Lancet.* 2000;356(9237):1232–1235.
33. Grigsby PW, Pilepich MV, Parsons CL. Preliminary results of a phase I/II study of sodium pentosanpolysulfate in the treatment of chronic radiation-induced proctitis. *Am J Clin Oncol.* 1990;13(1):28–31.
34. Pilepich MV, Paulus R, St Clair W, et al. Phase III study of pentosanpolysulfate (PPS) in treatment of gastrointestinal tract sequelae of radiotherapy. *Am J Clin Oncol.* 2006;29(2):132–137.
35. Kennedy M, Bruninga K, Mutlu EA, et al. Successful and sustained treatment of chronic radiation proctitis with antioxidant Vitamins E and C. *Am J Gastroenterol.* 2001;96(4):1080–1084.
36. Venkitaraman R, Price A, Coffey J, et al. Pentoxifylline to treat radiation proctitis: a small and inconclusive randomised trial. *Clin Oncol (R Coll Radiol).* 2008;20(4):288–292. doi:10.1016/j.clon.2008.01.012. Erratum in: *Clin Oncol (R Coll Radiol).* 2008;20(5):386. Price, A [added].
37. Clarke RE, Tenorio LM, Hussey JR, et al. Hyperbaric oxygen treatment of chronic refractory radiation proctitis: a randomized and controlled double-blind crossover trial with long-term follow-up. *Int J Radiat Oncol Biol Phys.* 2008;72(1):134–143.
38. Smit SG, Heyns CF. Management of radiation cystitis. *Nat Rev Urol.* 2010;7(4): 206–214. doi:10.1038/nrurol.2010.23
39. Denton AS, Clarke NW, Maher EJ. Non-surgical interventions for late radiation cystitis in patients who have received radical radiotherapy to the pelvis. *Cochrane Database Syst Rev.* 2002;(3):CD001773. doi:10.1002/14651858.CD001773
40. Crook J, Esche B, Futter N. Effect of pelvic radiotherapy for prostate cancer on bowel, bladder, and sexual function: the patient's perspective. *Urology.* 1996;47(3):387–394.
41. Al Hussein Al Awamlh B, Lee DJ, Nguyen DP, et al. Assessment of the quality-of-life and functional outcomes in patients undergoing cystectomy and urinary diversion for the management of radiation-induced refractory benign disease. *Urology.* 2015;85(2):394–401.
42. Liberman D, Mehus B, Elliott SP. Urinary adverse effects of pelvic radiotherapy. *Transl Androl Urol.* 2014;3(2):186–195.
43. Díez P, Mullassery V, Dankulchai P, et al. Dosimetric analysis of urethral strictures following HDR (192)Ir brachytherapy as monotherapy for intermediate- and high-risk prostate cancer. *Radiother Oncol.* 2014;113(3):410–413.
44. Rubin P, Constine LS, Marks LB. *ALERT - adverse late effects of cancer treatment. Vol. 2: normal tissue specific sites and systems.* Heidelberg: Springer-Verlag; 2014:488.
45. Gould, S. Urinary tract disorders. Clinical comparison of flavoxate and phenazopyridine. *Urology.* 1975;5(5):612–615.
46. Rigaud, J, Hetet JF, Bouchot O. Management of radiation cystitis. *Prog Urol.* 2004;14(4):568–572.
47. Hampson SJ, Woodhouse CR. Sodium pentosanpolysulphate in the management of haemorrhagic cystitis: experience with 14 patients. *Eur Urol.* 1994;25(1):40–42.
48. Sandhu SS, Goldstraw M, Woodhouse CR. The management of haemorrhagic cystitis with sodium pentosan polysulphate. *BJU Int.* 2004;94(6):845–847.

49. Liu YK, Harty JI, Steinbock GS, et al. Treatment of radiation or cyclophosphamide induced hemorrhagic cystitis using conjugated estrogen. *J Urol*. 1990;144(1):41–43.

50. Veerasarn V, Khorprasert C, Lorvidhaya V, et al. Reduced recurrence of late hemorrhagic radiation cystitis by WF10 therapy in cervical cancer patients: a multicenter, randomized, two-arm, open-label trial. *Radiother Oncol*. 2004;73(2):179–185.

51. Veerasarn V, Boonnuch W, Kakanaporn C. A Phase II study to evaluate WF10 in patients with late hemorrhagic radiation cystitis and proctitis. *Gynecol Oncol*. 2006;100(1):179–184.

52. Dewan AK, Mohan GM, Ravi R. Intravesical formalin for hemorrhagic cystitis following irradiation of cancer of the cervix. *Int J Gynaecol Obstet*. 1993;42(2):131–135.

53. Lojanapiwat B, Sripralakrit S, Soonthornphan S, et al. Intravesicle formalin instillation with a modified technique for controlling haemorrhage secondary to radiation cystitis. *Asian J Surg*. 2002;25(3):232–235.

54. Shao Y, Lu GL, Shen ZJ. Comparison of intravesical hyaluronic acid instillation and hyperbaric oxygen in the treatment of radiation-induced hemorrhagic cystitis. *BJU Int*. 2012;109(5):691–694.

55. Arrizabalaga M, Extramiana J, Parra JL, et al. Treatment of massive haematuria with aluminous salts. *Br J Urol*. 1987;60(3):223–226.

56. Hemal AK, Praveen BV, Sankaranarayanan A, Vaidyanathan S. Control of persistent vesical bleeding due to radiation cystitis by intravesical application of 15 (S) 15-methyl prostaglandin F2-alpha. *Indian J Cancer*. 1989;26(2):99–101.

57. Eifel PJ, Levenback C, Wharton JT, et al. Time course and incidence of late complications in patients treated with radiation therapy for FIGO stage IB carcinoma of the uterine cervix. *Int J Radiat Oncol Biol Phys*. 1995;32(5):1289–1300.

58. Kaplan JR, Wolf JS Jr. Efficacy and survival associated with cystoscopy and clot evacuation for radiation or cyclophosphamide induced hemorrhagic cystitis. *J Urol*. 2009;181(2):641–646. doi:10.1016/j.juro.2008.10.037

59. Kuo YC, Kuo HC. O'Leary-Sant symptom index predicts the treatment outcome for OnabotulinumtoxinA injections for refractory interstitial cystitis/bladder pain syndrome. *Toxins*. 2015;7(8):2860–2871.

60. Chuang YC, Kim DK, Chiang PH, et al. Bladder botulinum toxin A injection can benefit patients with radiation and chemical cystitis. *BJU Int*. 2008;102(6):704–706.

61. Ravi R. Endoscopic neodymium: YAG laser treatment of radiation-induced hemorrhagic cystitis. *Lasers Surg Med*. 1994;14(1):83–87.

62. Wines MP, Lynch WD. A new minimally invasive technique for treating radiation cystitis: the argon-beam coagulator. *BJU Int*. 2006;98(3):610–612.

63. Zhu J, Xue B, Shan Y, et al. Transurethral coagulation for radiation-induced hemorrhagic cystitis using Greenlight™ potassium-titanyl-phosphate laser. *Photomed Laser Surg*. 2013;31(2):78–81.

64. Kaushik D, Teply BA, Hemstreet GP 3rd. Novel treatment strategy for refractory hemorrhagic cystitis following radiation treatment of genitourinary cancer: use of 980-Nm diode laser. *Lasers Med Sci*. 2012;27(5):1099–1102.

65. Mendenhall WM, Henderson RH, Costa JA, et al. Hemorrhagic radiation cystitis. *Am J Clin Oncol*. 2015;38:331–336. http://journals.lww.com/amjclinicaloncology/Abstract/2015/06000/Hemorrhagic_Radiation_Cystitis.18.aspx

66. Vistad I, Cvancarova M, Fosså SD, Kristensen GB. Postradiotherapy morbidity in long-term survivors after locally advanced cervical cancer: how well do physicians' assessments agree with those of their patients? *Int J Radiat Oncol Biol Phys*. 2008;71(5):1335–1342. doi:10.1016/j.ijrobp.2007.12.030

67. Flay LD, Matthews JH. The effects of radiotherapy and surgery on the sexual function of women treated for cervical cancer. *Int J Radiat Oncol Biol Phys*. 1995;31(2):399–404.

68. Bergmark K, Avall-Lundqvist E, Dickman PW, et al. Vaginal changes and sexuality in women with a history of cervical cancer. *N Engl J Med*. 1999;340(18): 1383–1389.

69. Jensen PT, Froeding LP. Pelvic radiotherapy and sexual function in women. *Transl Androl Urol*. 2015;4(2):186–205. doi:10.3978/j.issn.2223-4683.2015.04.06

70. Townamchai K, Lee L, Viswanathan AN. A novel low dose fractionation regimen for adjuvant vaginal brachytherapy in early stage endometrioid endometrial cancer. *Gynecol Oncol*. 2012;127(2):351–355. doi:10.1016/j.ygyno.2012.07.111

71. Bradley KA, McHaffie DR. Treatment-related toxicity from the use of radiation therapy for gynecologic malignancies. In Vora SR, ed. *UpToDate*. https://www.uptodate.com/contents/treatment-related-toxicity-from-the-use-of-radiation-therapy-for-gynecologic-malignancies. Updated January 28, 2015.

72. Denton AS, Maher EJ. Interventions for the physical aspects of sexual dysfunction in women following pelvic radiotherapy. *Cochrane Database of Systematic Reviews*. 2003;(1). doi:10.1002/14651858.CD003750

73. Miles T, Johnson N. Vaginal dilator therapy for women receiving pelvic radiotherapy. *Cochrane Database Syst Rev*. 2014;(9):CD007291. doi:10.1002/14651858.CD007291.pub3

74. Robinson JW, Faris PD, Scott CB. Psychoeducational group increases vaginal dilation for younger women and reduces sexual fears for women of all ages with gynecological carcinoma treated with radiotherapy. *Int J Radiat Oncol Biol Phys*. 1999;44(3):497–506.

75. Miles TP. *Evaluating vaginal dilator therapy after pelvic radiotherapy* [PhD thesis]. Bristol, UK: The University of the West of England Bristol, Faculty of Health and Social Care; 2012.

76. Sobotkowski J, Markowska J, Fijuth J, Pietraszek A. Preliminary results of mitomycin C local application as post-treatment prevention of vaginal radiation-induced morbidity in women with cervical cancer. *Eur J Gynaecol Oncol*. 2006;27(4):356–358.

77. Fawaz ZS, Barkati M, Beauchemin MC, et al. Cervical necrosis after chemoradiation for cervical cancer: case series and literature review. *Radiat Oncol*. 2013;8:220. doi:10.1186/1748-717X-8-220

78. Williams JA Jr, Clarke D, Dennis WA, et al. The treatment of pelvic soft tissue radiation necrosis with hyperbaric oxygen. *Am J Obstet Gynecol*. 1992;167(2):412–415; discussion 415–416.

79. Dion MW, Hussey DH, Doornbos JF, et al. Preliminary results of a pilot study of pentoxifylline in the treatment of late radiation soft tissue necrosis. *Int J Radiat Oncol Biol Phys*. 1990;19(2):401–407.

80. Safra T, Gutman G, Fishlev G, et al. Improved quality of life with hyperbaric oxygen therapy in patients with persistent pelvic radiation-induced toxicity. *Clin Oncol*. 2008;20(4):284–287.

81. Moore KN, Gold MA, Mcmeekin DS, et al. Vesicovaginal fistula formation in patients with Stage IVA cervical carcinoma. *Gynecol Oncol*. 2007;106(3):498–501.

82. Wallace WH, Thomson AB, Saran F, et al. Predicting age of ovarian failure after radiation to a field that includes the ovaries. *Int J Radiat Oncol Biol Phys*. 2005;62(3):738–744.

83. Skaznik-Wikiel ME, Gilbert SB, Meacham RB, et al. Fertility preservation options for men and women with cancer. *Rev Urol*. 2015;17(4):211–219.

84. Lambertini M, Del Mastro L, Pescio MC, et al. Cancer and fertility preservation: international recommendations from an expert meeting. *BMC Med*. 2016;14:1. doi:10.1186/s12916-015-0545-7

85. Lee SJ, Schover LR, Partridge AH, et al. American Society of Clinical Oncology recommendations on fertility preservation in cancer patients. *J Clin Oncol*. 2006;24(18):2917–2931.

86. Mahran YF, El-Demerdash E, Nada AS, et al. Growth hormone ameliorates the radiotherapy-induced ovarian follicular loss in rats: impact on oxidative stress, apoptosis and IGF-1/IGF-1R axis. *PLOS ONE*. 2015;10(10):e0140055. doi:10.1371/journal.pone.0140055

87. Macdonald AG, Keyes M, Kruk A, et al. Predictive factors for erectile dysfunction in men with prostate cancer after brachytherapy: is dose to the penile bulb important? *Int J Radiat Oncol Biol Phys*. 2005;63(1):155–163.

88. Mendenhall WM, Henderson RH, Indelicato DJ, et al. Erectile dysfunction after radiotherapy for prostate cancer. *Am J Clin Oncol*. 2009;32(4):443–447.

89. Mantz CA, Song P, Farhangi E, et al. Potency probability following conformal megavoltage radiotherapy using conventional doses for localized prostate cancer. *Int J Radiat Oncol Biol Phys*. 1997;37(3):551–557.

90. Potosky AL, Legler J, Albertsen PC, et al. Health outcomes after prostatectomy or radiotherapy for prostate cancer: results from the prostate cancer outcomes study. *J Natl Cancer Inst*. 2000;92(19):1582–1592.

91. Hamilton AS, Stanford JL, Gilliland FD, et al. Health outcomes after external-beam radiation therapy for clinically localized prostate cancer: results from the Prostate Cancer Outcomes Study. *J Clin Oncol*. 2001;19(9):2517–2526.

92. Talcott JA, Rieker P, Clark JA, et al. Patient-reported symptoms after primary therapy for early prostate cancer: results of a prospective cohort study. *J Clin Oncol*. 1998;16(1):275–283.

93. Alemozaffar M, Regan MM, Cooperberg MR, et al. Prediction of erectile function following treatment for prostate cancer. *JAMA*. 2011;306(11):1205–1214.

94. Buyyounouski MK, Horwitz EM, Price RA, et al. Intensity-modulated radiotherapy with MRI simulation to reduce doses received by erectile tissue during prostate cancer treatment. *Int J Radiat Oncol Biol Phys*. 2004;58(3):743–749.

95. Roach M 3rd, Nam J, Gagliardi G, et al. Radiation dose-volume effects and the penile bulb. *Int J Radiat Oncol Biol Phys*. 2010;76(3, Suppl):S130–S134.

96. Peters CA, Stock RG, Cesaretti JA, et al. TGFB1 single nucleotide polymorphisms are associated with adverse quality of life in prostate cancer patients treated with radiotherapy. *Int J Radiat Oncol Biol Phys*. 2008;70(3):752–759.

97. Watkins Bruner D, James JL, Bryan CJ, et al. Randomized, double-blinded, placebo-controlled crossover trial of treating erectile dysfunction with sildenafil after radiotherapy and short-term androgen deprivation therapy: results of RTOG 0215. *J Sex Med*. 2011;8(4):1228–1238.

98. Hanisch LJ, Bryan CJ, James JL, et al. Impact of sildenafil on marital and sexual adjustment in patients and their wives after radiotherapy and short-term androgen suppression for prostate cancer: analysis of RTOG 0215. *Support Care Cancer*. 2012;20(11):2845–2850.

99. Pisansky TM, Pugh SL, Greenberg RE, et al. Tadalafil for prevention of erectile dysfunction after radiotherapy for prostate cancer: the Radiation Therapy Oncology Group [0831] randomized clinical trial. *JAMA*. 2014;311(13):1300–1307.

100. Zelefsky MJ, Shasha D, Branco RD, et al. Prophylactic sildenafil citrate improves select aspects of sexual function in men treated with radiotherapy for prostate cancer. *J Urol*. 2014;192(3):868–874.

101. Shalet SM. Effect of irradiation treatment on gonadal function in men treated for germ cell cancer. *Eur Urol*. 1993;23(1):148, 151; discussion 152.

102. Rowley MJ, Leach DR, Warner GA, et al. Effect of graded doses of ionizing radiation on the human testis. *Radiat Res*. 1974;59(3):665–678.

103. Feldschuh J, Brassel J, Durso N, et al. Successful sperm storage for 28 years. *Fertil Steril*. 2005;84(4):1017.e3–1017.e4.

104. Hsiao W, Stahl PJ, Osterberg EC, et al. Successful treatment of postchemotherapy azoospermia with microsurgical testicular sperm extraction: the weill cornell experience. *J Clin Oncol*. 2011;29(12):1607–1611.

105. Dunberger G, Lindquist H, Waldenström AC, et al. Lower limb lymphedema in gynecological cancer survivors—effect on daily life functioning. *Support Care Cancer*. 2013;21(11):3063–3070.

106. Pieterse QD, Kenter GG, Maas CP, et al. Self-reported sexual, bowel and bladder function in cervical cancer patients following different treatment modalities: longitudinal prospective cohort study. *Int J Gynecol Cancer*. 2013;23(9):1717–1725.

107. Beesley V, Janda M, Eakin E, et al. Lymphedema after gynecological cancer treatment: prevalence, correlates, and supportive care needs. *Cancer*. 2007;109(12):2607–2614.

108. Baxter NN, Habermann EB, Tepper JE, et al. Risk of pelvic fractures in older women following pelvic irradiation. *JAMA*. 2005;294(20):2587–2593.

109. Ikushima H, Osaki K, Furutani S, et al. Pelvic bone complications following radiation therapy of gynecologic malignancies: clinical evaluation of radiation-induced pelvic insufficiency fractures. *Gynecol Oncol*. 2006;103(3):1100–1104.

110. Oh D, Huh SJ, Nam H, et al. Pelvic insufficiency fracture after pelvic radiotherapy for cervical cancer: analysis of risk factors. *Int J Radiat Oncol Biol Phys*. 2008;70(4):1183–1188.

111. Klopp AH, Moughan J, Portelance L, et al. Hematologic toxicity in RTOG 0418: a phase 2 study of postoperative IMRT for gynecologic cancer. *Int J Radiat Oncol Biol Phys*. 2013;86(1):83–90.

112. Rose BS, Aydogan B, Liang Y, et al. Normal tissue complication probability modeling of acute hematologic toxicity in cervical cancer patients treated with chemoradiotherapy. *Int J Radiat Oncol Biol Phys*. 2011;79(3):800–807.

113. Lee AY, Bazan JG, Pelizzari CA, et al. Lower pelvis bone marrow dose constraints to reduce hematologic toxicity in the treatment of anal cancer. *Int J Radiat Oncol Biol Phys*. 2014;90(1):S33.

114. Bray FN, Simmons BJ, Wolfson AH, Nouri K. Acute and chronic cutaneous reactions to ionizing radiation therapy. *Dermatol Ther (Heidelb)*. 2016;6(2):185–206. doi:10.1007/s13555-016-0120-y

115. Gosselin TK, Schneider SM, Plambeck MA, et al. A prospective randomized, placebo-controlled skin care study in women diagnosed with breast cancer undergoing radiation therapy. *Oncol Nurs Forum*. 2010;37(5):619–626.

116. Heggie S, Bryant GP, Tripcony L, et al. A phase III study on the efficacy of topical aloe vera gel on irradiated breast tissue. *Cancer Nurs.* 2002;25(6):442–451.
117. Fenig E, Brenner B, Katz A, et al. Topical biafine and lipiderm for the prevention of radiation dermatitis: a randomized prospective trial. *Oncol Rep.* 2001;8(2):305–309.
118. Pommier P, Gomez F, Sunyach MP, et al. Phase III randomized trial of calendula officinalis compared with trolamine for the prevention of acute dermatitis during irradiation for breast cancer. *J Clin Oncol.* 2004;22(8):1447–1453.
119. Omidvari S, Saboori H, Mohammadianpanah M, et al. Topical betamethasone for prevention of radiation dermatitis. *Indian J Dermatol Venereol Leprol.* 2007;73(3):209.
120. Wells M, Macmillan M, Raab G, et al. Does aqueous or sucralfate cream affect the severity of erythematous radiation skin reactions? A randomised controlled trial. *Radiother Oncol.* 2004;73(2):153–162.
121. McQuestion M. Evidence-based skin care management in radiation therapy: clinical update. *Semin Oncol Nurs.* 2011;27(2):e1–e17.
122. Kassab S, Cummings M, Berkovitz S, et al. Homeopathic medicines for adverse effects of cancer treatments. *Cochrane Database Syst Rev.* 2009;(2):CD004845. doi:10.1002/14651858.CD004845.pub2
123. Murray L, Henry A, Hoskin P, et al. Second primary cancers after radiation for prostate cancer: a systematic review of the clinical data and impact of treatment technique. *Radiother Oncol.* 2014;110(2):213–228.

## RECOMMENDED READING

Anserini P, Chiodi S, Spinelli S, et al. Semen analysis following allogeneic bone marrow transplantation. Additional data for evidence-based counselling. *Bone Marrow Transplant.* 2002;30(7):447–451.

Babb RR. Radiation proctitis: a review. *Am J Gastroenterol.* 1996;91(7):1309–1311.

Bradley KA., McHaffie DR. Treatment-related toxicity from the use of radiation therapy for gynecologic malignancies. https://www.uptodate.com/contents/treatment-related-toxicity-from-the-use-of-radiation-therapy-for-gynecologic-malignancies. Published 2015.

Dalkin BL. Re: health outcomes after prostatectomy or radiotherapy for prostate cancer: results from the prostate cancer outcomes study. *J Natl Cancer Inst.* 2001;93(5):401–402.

Erickson VS, Pearson ML, Ganz PA, et al. Arm edema in breast cancer patients. *J Natl Cancer Inst.* 2001;93(2):96–111.

Feldmeier JJ, Jelen I, Davolt DA, et al. Hyperbaric oxygen as a prophylaxis for radiation-induced delayed enteropathy. *Radiother Oncol.* 1995;35(2):138–144.

Fiorino C, Valdagni R, Rancati T, et al. Dose-volume effects for normal tissues in external radiotherapy: pelvis. *Radiother Oncol.* 2009;93(2):153–167.

Freedman GM, Anderson PR, Li J, et al. Intensity modulated radiation therapy (IMRT) decreases acute skin toxicity for women receiving radiation for breast cancer. *Am J Clin Oncol.* 2006;29(1):66–70.

Fuentes-Raspall R, Inoriza JM, Martí-Utzet MJ, et al. Hyperbaric oxygen therapy for late rectal and bladder toxicity after radiation in prostate cancer patients. A symptom control and quality-of-life study. *Clin Oncol.* 2012;24(8):e126.

Gothard L, Cornes P, Brooker S, et al. Phase II study of vitamin e and pentoxifylline in patients with late side effects of pelvic radiotherapy. *Radiother Oncol.* 2005;75(3):334–341.

Karamanolis G, Triantafyllou K, Tsiamoulos Z, et al. Argon plasma coagulation has a long-lasting therapeutic effect in patients with chronic radiation proctitis. *Endoscopy Endoscopy.* 2009;41(6):529–531.

Lagrange JL, Bascoul-Mollevi C, Geoffrois L, et al. Quality of life assessment after concurrent chemoradiation for invasive bladder cancer: results of a multicenter prospective study (GETUG 97-015). *Int J Radiat Oncol Biol Phys.* 2011;79(1):172–178.

Maggio A, Magli A, Rancati T, et al. Daily sodium butyrate enema for the prevention of radiation proctitis in prostate cancer patients undergoing radical radiation therapy: results of a multicenter randomized placebo-controlled dose-finding phase 2 study. *Int J Radiat Oncol Biol Phys.* 2014;89(3):518–524.

Marks LB, Carroll PR, Dugan TC, Anscher MS. The response of the urinary bladder, urethra, and ureter to radiation and chemotherapy. *Int J Radiat Oncol Biol Phys.* 1995;31(5):1257–1280.

Niewald M, Wenzlawowicz KV, Fleckenstein J, et al. Results of radiotherapy for Peyronie's disease. *Int J Radiat Oncol Biol Phys.* 2006;64(1):258–262.

Ozden TA, Uzun H, Bohloli M, et al. The effects of hyperbaric oxygen treatment on oxidant and antioxidants levels during liver regeneration in rats. *Tohoku J Exp Med.* 2004;203(4):253–265.

Silva RA, Correia AJ, Dias LM, et al. Argon plasma coagulation therapy for hemorrhagic radiation proctosigmoiditis. *Gastrointest Endosc.* 1999;50(2):221–224.

Taïeb S, Rolachon A, Cenni JC, et al. Effective use of argon plasma coagulation in the treatment of severe radiation proctitis. *Dis Colon Rectum.* 2001;44(12):1766–1771.

Tjandra JJ, Sengupta S. Argon plasma coagulation is an effective treatment for refractory hemorrhagic radiation proctitis. *Dis Colon Rectum.* 2001;44(12):1759, 1765; discussion 1771.

Tunio MA, Hashmi A, Rafi M. Need for a new trial to evaluate postoperative radiotherapy in renal cell carcinoma: a meta-analysis of randomized controlled trials. *Annals of Oncology.* 2010;21(9):1839–1845.

Vistad I, Cvancarova M, Fosså SD, Kristensen GB. Postradiotherapy morbidity in long-term survivors after locally advanced cervical cancer: how well do physicians' assessments agree with those of their patients? *Int J Radiat Oncol Biol Phys.* 2008;71(5):1335–1342.

Wong SS, Aboumarzouk OM, Narahari R, et al. Simple urethral dilatation, endoscopic urethrotomy, and urethroplasty for urethral stricture disease in adult men. *Cochrane Database Syst Rev.* 2012;(12):CD006934. doi:10.1002/14651858.CD006934.pub2

Wortel RC, Incrocci L, Pos FJ. Acute toxicity after image-guided intensity modulated radiation therapy compared to 3D conformal radiation therapy in prostate cancer patients. *Int J Radiat Oncol Biol Phys.* 2015;91(4):737–744.

# 7

# Radiation Therapy Effects on Skin and Extremities

*Adam A. Garsa and Alexander R. Gottschalk*

## OVERVIEW

- Skin cancers are very common, with 76,000 cases of melanoma and 3.5 million nonmelanomatous skin cancers (NMSCs) every year in the United States.
- While predominantly treated surgically, radiation can be very effective as curative treatment for NMSCs and to prevent recurrence after surgery for high-risk melanomas and NMSCs.
- While high-energy photons used for deep-seated tumors "spare" skin from high dose, radiation for cancers near or involving the skin can cause significant skin toxicity (eg, breast, anal, head and neck cancers).
- Skin toxicity from radiation includes both near-immediate acute toxicity driven by inflammation, and late toxicity consisting of fibrosis.

In the United States, there were approximately 76,000 cases of melanoma and 10,000 deaths due to melanoma in 2016, with a rising incidence (1). There are as many as 3.5 million cases of NMSC per year in the United States (2). Ultraviolet radiation exposure is a major risk factor for both melanoma and NMSCs. Although skin cancers can occur anywhere on the body, they are most common on sun-exposed areas, including the face, ears, scalp, neck, and arms (3,4). Immunosuppression due to organ transplantation or chronic lymphocytic leukemia (CLL) is also a risk factor for all types of skin cancer (5,6).

Early stage melanoma and NMSCs are typically treated with surgery alone. If adverse pathologic features are present, postoperative radiation therapy (RT) is considered. Merkel cell carcinomas have a high rate of local recurrence when treated with surgery alone, so postoperative radiation therapy is routinely administered. Curative radiation therapy alone can be used with excellent results for NMSCs if patients are not candidates for surgery or if they decline surgery (7,8).

For advanced stage skin cancers, postoperative radiation therapy is commonly indicated. In patients with metastatic disease, radiation therapy may be used for palliation.

Skin is commonly irradiated for other cancers as well. With current technology allowing skin sparing through high-energy photons, skin toxicity is most common when treating malignancies close to or potentially involving the skin, such as breast cancer, head and neck cancers, and anal cancer. Skin toxicity has two phases: an initial acute toxicity phase predominantly driven by inflammation and temporary cessation in stem cell proliferation, and a late or chronic toxicity effect characterized by fibrosis and its effects. This includes reduced lymphovascular functioning resulting in lymphedema, poor wound healing from reduced vascularity, and/or joint stiffness.

## ACUTE TOXICITY

- *Symptoms:* erythema, hyperpigmentation, dry desquamation, moist desquamation
- *Timing:* with conventionally fractionated radiation therapy, erythema and hyperpigmentation develop approximately during the third week of treatment and become more pronounced through the remainder of treatment. Dry and/or moist desquamation may develop during the fourth to sixth weeks of treatment. Desquamation is more likely to occur along skin folds or creases. With hypofractionated schedules these reactions can occur earlier.
- *Prevention:*
  - Avoid application of lotion or ointment within 3 hours prior to radiation treatment.
  - Remove all dressings prior to radiation treatment.
  - Do not use tape or adhesives on skin receiving radiation.
  - If the treatment site is in a location covered by clothing, patients should wear loose, soft clothing to minimize friction and irritation.
  - Patients should avoid scratching or rubbing the radiated skin.
  - If treating involves the neck or face of a male patient, electric razors are preferable to blade razors to minimize the risk of cuts to the skin.
  - Protect the radiated site from sun exposure (eg, use wide-brimmed hat, scarf, SPF 30 or higher sunscreen).
- Treatment for skin erythema and hyperpigmentation
  - Calendula or light hypoallergenic moisturizer. Apply a thin layer twice a day.
  - Cleanse daily with mild nonperfumed soap and water.
  - Cooling compresses may be applied to inflamed sites twice a day. Use a cool towel or a thick towel covering an ice pack. Use caution to avoid cold thermal trauma to the skin.
- Treatment for dry desquamation
  - Aquaphor or A+D ointment twice a day.
  - Skintegrity, Domeboro, or similar wound cleanser daily. Spray liberally on the radiation site, rinse off after 1 to 2 minutes.
  - Consider a dressing, such as Mepilex Lite, to protect the skin and allow healing.
- Treatment for moist desquamation
  - Skintegrity, Domeboro, or similar wound cleanser daily. Spray liberally on the radiation site, rinse off after 1 to 2 minutes.
  - Manually debride dry, peeling skin once a day if needed (the patient should not do this).
  - Wound dressing (eg, Aquacel Ag, Algicel Ag, Mepitel Ag), change every 1 to 2 days.

- Pentoxifylline 400 mg three times a day and topical purified honey ointment showed promise at reducing pain and desquamation interval for breast cancer patients in a small trial (9).
- Topical or oral pain medication as required.

## LATE TOXICITY
### Skin

- *Symptoms:* alopecia, telangiectasias, pigmentation change, fibrosis, poor wound healing, ulceration, cartilage or bone necrosis
- *Timing:* months to years after radiation. Typically occurs after a latency period
- *Prevention:*
  - Reduced dose per fraction may lower the risk of cartilage necrosis. For skin cancers of the pinna, Hayter et al (10) reported that a fraction size more than 6 Gy was associated with a higher rate of necrosis (16% versus 2%). Similarly, Silva et al (11) found that fraction size more than 4 Gy was a significant predictor of necrosis or ulceration.
  - Oral pentoxifylline 400 mg three times daily and oral vitamin E (tocopherol) 400 IU daily for 6 months after radiation reduced fibrosis in breast cancer patients (12).
- *Treatment:*
  - Physical therapy for fibrosis to improve circulation
  - Dermatology treatments (such as pulsed dye laser) for telangiectasias and hyperpigmentation (13)
  - Pentoxifylline/tocopherol: this combination has been studied with some ability to reduce fibrosis (14).

### Extremity
#### *Edema*

- *Symptoms:* pain, swelling
- *Timing:* typically begins months after radiation, although can present several years later
  - Predictors of lymphedema include tumor size larger than 5 cm and deep location (15). In patients with thigh soft tissue sarcoma (STS), the rate of lymphedema was found to be higher in medial compartment tumors (25.7%) compared with tumors of the anterior and posterior compartments (9%), likely due to the rich lymphatics in the medial compartment (16).
- *Prevention:*
  - To minimize risk of lymphedema, at least a 1-cm thick strip of skin and subcutaneous tissue should be spared. With three-dimensional conformal techniques, this portion of the limb can usually be entirely excluded from the radiation fields. With intensity-modulated radiation therapy (IMRT), dose to this region should be minimized to less than 20 Gy.

- Patients should:
  - Wear properly fitting shoes and avoid walking barefoot.
  - Avoid tight, constrictive clothing.
  - Avoid or limit time in extreme hot or cold temperatures (ie, hot tub or sauna).
  - Do exercises and stretching of the affected limb.
  - Maintain ideal body weight.
- Use of preventative physical therapy (PT)/compression garment has not been shown to be effective in a randomized trial (17).
- *Treatment:*
  - Consider referral to lymphedema therapist. Treatment options include compression stockings, bandaging, and manual lymphatic drainage. Patients should protect the affected limb from cuts and scratches to minimize risk of infection. Cuts and scratches should be cleaned thoroughly with soap and water, treated with an antibiotic ointment, and covered with a bandage.
  - Cellulitis should be treated with antibiotics (eg, cephalexin, trimethoprim-sulfamethoxazole, or clindamycin).

## *Joint stiffness*

- *Timing:* months to years
- *Prevention:*
  - To minimize the risk of joint fibrosis, limit the whole joint dose to less than 40 to 45 Gy.
  - Risk of developing late toxicity may be reduced with the use of reduced target volumes and, when possible, prevent inclusion of the whole joint. Radiation Therapy Oncology Group (RTOG) 0630 utilized image-guided radiation therapy (IGRT) and reduced target volumes in a phase II preoperative radiation trial (18). Compared with historical controls from the National Cancer Institute of Canada (NCIC) trial, there was a significant reduction in the rate of grade 2 or higher late toxicity (10.5% versus 37%), with no marginal recurrences. Institutional phase II studies using IMRT and IGRT have also demonstrated a significant reduction in late toxicities (19,20).
- *Treatment:* evaluation and treatment by physical therapy.

## *Bone fracture*

- *Timing:* years after RT
  - Radiation-induced fractures occur within the previous radiation field. Associated with minimal or no trauma. More common in the lower extremity (2%–10% risk).
- *Prevention:*
  - Risk may be minimized with careful radiation therapy planning to minimize high dose to the bone. Dickie et al (21) found that radiation-related bone fractures were reduced when volume of bone

receiving 40 Gy (V40) or higher was less than 64%, mean dose to bone less than 37 Gy, and maximum dose to bone less than 59 Gy.
- ○ Risk factors include female gender, age over 50 years, and thigh tumor location (22,23). A nomogram has been developed to predict the risk of pathologic fracture of the femur (24).
- *Treatment:* typically requires surgical fixation.

# REFERENCES

1. Siegel RL, Miller KD, Jemal A. Cancer statistics, 2016. *CA Cancer J Clin*. 2016;66(1):7–30.
2. Rogers HW, Weinstock MA, Harris AR, et al. Incidence estimate of nonmelanoma skin cancer in the United States, 2006. *Arch Dermatol*. 2010;146:283–287.
3. Elwood JM, Gallagher RP. Body site distribution of cutaneous malignant melanoma in relationship to patterns of sun exposure. *Int J Cancer*. 1998;78:276–280.
4. Youl PH, Janda M, Aitken JF, et al. Body-site distribution of skin cancer, pre-malignant and common benign pigmented lesions excised in general practice. *Br J Dermatol*. 2011;165:35–43.
5. Zwald FO, Brown M. Skin cancer in solid organ transplant recipients: advances in therapy and management: part I. Epidemiology of skin cancer in solid organ transplant recipients. *J Am Acad Dermatol*. 2011;65:253–261.
6. Brewer JD, Habermann TM, Shanafelt TD. Lymphoma-associated skin cancer: incidence, natural history, and clinical management. *Int J Dermatol*. 2014;53(3):267–274.
7. Locke J, Karimpour S, Young G, et al. Radiotherapy for epithelial skin cancer. *Int J Radiat Oncol Biol Phys*. 2001;51(3):748–755.
8. Mendenhall WM, Parsons JT, Mendenhall NP, et al. T2-T4 carcinoma of the skin of the head and neck treated with radical irradiation. *Int J Radiat Oncol Biol Phys*. 1987;13(7):975–981.
9. Shoma A, Eldars W, Noman N, et al. Pentoxifylline and local hone for radiation-induced burn following breast conservative surgery. *Curr Clin Pharmacol*. 2010;5(4):251–256.
10. Hayter CR, Lee KH, Groome PA, et al. Necrosis following radiotherapy for carcinoma of the pinna. *Int J Radiat Oncol Biol Phys*. 1996;36(5):1033–1037.
11. Silva JJ, Tsang RW, Panzarella T, et al. Results of radiotherapy for epithelial skin cancer of the pinna: the Princess Margaret Hospital experience, 1982–1993. *Int J Radiat Oncol Biol Phys*. 2000;47(2):451–459.
12. Jacobson G, Bhatia S, Smith BJ, et al. Randomized trial of pentoxifylline and vitamin E vs standard follow-up after breast irradiation to prevent breast fibrosis, evaluated by tissue compliance meter. *Int J Radiat Oncol Biol Phys*. 2013;85(3): 604–608.
13. Rossi AM, Nehal KS, Lee EH. Radiation-induced breast telangiectasias treated with pulsed dye laser. *J Clin Aesthet Dermatol*. 2014;7(12):34–37.
14. Haddad P, Kalaghchi B, Amouzegar-Hashemi F. Pentoxifylline and Vitamin E combination for superficial radiation-induced fibrosis: a phase II clinical trial. *Radiother Oncol*. 2005;77(3):324–326.
15. Friedmann D, Wunder JS, Ferguson P, et al. Incidence and severity of lymphoedema following limb salvage of extremity soft tissue sarcoma. *Sarcoma*. 2011;2011:289673. doi:10.1155/2011/289673

16. Rimner A, Brennan MF, Zhang Z, et al. Influence of compartmental involvement on the patterns of morbidity in soft tissue sarcoma of the thigh. *Cancer.* 2009;115(1):149–157.
17. Paskett E, Le-Rademacher J, Oliveri J, et al. Prevention of lymphedema in women with breast cancer: results of CALGB (Alliance) 70305. *J Clin Oncol.* 2017;35 (5 Suppl.):104.
18. Wang D, Zhang Q, Eisenberg BL, et al. Significant reduction of late toxicities in patients with extremity sarcoma treated with image-guided radiation therapy to a reduced target volume: results of radiation therapy oncology group RTOG-0630 trial. *J Clin Oncol.* 2015;33(20):2231–2338.
19. Alektiar KM, Brennan MF, Healey JH, et al. Impact of intensity-modulated radiation therapy on local control in primary soft-tissue sarcoma of the extremity. *J Clin Oncol.* 2008;26:3440–3444.
20. O'Sullivan B, Griffin AM, Dickie CI, et al. Phase 2 study of preoperative image-guided intensity-modulated radiation therapy to reduce wound and combined modality morbidities in lower extremity soft tissue sarcoma. *Cancer.* 2013;119:1878–1884.
21. Dickie CI, Parent AL, Griffin AM, et al. Bone fractures following external beam radiotherapy and limb-preservation surgery for lower extremity soft tissue sarcoma: relationship to irradiated bone length, volume, tumor location and dose. *Int J Radiat Oncol Biol Phys.* 2009;75(4):1119–1124.
22. Livi L, Santoni R, Paiar F, et al. Late treatment-related complications in 214 patients with extremity soft-tissue sarcoma treated by surgery and postoperative radiation therapy. *Am J Surg.* 2006;192(2):230–234.
23. Holt GE, Griffin AM, Pintilie M, et al. Fractures following radiotherapy and limb-salvage surgery for lower extremity soft-tissue sarcomas. A comparison of high-dose and low-dose radiotherapy. *J Bone Joint Surg Am.* 2005;87(2):315–319.
24. Gortzak Y, Lockwood GA, Mahendra A, et al. Prediction of pathologic fracture risk of the femur after combined modality treatment of soft tissue sarcoma of the thigh. *Cancer.* 2010;116(6):1553–1559.

# 8

# Radiation Toxicity Management in Children

*Clayton B. Hess and Torunn I. Yock*

## OVERVIEW

Radiation toxicity is of great concern in children. Acute toxicity can limit delivery of life-saving therapies while late toxicity can impair quality of life and shorten life spans in childhood cancer survivors. This has catalyzed intense efforts to improve late radiation effects in children, including large financial investment in treatments that improve radiation conformality.

This chapter is designed for radiation oncologists throughout the treatment and follow-up period, as an aid to predict and manage acute and late toxicities in irradiated children. Some toxicity management in children is analogous to that of adults and addressed in other chapters of this text, but many concerns are unique to children, including altered development and maturation, shortened stature from stalled bone growth, delayed neurocognitive development, and so forth. The purpose of this chapter is to:

1. identify organ-specific acute and late radiation toxicity concerns in children in the context of the other therapies received.
2. provide bullet point recommendations tailored to children for:
   a. Management of acute toxicities
   b. Follow-up and survivorship care for late toxicities.

## BONE

The multiple toxicities listed in the following all occur in irradiated bone, but result from distinct etiologies that are dependent on the area of bone treated and dose delivered.

### Avascular Necrosis

Bone marrow transplantation, whole-body radiation, focal radiation therapy (RT) to bone or gonads, and chronic use of glucocorticoids increase the risk of osteoclast and osteoblast cell death, a condition also known as joint avascular necrosis (AVN), osteoradionecrosis or aseptic osteonecrosis (1). AVN is a late toxicity, has a poorly understood etiology, occurs with an estimated incidence around 0.5% to 1% in childhood cancer patients, but more frequently in adolescents (period of rapid bone growth), and can lead to a range of symptoms from arthritic pain and loss of range of motion to articular collapse and need for surgical intervention, especially in weight-bearing joints (1–3). Prolonged glucocorticoid therapy for leukemia treatment has been implicated in the development of AVN, as well as older age

(9–18 years), exposure to alkylating agents, methotrexate, obesity, genetic factors, and bone/joint radiation therapy (2,4). Bone necrosis is commonly treated with analgesia supplemented by therapies aimed at improving vascular oxygen delivery to surrounding tissues, including hyperbaric oxygen, pentoxifylline, antioxidants like vitamin E, bevacizumab, the antivascular endothelial growth factor (VEGF) monoclonal antibody, and when required, surgical intervention (5,6). Consensus about classification of AVN, its treatment, and need for screening imaging is lacking (7,8).

- Consider screening imaging of irradiated joints, conservative therapies for joint pain or radiographic AVN, and orthopedic referral for refractory pain and joint dysfunction.

[See "Bone joint" row in Table 8.1]

## Bone Marrow

Like adults, acute hematologic toxicities from bone marrow irradiation occur in children as a multifaceted function of age, preirradiation blood indices, radiation dose, dynamic rates of blood flow in and out of radiation fields throughout the total treatment time, amount of bone marrow irradiated, and contributing toxicities from systemic therapy (9). The order of hematopoietic decline is a function of half-life: granulocytes (6–8 hours), platelets (5–7 days), and red blood cells (120 days) (10,11). Bone marrow blood production in adults typically comes from the following anatomic locations: pelvis (23%), thoracic spine (18%), ribs/clavicles/scapulae (17%), lumbar spine (15%), sacrum (7%), skull and facial bones (6%), bilateral proximal femurs (6%), cervical spine (4%), bilateral proximal humeri (4%), and sternum (2%), while long bones (including femur and tibia) are more important centers of hematopoiesis in children (12). Therefore, about 43% of the bone marrow reserve is contained in typical craniospinal irradiation (CSI) volumes (12). Lymphopenia occurs almost immediately following RT delivery, whereas neutropenia occurs within 10 days, thrombocytopenia in 2 to 3 weeks, and anemia toward the end of treatment (11,13). Brief treatment interruptions due to hematologic toxicity in CSI have been reported at rates of around 23% to 47% historically, following multiagent pre-CSI chemotherapy, but treatment breaks of over 3 days are less common (9,14,15). Treatment interruptions extending total radiation time beyond 45 days, or delays between surgery and RT completion beyond 90 days, can decrease radiation efficacy (16–19). Treatment interruptions should only be given when the patients are symptomatic. Other supportive measures can be employed, such as giving growth colony stimulating factor, transfusing blood products, or switching to boost volumes to spare marrow and allow blood count recovery (9,14,15). Following treatment, diminished marrow cellularity can persist for 6 months to 1 year before recovery, and fatty replacement of the spinal marrow can be seen radiographically out to 30 or 40 months posttreatment (20,21). Lowered blood counts have been negatively associated with tumor outcomes, possibly related to diminished host immune response and tumor surveillance (22–25).

### *Acute Toxicity Management*

- Design marrow-sparing treatment (most easily done with proton RT), if feasible, especially when preradiation chemotherapy is used. Vertebral

(*text continues on page 179*)

## Table 8.1 Management of Acute and Late Toxicity by Organ Site in Children

| Organ | Ailment | Usual timing | Mild | Moderate/severe | Preventative strategies |
|---|---|---|---|---|---|
| Bone joint | AVN | Late effect | Analgesia | Reoxygenation therapies Orthopedic referral | Lack of consensus |
| Bone marrow | Cytopenia | Acute/subacute | Infusion. Treat boost volumes first | Treatment interruption | Spare mature marrow GCSF support and deliberate timing |
| Growth plates | Skeletal abnormalities | Late effect | Growth monitoring | Orthopedic and/or endocrine referral Compensatory intervention or delay of epiphyseal closure | Symmetric irradiation of vertebral bodies Growth plate avoidance |
| Cortical bone | Loss of bone density | Late effect | Calcium, bisphosphonates, vitamin D, endocrine hormones | Endocrinology referral Orthopedic fracture management | Surveillance for osteoporosis in patients with known GH deficiency |
| Brainstem | Necrosis | Late effect | Follow radiographic changes and consider reoxygenation and anti-inflammatory therapy | Neurologic and respiratory support, as needed | Controversial. Consider limiting dose to surface of brainstem, decreasing prescription dose |
| Cochlea | Hearing loss | Late effect (RT) Early effect (chemotherapy) | Serial audiograms | Cochlear implant Hearing aid Referral to audiology | Cochlea avoidance Early screening Ototoxic chemotherapy dose modification |

(*continued*)

Table 8.1 Management of Acute and Late Toxicity by Organ Site in Children (continued)

| Organ | Ailment | Usual timing | Mild | Moderate/severe | Preventative strategies |
|---|---|---|---|---|---|
| Gonads | Infertility Pubertal abnormalities Hormonal dysfunction | Acute and late effect | Asymptomatic laboratory abnormalities Consider replacement for prevention | Hormonal replacement Endocrinology referral | Gonad harvesting Shielding Oophoropexy |
| Heart | Heart disease | Late effect | Early evaluation of risk factors | Referral to cardiology Medical and invasive interventions | Heart avoidance Risk factor optimization |
| Brain | Cognitive decline More loss of IQ with higher baseline | Late effect | Serial monitoring Neuropsychological examination every 2–3 years | IEP Psychiatric referral | Temporal lobe and hippocampal avoidance, theoretically |
| Hypothalamic-pituitary axis | Endocrinopathies and obesity | Late effect | Endocrine replacement | Close nutritional and exercise monitoring for obesity management, consider surgical intervention Psychiatric referral for behavioral management | Maximally safe resection of craniopharyngiomas Obesity risk factor management BMI, growth curve, and endocrine monitoring |

(*continued*)

Table 8.1 Management of Acute and Late Toxicity by Organ Site in Children (continued)

| Organ | Ailment | Usual timing | Mild | Moderate/severe | Preventative strategies |
|---|---|---|---|---|---|
| Kidney | Renal injury | Pericontrast or late effect | Avoidance of nephrotoxic agents and monitoring pre- and postcontrast administration | Nephrology referral | Assessment of baseline injury or genetic predisposition Rule out renal artery stenosis |
| Lung | Pneumonitis | Subacute | Radiographic changes alone | Symptomatic; high-dose steroids Can be fatal | Be aware of pulmonary toxicity from chemotherapy Lung avoidance Lung blocks and low-dose rate during TBI |
| Posterior fossa | Posterior fossa syndrome | Within days of posterior fossa surgery | Self-limiting Do not delay radiation therapy | Severe cases are those in which children do not recover normal function | Not a radiation therapy–related toxicity |
| Whole body | Second malignancy | Late effect | Benign tumors | Malignant tumors | Screening based on genetic predisposition and site of radiation |
| Hair follicles | Epilation Alopecia | Acute effect Late effect | Temporary Topical skin care | Permanent alopecia Prosthesis | Follicle avoidance 40 Gy line predictive of permanent alopecia |

(continued)

**Table 8.1** Management of Acute and Late Toxicity by Organ Site in Children (*continued*)

| Organ | Ailment | Usual timing | Mild | Moderate/severe | Preventative strategies |
|---|---|---|---|---|---|
| Thyroid glands | Endocrinopathy | Late effect | Asymptomatic Replace deficiency | Symptomatic Endocrine referral and replacement | Thyroid avoidance or radiation Screening TSH and free T4 levels |
| Vasculature | Aneurysm Moyamoya Stenosis Stroke SMART HTN Peripheral vascular disease Arteritis | Late effect | Radiographic changes Risk factor reduction | Invasive intervention Neovascularization Endarterectomy Antihypertensives Antiplatelet therapy | Screening for vascular changes with carotid ultrasound, MRA Reduction of atherosclerotic risk factors Evaluation of personal and family history of stroke risk |
| Eye Visual apparatus Lacrimal gland Retina | Visual acuity Dry eye Field cut Keratitis Cataracts Retinopathy | Late effect | Asymptomatic cataract Elective surgical lens replacement Dry eye Artificial tears Ophthalmologic referral | Ophthalmologic intervention | Early ophthalmologic referral for screening and management Lens, eyelid, lacrimal gland, and retinal avoidance |

AVN, avascular necrosis; BMI, body mass index; GCSF, granulocyte colony stimulating factor; GH, growth hormone; HTN, hypertension; IEP, individual education plans; MRA, MR angiogram; RT, radiation therapy; TBI, total body irradiation; TSH, thyroid-stimulating hormone.

body–sparing CSI is currently only recommended for patients who are at or near skeletal maturity, with bone age typically determined by growth plate evaluation on x-rays of the hand.
- Consider platelet and/or red blood cell transfusion as supportive care, as well as colony growth factor stimulation to avoid treatment delays in the acute setting.
- Although some prior protocols have recommended a treatment break if the absolute neutrophil count (ANC) drops below 500/mcL (Children's Oncology Group ACNS 0331), we recommend avoiding treatment break, if at all possible, by using supportive measures, and particularly by switching to a few fractions of the smaller boost volumes during CSI fields to allow for blood count recovery. We recommend only interrupting treatment if children are acutely ill.

[See "Bone marrow" row in Table 8.1]

## Bone Growth Abnormalities

Osseous growth decline following radiation is related to arrested epiphyseal growth plate function, which is most potent in the rapidly growing bones of children from birth through age 6 years (26). Stunted vertebral body growth following radiation can lead to shortened sitting height, kyphosis/lordosis, and deformity of paraspinal skeletal muscle. Bone abnormalities begin to appear radiographically after 10 Gy of radiation. Bone tolerance for clinical abnormalities is 20 Gy for children less than 6 years of age. At age 6 years and older, only doses over 35 Gy result in significant skeletal or soft tissue changes. Skeletal abnormalities are unlikely to occur when irradiated at age older than 12 years (27). The effect of fraction size and the correct alpha/beta ratio of growing bone is a topic of ongoing controversy (28,29). Precocious puberty in girls and growth hormone (GH) deficiency may also affect small stature (30). Artificial endocrine prevention of bone plate fusion can counter delayed bone growth (31).

- Refer for endocrinology evaluation for consideration of delaying epiphysis fusion using estrogen therapy and GH replacement for optimized growth.
- Identify patients at additive musculoskeletal risk from combined growth plate irradiation and hypothalamus-pituitary secretion dysfunction.
- Consider orthopedic evaluation for management of skeletal abnormalities; however, shortened stature from craniospinal irradiation alone does not typically merit orthopedic evaluation.

[See "Growth plates" row in Table 8.1]

## Bone Density

Radiation can diminish bone mineral density (BMD), which is sometimes used as a marker of response to RT in adults (32). In children with leukemia, both chemotherapy and radiation have been implicated in low BMD and vitamin deficiency years following treatment (33,34). Radiation can also indirectly induce low BMD by affecting gonadal hormone production either through irradiation of the ovaries or testes, or more commonly, of the hypothalamic-pituitary axis causing secondary central gonadal dysfunction. Preventative or reparative therapies such as hormonal replacement, calcium and vitamin D supplementation, denosumab, and bisphosphonates can help prevent decline in BMD and avoid fractures (34,35).

- Perform surveillance evaluation of BMD in the setting of GH deficiency from radiation or chemotherapy, and refer to endocrinology for management (34,36).

[See "Cortical bone" row in Table 8.1]

## BRAINSTEM OR CENTRAL NERVOUS SYSTEM INJURY

Late toxicity to the brainstem and brain parenchyma includes radiation necrosis, a sinister complication that can lead to focal deficits and even death. Brainstem necrosis with photon and proton therapy has been reported at slightly discrepant rates of around 3% to 5% at doses between 50.4 and 59.4 Gy. There is ongoing controversy about brainstem dose tolerance thresholds and injury risk factors, such as prior posterior fossa surgery, photons versus proton therapy, chemotherapy exposures, vascular adequacy, and location within the brainstem (37–39).

- Discuss the risk of brainstem necrosis with patients/parents in terms of the anticipated treatment modality and maximum brainstem dose, as well as age, degree and location of prior surgery, and adjuvant/concurrent treatments.
- Consider hyperbaric oxygen, steroids, and bevacizumab as management (see earlier discussion of avascular necrosis) (40).

[See "Brainstem" row in Table 8.1.]

## COCHLEA

Hearing loss during and after childhood cancer treatment to the head and neck region can be due to serous otitis media, a common acute reaction wherein mucositis causes blockage of the Eustachian tube/external ear canal due to thickened cerumen or damage to the inner ear structures themselves (41,42). Doses over 30 Gy increase risk for cerumen impaction/secretion thickening leading to acute mastoiditis/mucositis that can block the Eustachian tube and reduce hearing (42). Sensorineural hearing loss (SNHL) caused by damage to the cochlea and auditory nerve occurs late (after 2–4 or more years) when induced by radiation and early when caused by ototoxic chemotherapy, although it is now recognized that chemotherapy injury can manifest later as well (43). Each cycle of ototoxic chemotherapy (cisplatin or carboplatin) should be preceded by an audiogram to appropriately dose reduce to minimize the adverse hearing outcomes. In the setting of radiation alone without chemotherapy, the threshold dose where ototoxicity appears to manifest is above 30 Gy (44). Little is known what the threshold dose is in the setting of cisplatin or carboplatin chemotherapy as both agents can cause hearing loss on their own, but the risk is additive if not synergistic. All patients exposed to either ototoxic chemotherapy or cochlear radiation should be followed with annual audiograms (45,46).

- Audiogram prior to each cycle of cisplatin or carboplatin chemotherapy, as well as before (or during) radiation, and then annually thereafter for any patient receiving any ototoxic drug or radiation.

[See "Cochlea" row in Table 8.1]

## CRANIOSPINAL AXIS

Acute toxicity from CSI combines risk from multiple anatomic sites and includes the following: bone marrow myelosuppression, dermatitis, fatigue, alopecia, nausea, weight loss, vomiting, anorexia, otitis media, otitis externa, laryngitis, pharyngitis, esophagitis, gastritis, acute pericarditis, enteritis, cystitis, and temporary worsening of tumor-associated neurological symptoms. Decreased bone marrow reserve may limit the ability to give chemotherapy after CSI, although it is typically sequenced this way for medulloblastoma. Data suggest higher grades of acute anorexia, nausea, and alopecia associated with CSI, compared to involved-field radiation for central nervous system malignancies (47). Proton therapy decreases acute thrombocytopenia and diarrhea in children undergoing CSI (48). Mild dermatitis and alopecia are common with historical techniques, and about 1 in 4 patients experienced grade 3 to 5 hematologic toxicity (49). Onset of headache and vomiting usually occur within the first 24 to 72 hours of embarking on CSI. Bowel changes (ie, loosening of stool) take longer to manifest and may not appear if concurrent agents such as vincristine are used, which can be profoundly constipating. Bowel changes should be managed supportively with laxatives or Imodium, as needed, depending on symptoms (50). Radiation somnolence syndrome is a subacute reaction that has been observed following whole-brain irradiation in children. It is thought to be an inflammatory or demyelinating process, with symptoms including somnolence, fever, nausea, and headache typically occurring within 4 to 8 weeks after RT and self-limited lasting 2 to 4 weeks (51,52).

Long-term complications of CSI typically occur 3 months or more following completion of CSI and tend to be permanent. Complications arising from irradiation of the cranial portion of CSI include induction of second malignancy, permanent hair loss, cataract formation, retinopathy, SNHL, neuroendocrine dysfunction, and neurocognitive sequelae. The patient's age and dose of radiation delivered to the brain largely determine the degree of neurocognitive outcome. Adverse long-term effects from irradiation of the spinal portion include induction of second malignancy, stunting of growth of vertebral bodies, and hypoplasia of paraspinal muscles and connective tissue resulting in shortened sitting height, spinal cord or nerve root damage (rare at doses <39 Gy), primary hypothyroidism, adverse effects on the heart, pneumonitis, peptic ulcer disease, small and large bowel enteritis, primary ovarian failure, and decreased marrow reserve.

### *Acute Toxicity Management*

- See site-specific recommendations for sites within CSI fields.
- Educate patients/parents about subacute symptoms of somnolence syndrome.

*Late Toxicity Management*

- See site-specific recommendations for sites within CSI fields.

## GASTROINTESTINAL TRACT

Acute gastrointestinal tract toxicity in children is similar to adults and can be managed supportively. Nausea, anorexia, esophagitis, reflux, and change in bowel habits are very common with spinal irradiation, especially when concurrent chemotherapy is given (53). Late toxicity is also similar to that of adults, with the notable exception of heightened second gastrointestinal tract malignancies, the risk of which is larger in children than in adults. Radiation to the pancreas can lead to late onset of diabetes mellitus in childhood cancer survivors (54,55).

*Acute Toxicity Management*

- Antiemetic, antidiarrheal, antireflux medications similar to adults.

*Late Toxicity Management*

- Late toxicity management similar to adults.
- Referral to endocrinology for diabetes work-up when clinically indicated.

## GONADS (TESTES AND OVARIES)

Reproductive function in children is dose and age dependent. Prepubescent and adolescent girls are at risk for infertility and premature menopause. Irreversible ovarian failure is seen in women over 40 years of age, treated with 4 to 7 Gy of fractionated radiation to both ovaries, while onset of amenorrhea requires doses up to 12 or 15 Gy (10). The ovaries of younger females are more radioresistant and can tolerate higher doses of radiation, resulting in delayed, rather than omitted, puberty. Also, as age increases, the oocyte reserve diminishes and the risk of sterility increases. Oophoropexy can move the ovaries away from treatment beams. Boys are at risk for low testosterone and low sperm count, leading to infertility as well. Doses as low as 0.15, 0.30, and 2 to 3 Gy can induce decreased sperm count, temporary azoospermia, and spermatocyte death, with decline in spermatid count, respectively. Permanent azoospermia tends to occur after exposure to 4 to 6 Gy (10,56).

- Refer patients to fertility specialist for sperm and egg harvesting prior to initiating radiation.
- Shield (clam shell) testicles during RT when possible.
- Be aware of image-guided radiation therapy dose contributions in relation to gonadal thresholds (especially daily cone-beam CT) that can contribute substantial relative gonadal dose in certain clinical situations (57).
- Refer to endocrinology for monitoring and replacement, as needed, in patients who have received a significant dose of radiation.

[See "Gonads" row in Table 8.1]

## HEART

Cardiac radiation is associated with coronary heart disease (CHD), myocardial infarction (MI), pericarditis, valvular heart disease, cardiomyopathy, and congestive heart failure in a dose-dependent manner (58). Mean heart doses over 20 Gy convey a 2.5-fold increased risk of CHD (58). Use of anthracycline chemotherapy increases risk, is dose dependent, and can confound radiation risk estimations. Doxorubicin-induced cardiac toxicity is also dose dependent and can approach 20% to 50% in some patients. Ninety-seven percent of cases of radiation-related pericarditis occur at doses over 40 Gy. Valvular heart disease is less likely when dose maximums are less than 40 Gy, with incidence occurring at a range of 5 to 13 years (59). Risk of MI is thought to be related to acceleration of the atherosclerotic process from endothelial damage and fibrosis of the intima, which leads to formation of occlusive plaques (60). Metrics for reducing radiation-induced cardiac toxicity are ongoing.

- Referral to cardiology for any patient with significant radiation dose for monitoring and treatment. Consider enalapril therapy for left ventricular dysfunction in doxorubicin-treated survivors of childhood cancer and cardiac function monitoring (61).
- Early intervention for risk factors that contribute to MI, such as elevated blood pressure, increased body mass index (BMI), positive smoking history, diabetes mellitus, hypercholesterolemia, and family history of MI (58).

[See "Heart" row in Table 8.1]

## HIPPOCAMPUS AND TEMPORAL LOBES

Cognitive impairment and memory decline have been well documented following cranial irradiation, improved following hippocampal sparing whole-brain radiation in adults (62), in terms of spatial learning, working memory, decreased verbal memory, and intellectual decline (63,64). Retrospective data has similarly correlated hippocampal and left temporal lobe dose to decline in longitudinal IQ in irradiated children, suggesting that dose reduction to this cerebral region, when possible, may similarly mitigate toxicity in children (65,66). The most rapid period of brain development and myelination occurs during the first 3 years of life, with maturation extending into adolescence and beyond age 20 years. Demyelination is thought to be the major mechanism for radiation injury, together with activation of transcription factors, signal transduction, vascular and glial cell proliferation, neurogenesis, and neuronal dysfunction. A full neuropsychological assessment of specific functional domains is recommended for all children undergoing cranial irradiation. Processing speed is typically the most affected, but academic accommodations based on the testing (such as increased time on standardized tests and assignments) can allow the child to achieve more in school. Neuropsychological referral is of utmost importance in the follow-up and care of these children to maximize their potential after treatment (67).

- Refer all children undergoing cranial irradiation for comprehensive neuropsychological evaluation at baseline and to inform school

interventions and individual education plans (IEP). Repeat every 2 to 3 years until late teen years or until no new symptoms of neuropsychological problems.
- Childhood survivors of brain tumors are at higher risk for psychological disorders, such as depression, and early referral to psychiatrists for any warning signs is helpful (68). Refer for psychological services for dramatic changes in parental report, school records, variability in IQ profile, gross inattention or lack of motivation/cooperation, and/or concurrent functional illness (eg, depression). Inform psychologist immediately of known psychological red-flag risk factors (identified in protocol ALTE07CI, Appendix V).

[See "Brain" row in Table 8.1]

## HYPOTHALAMIC-PITUITARY AXIS

Dose-dependent neuroendocrine dysfunction is common after cranial irradiation in children (69). Dysfunction has been seen to begin at doses of approximately 22 to 30 Gy to the pituitary and hypothalamus, with GH deficiencies being the most common, followed by hyperprolactinemia, diminished gonadal hormones, and low morning cortisol (70,71). Lack of an adrenal stress response is notably the only life-threatening endocrinopathy. Lifelong monitoring for hypopituitarism with hormone replacement is indicated.

Hypothalamic obesity can result from surgical manipulation of the hypothalamus, and is characterized by intractable weight gain and insatiable appetite. Unfortunately, it is a relatively common complication of craniopharyngioma resection or other hypothalamic manipulation. It typically appears immediately following surgery and can be associated with behavioral changes (72). Cranial irradiation, without hypothalamic surgery, has also been implicated in obesity following childhood cancer treatments. Children with acute lymphoblastic leukemia treated with cranial irradiation without hypothalamic manipulation were at risk for increased obesity of (contrastingly) late onset (73). The mechanism of radiation-induced obesity is hypothesized to include interruption of leptin signaling pathway but is incompletely understood (74).

- Evaluate endocrine function prior to treatment and annually thereafter whenever the dose to the hypothalamus or pituitary axis is 20 Gy or more, including prolactin, thyroid-stimulating hormone (TSH)/free T4, GH, insulin-like growth factor (IGF)-1, IGF-binding protein 3 (BP3), luteinizing hormone (LH)/follicle-stimulating hormone (FSH) and estradiol/testosterone (if child has delayed or precocious puberty [defined as onset before age 8 in girls or 9 in boys]), and morning cortisol level (recommendations from ACNS 0831).
- Prioritize maximally safe resection over gross-total resection for hypothalamic tumors and craniopharyngiomas (72). Postoperative radiation is effective in disease control and is often less morbid than a gross total resection.
- Follow BMI and growth curves for children following cranial irradiation or hypothalamic manipulation. Monitor cholesterol and

triglyceride levels and screen for cardiovascular risk factors. Establish exercise programs and nutritional diaries with nutritionist, social work, and nursing support staff, if persistent weight gain occurs. Some children with extreme obesity have benefited from a gastric bypass (75).

[See "Hypothalamic pituitary axis" row in Table 8.1]

## KIDNEYS

Volume of radiation dose as well as genetic propensities can affect risk of renal failure in children undergoing radiation therapy. Patients with the Denys-Drash syndrome, for example, have a presusceptibility for severe nephropathy believed to be due to a dominant negative effect of the WT1 mutation (76). Hypertension may be a surrogate marker for some degree of renal dysfunction. Radiation-induced renal artery stenosis can be a confounding problem (see section on vascular effects) (77). Current COG protocols typically call for renal scintigraphy to confirm bilateral kidney flow and function when kidneys are at risk for radiation toxicity. Ipsilateral constraints are often used with nephrogenic or peri-nephric tumors.

- Obtain preradiation blood pressure, as hypertension may be a sign of underlying kidney injury.
- Monitor renal function in children who undergo nephrectomy, especially those with genetic predisposition for kidney injury.
- Hydrate before and after contrast administration to avoid nephrotoxicity.
- Perform imaging to rule out renal artery stenosis, if dosimetrically and clinically indicated.

[See "Kidney" row in Table 8.1]

## LUNGS

A number of factors influence the incidence and severity of pulmonary toxicity, including total dose and volume of lung irradiated, fraction size, dose rate, concomitant use of chemotherapeutic agents, tobacco use, and previous coexisting lung disease. Radiation pneumonitis commonly presents with a pneumonia-like picture of fever, cough, and shortness of breath, lacking an infectious stimulus, with radiation injury to the lung parenchyma inducing an inflammatory response. A volume of normal lung receiving 20 Gy of around 30% in adults and a mean lung dose in children around 16 Gy have been prognostic for symptomatic pneumonitis (78,79). Total body irradiation (TBI) is low-dose treatment typically administered within stem-cell transplant regimens. This low-dose radiation, jointly with chemotherapies, contribute to a peritransplant toxicity profile affecting bone, lung, parotid glands, skin/nails, and gastrointestinal tract.

- Use lung blocks to limit lung dose to 10 Gy with partial transmission blocks for TBI (80).
- Use a dose rate of less than 15 cGy/min to diminish the risk of pneumonitis for TBI (80).

- Carefully consider concurrent use of chemotherapies with radiation, especially adriamycin, actinomycin D, bleomycin, and busulfan to avoid synergistic pulmonary toxicity.

[See "Lung" row in Table 8.1]

## POSTERIOR FOSSA (SYNDROME)

About 30% of children with medulloblastoma develop a postoperative constellation of debilitating symptoms known as posterior fossa syndrome (PFS) (81). While it lacks a well-understood etiology, it is most commonly seen after posterior fossa resections in children, and consists of mutism within 1 to 2 days that can last over 4 weeks in the majority of cases, with occasional dysarthria, ataxia, hypotonia, cranial neuropathies, lability of mood, or long tract signs (81,82). While not technically a radiation-related toxicity, radiation providers should be aware of the syndrome as it can often persist into periods when delivery of adjuvant radiation therapy may be indicated. The syndrome can be self-limited and long-term prognosis is not affected by adjuvant radiation, which should not be delayed (81).

- Radiation therapy need not be delayed for PFS, if logistically feasible. Mutism, dystonia, and ataxia can inhibit transportation to treatment centers, but in and of itself is not an indication to delay radiation therapy.
- Patients with PFS often have issues with swallowing and may need to be evaluated by an ENT doctor to determine if safe to put under sedation for daily radiation treatment.
- Referral to psychiatry can be helpful as patients often have behavioral manifestations that inhibit rehabilitation, which can be managed with pharmaceutical interventions (81).

[See "Posterior fossa" row in Table 8.1]

## SECOND MALIGNANCY

Cumulative risk of second malignancies following childhood radiation is on the decline compared to prior decades, is site specific, is primary tumor histology–specific, and is modified by the use of chemotherapeutic agents. The risk varies roughly between 1% and 3% at 5 years to 15% to 20% at 30 years, and is thought to be both age and radiation dose dependent in most instances (83–85). Based on survivors of the atomic bombings, the latency period between diagnosis and treatment is shorter for leukemia and longer for solid tumors and risk is dose dependent with linear-no-threshold modeling. Younger age at diagnosis and female gender are associated with an increased risk (86,87). Children have increased carcinogenic susceptibility because of rapid cell proliferation, or specific genetic predispositions, such as familial retinoblastoma, Lynch syndrome, or other genetic markers that can result in third or even fourth subsequent malignancies (87). Germline mutations, specifically, have been identified more commonly in pediatric cancer patients not predicted by family history (88).

- Inquire after genetic risk factors and refer for genetic counselling if there is a family history or predisposing genetic abnormality suspected (86,89).

[See "Whole body" row in Table 8.1]

## SKIN AND HAIR FOLLICLES

Temporary hair loss following cranial irradiation is universal above single-fraction doses of around 300 to 400 cGy, a range used therapeutically in the 1950s for intentional epilation in children with tinea capitis (90,91). Temporary alopecia has been reported in low-risk lymphoma treated with two fractions of radiation at the standard dose of 200 cGy each (92). Permanent alopecia is also dose dependent and a higher incidence has been correlated with hair follicle doses above 40 to 43 Gy in adults (93). In children with medulloblastoma, permanent alopecia following craniospinal irradiation has been reported after doses of 21 to 30 Gy with and without high-dose chemotherapy. Concurrent chemotherapy reduces follicular tolerance, and clearly host factors also play a role (94). Radiation dermatitis can be severe enough to mandate a break. Typically, this occurs in patients getting chemotherapy and is commonly seen in Ewing's patients with tumors close to the skin (such as the iliac crest) and who are receiving chemotherapy every 2 weeks. Sometimes, stretching the interval between chemotherapy cycles can also help modulate radiation skin toxicity. Recall reactions of radiation dermatitis and mucositis can occur with certain chemotherapies (most classically actinomycin D and doxorubicin) weeks to months after radiation completion (95,96).

- Consider skin-sparing techniques to minimize acute dermatitis that can lead to treatment interruptions.
- Consider psychosocial impact of permanent scalp alopecia in social childhood development, and refer to cranial hair prostheses if desired.

[See "Hair follicles" row in Table 8.1]

## THYROID

Thyroid cancer and nodules were reported following low-dose x-ray epilation for tinea capitis (97). Irradiating the neuroaxis with photon irradiation for medulloblastoma historically induced 58% decompensated thyroid function (98). The effect has been shown to be dose dependent in in vivo animal-models (99), irradiated adults (100,101), and children, with prevalence in the latter also being determined by younger age and chemotherapy administration (102,103). Wide incident ranges of thyroid dysfunction have been reported between studies, between 17% and 78%, depending on the dose delivered and other clinical factors (104,105). The incidence of thyroid neoplasm is reported around 1% to 2% in 5-year survivors (106).

- Minimize dose to the thyroid gland.
- Screen for hypothyroidism.
- Perform annual clinical thyroid examinations for carcinogenesis and nodule growth.

[See "Thyroid glands" row in Table 8.1]

## TOTAL BODY IRRADIATION

Similar to CSI, toxicity from TBI in children can span numerous anatomic sites and is based on the volume and dose treated. Commonly, because TBI are low-dose treatments and typically administered within stem-cell transplant regimens and algorithms, radiation is often only one of numerous contributing factors to a toxicity profile dominated by the peritransplant chemotherapies and hospital admission. Radiation-specific toxicities from TBI include immunosuppression, pneumonitis, and nausea, as related to bone, lung, and gastrointestinal tract irradiation, respectively.

- Use lung blocks to limit lung dose to 10 Gy with partial transmission blocks and use a dose rate of less than 15 cGy/min to avoid pneumonitis (80).
- See guidelines for "bone marrow," "lungs," and "gastrointestinal tract."

## VASCULATURE

Radiation therapy can increase the thickness of the arterial intima and media (107). The clinical significance of vascular changes following childhood irradiation is not well understood and literature is generally limited to case reports. Potential late vascular toxicity are anatomic site specific. Within the brain, these include moyamoya syndrome (108–111), ischemic stroke (112,113), cerebral AVN (114), astrogliosis and resulting permeability of the blood-brain barrier (115–117), and stroke-like migraine attacks after radiation therapy (SMART) syndrome (118–120). Aneurysmal wall defects are less common than arterial occlusive disease, but have been reported up to 20 years following radiation therapy, but also usually involve surgical manipulation of the area as well (121–123). Moyamoya syndrome is an obstructive cerebrovascular disease with typical symptoms of transient focal ischemic attacks, as well as global intellectual and psychological decline, which can be treated with revascularization surgery and antiplatelet therapy, but can also be fatal in its most severe forms (110,111,124). Permanent ischemic strokes have been observed and are thought to be of similar etiology, with fusiform dilatations and narrowing of cerebral vasculature (112). SMART syndrome is a rare and historically reversible diagnosis of focal neurologic deficits or seizures combined with T2-weighted cerebral enhancement in irradiated patients years into the follow-up period (118).

Outside of the brain, radiation therapy has been associated with vascular changes including renal artery stenosis (77), resulting hypertension (125), peripheral vascular disease (PVD), and radiation arteritis (126,127). Well-informed consent of children and parents should include a discussion of vascular toxicity and appropriate follow-up.

- Provide education regarding signs of cerebral infarct and altered vascularization. In patients with tumors around vasculature and most notably the circle of Willis, obtain a baseline MR angiogram (MRA) to evaluate for tumor- or surgical-related preexisting vasculopathy and to serve as a baseline for future follow-up.
- Evaluate stroke risk including coagulopathies, cholesterol, triglycerides, lifestyle.
- For patients with tumors in the suprasellar region, consider adding an MR angiogram to surveillance MRIs every other year.
- Screen patients for carotid artery stenosis, atherosclerosis, and PVD when clinically indicated with ultrasound, noting that radiation-induced plaques tend to be more widely distributed.

[See "Vasculature" row in Table 8.1]

## VISION

Visual decline from radiation-induced damage is rare under 54 Gy to the optic chiasm and nerves and 45 to 50 Gy to the retina (128). However, radiation has a more pronounced effect when visual apparatus fibers have been stretched or otherwise compromised by intervention or pathology. Cataracts are commonly induced by radiation and are treated with lens replacement, similar to adult patients. Lacrimal gland damage, in children as in adults, can lead to decreased tearing, chronic dry eye syndrome, resulting in corneal damage and acuity decline. However, sparing the meibomian accessory glands in the lids can be helpful in diminishing the risk of dry eye. These glands of the corneal surface of the eyelid are oriented parallel to the eyelashes and positioned serially along the eyelid. They contain mucin-rich goblet cells that prevent evaporative dry eye and have been correlated to tear film instability following proton beam therapy (129). In rare cases, dry eye can result in need for enucleation, but is most commonly well managed conservatively with artificial tears and lubrication. Ophthalmologic follow-up is typically recommended when 54 Gy or 45 to 50 Gy or higher are delivered to visual structures and the retina, respectively.

- Ophthalmologic examination prior to treatment and annually thereafter for patients with or at risk for field cuts, acuity decline, or dry eye (recommendation from ACNS 0831).

[See "Eye" row in Table 8.1]

## CONCLUSION

Radiation-related toxicity is common in children exposed to radiation therapy. The management of acute and late radiation toxicity in children is an area requiring a multidisciplinary team of providers, educators, support staff, and parents. The optimal management and prevention of many radiation late effects in children is still evolving but the long-term follow-up guidelines published on the Children's Oncology Group website are periodically updated and is a good source for how to follow patients during their survivorship from childhood cancers (36).

## REFERENCES

1. Kadan-Lottick NS, Dinu I, Wasilewski-Masker K, et al. Osteonecrosis in adult survivors of childhood cancer: a report from the childhood cancer survivor study. *J Clin Oncol*. 2008;26(18):3038–3045.
2. Michalecki L, Gabrys D, Kulik R, et al. Radiotherapy induced hip joint avascular necrosis-Two cases report. *Rep Pract Oncol Radiother*. 2011;16(5):198–201.
3. Bomelburg T, von Lengerke HJ, Ritter J. Aseptic osteonecroses in the treatment of childhood acute leukaemias. *Eur J Pediatr*. 1989;149(1):20–23.
4. Vora A. Management of osteonecrosis in children and young adults with acute lymphoblastic leukaemia. *Br J Haematol*. 2011;155(5):549–560.
5. Delanian S, Lefaix JL. Current management for late normal tissue injury: radiation-induced fibrosis and necrosis. *Semin Radiat Oncol*. 2007;17(2):99–107.
6. Hanif I, Mahmoud H, Pui CH. Avascular femoral head necrosis in pediatric cancer patients. *Med Pediatr Oncol*. 1993;21(9):655–660.

7. Niinimaki T, Harila-Saari A, Niinimaki R. The diagnosis and classification of osteonecrosis in patients with childhood leukemia. *Pediatr Blood Cancer.* 2014;62:198–203.

8. Li X, Brazauskas R, Wang Z, et al. Avascular necrosis of bone after allogeneic hematopoietic cell transplantation in children and adolescents. *Biol Blood Marrow Transplant.* 2014;20(4):587–592.

9. Chang EL, Allen P, Wu C, et al. Acute toxicity and treatment interruption related to electron and photon craniospinal irradiation in pediatric patients treated at the University of Texas M. D. Anderson Cancer Center. *Int J Radiat Oncol Biol Phys.* 2002;52(4):1008–1016.

10. Halperin EC. *Pediatric Radiation Oncology.* 5th ed. Philadelphia, PA: Lipincott Williams and Wilkins; 2011.

11. Kumar V, Abbas AK, Aster JC. *Robbins and Cotran Pathologic Basis of Disease.* 9th ed. Philadelphia, PA: Elsevier; 2015.

12. Campbell BA, Callahan J, Bressel M, et al. Distribution atlas of proliferating bone marrow in non-small cell lung cancer patients measured by FLT-PET/CT imaging, with potential applicability in radiation therapy planning. *Int J Radiat Oncol Biol Phys.* 2015;92(5):1035–1043.

13. Petersson K, Gebre-Medhin M, Ceberg C, et al. Haematological toxicity in adult patients receiving craniospinal irradiation—indication of a dose-bath effect. *Radiother Oncol.* 2014;111(1):47–51.

14. Marks LB, Cuthbertson D, Friedman HS. Hematologic toxicity during craniospinal irradiation: the impact of prior chemotherapy. *Med Pediatr Oncol.* 1995;25(1):45–51.

15. Jefferies S, Rajan B, Ashley S, et al. Haematological toxicity of cranio-spinal irradiation. *Radiother Oncol.* 1998;48(1):23–27.

16. Pai Panandiker AS, Wong JK, Nedelka MA, et al. Effect of time from diagnosis to start of radiotherapy on children with diffuse intrinsic pontine glioma. *Pediatr Blood Cancer.* 2014;61(7):1180–1183.

17. Putora PM, Schmuecking M, Aebersold D, et al. Compensability index for compensation radiotherapy after treatment interruptions. *Radiat Oncol.* 2012;7:208. doi:10.1186/1748-717X-7-208

18. del Charco JO, Bolek TW, McCollough WM, et al. Medulloblastoma: time-dose relationship based on a 30-year review. *Int J Radiat Oncol Biol Phys.* 1998;42(1):147–154.

19. Paulino AC, Jaboin JJ. Radiotherapy deferral in medulloblastoma. *JAMA Oncol.* 2016;2(12):1582.

20. Wilke C, Holtan SG, Sharkey L, et al. Marrow damage and hematopoietic recovery following allogeneic bone marrow transplantation for acute leukemias: effect of radiation dose and conditioning regimen. *Radiother Oncol.* 2016;118(1):65–71.

21. Cavenagh EC, Weinberger E, Shaw DW, et al. Hematopoietic marrow regeneration in pediatric patients undergoing spinal irradiation: MR depiction. *AJNR Am J Neuroradiol.* 1995;16(3):461–467.

22. D'Emic N, Engelman A, Molitoris J, et al. Prognostic significance of neutrophil-lymphocyte ratio and platelet-lymphocyte ratio in patients treated with selective internal radiation therapy. *J Gastrointest Oncol.* 2016 Apr;7(2):269–277.

23. Lu A, Li H, Zheng Y, et al. Prognostic significance of neutrophil to lymphocyte ratio, lymphocyte to monocyte ratio, and platelet to lymphocyte ratio in patients with nasopharyngeal carcinoma. *Biomed Res Int.* 2017;2017:3047802. doi:10.1155/2017/3047802

24. Tumturk A, Ozdemir MA, Per H, et al. Pediatric central nervous system tumors in the first 3 years of life: pre-operative mean platelet volume, neutrophil/lymphocyte count ratio, and white blood cell count correlate with the presence of a central nervous system tumor. *Childs Nerv Syst*. 2017 Feb;33(2):233–238.

25. Miljković MD, Grossman SA, Ye X, et al. Patterns of radiation-associated lymphopenia in children with cancer. *Cancer Invest*. 2016;34(1):32–38.

26. Probert JC, Parker BR. The effects of radiation therapy on bone growth. *Radiology*. 1975;114(1):155–162.

27. Dorr W, Kallfels S, Herrmann T. Late bone and soft tissue sequelae of childhood radiotherapy. Relevance of treatment age and radiation dose in 146 children treated between 1970 and 1997. *Strahlenther Onkol*. 2013;189(7):529–534.

28. Genc M, Aksu GM, Korcum AF, et al. Commentary on "late bone and soft tissue sequelae of childhood radiotherapy." *Strahlenther Onkol*. 2014;190(10):962.

29. Dorr W, Kallfels S, Herrmann T. Response to the letter to the editor by Genc et al. *Strahlenther Onkol*. 2014;190(10):963–964.

30. Smuel K, Kauli R, Lilos P, et al. Growth, development, puberty and adult height before and during treatment in children with congenital isolated growth hormone deficiency. *Growth Horm IGF Res*. 2015;25(4):182–188.

31. Shim KS. Pubertal growth and epiphyseal fusion. *Ann Pediatr Endocrinol Metab*. 2015;20(1):8–12.

32. Kouloulias V, Liakouli Z, Zygogianni A, et al. Bone density as a marker of response to radiotherapy in bone metastatic lesions: a review of the published data. *Int J Mol Sci*. 2016;17(9):1391. doi:10.3390/ijms17091391

33. Reisi N, Iravani P, Raeissi P, et al. Vitamin D and bone minerals status in the long-term survivors of childhood acute lymphoblastic leukemia. *Int J Prev Med*. 2015;6:87. doi:10.4103/2008-7802.164691

34. Ward LM, Konji VN, Ma J. The management of osteoporosis in children. *Osteoporos Int*. 2016;27(7):2147–2179.

35. Ottanelli S. Prevention and treatment of bone fragility in cancer patient. *Clin Cases Miner Bone Metab*. 2015;12(2):116–129.

36. Hudson MM, Landler W, Constine LS, et al. Children's Oncology Group long-term follow-up guidelines for survivors of childhood, adolescent, and young adult cancers 2013 [Version 4.0]. http://www.survivorshipguidelines.org/pdf/LTFUGuidelines_40.pdf

37. Indelicato DJ, Flampouri S, Rotondo RL, et al. Incidence and dosimetric parameters of pediatric brainstem toxicity following proton therapy. *Acta Oncol*. 2014;53(10):1298–1304.

38. Yock TI, Constine LS, Mahajan A. Protons, the brainstem, and toxicity: ingredients for an emerging dialectic. *Acta Oncol*. 2014;53(10):1279–1282.

39. Merchant TE, Li C, Xiong X, et al. Conformal radiotherapy after surgery for paediatric ependymoma: a prospective study. *Lancet Oncol*. 2009;10(3):258–266.

40. Rahmathulla G, Marko NF, Weil RJ. Cerebral radiation necrosis: a review of the pathobiology, diagnosis and management considerations. *J Clin Neurosci*. 2013;20(4):485–502.

41. Lockney NA, Friedman DN, Wexler LH, et al. Late toxicities of intensity-modulated radiation therapy for head and neck rhabdomyosarcoma. *Pediatr Blood Cancer*. 2016;63(9):1608–1614.

42. Walker GV, Ahmed S, Allen P, et al. Radiation-induced middle ear and mastoid opacification in skull base tumors treated with radiotherapy. *Int J Radiat Oncol Biol Phys*. 2011;81(5):e819–e823.

43. Bass JK, Hua CH, Huang J, et al. Hearing loss in patients who received cranial radiation therapy for childhood cancer. *J Clin Oncol*. 2016;34(11):1248–1255.

44. Hua C, Bass JK, Khan R, et al. Hearing loss after radiotherapy for pediatric brain tumors: effect of cochlear dose. International journal of radiation oncology, biology, physics. 2008;72(3):892–899.

45. Grewal S, Merchant T, Reymond R, et al. Auditory late effects of childhood cancer therapy: a report from the Children's Oncology Group. *Pediatrics*. 2010;125(4):e938–e950.

46. Bass JK, Knight KR, Yock TI, et al. Evaluation and management of hearing loss in survivors of childhood and adolescent cancers: a report from the Children's Oncology Group. *Pediatr Blood Cancer*. 2016;63(7):1152–1162.

47. Suneja G, Poorvu PD, Hill-Kayser C, et al. Acute toxicity of proton beam radiation for pediatric central nervous system malignancies. *Pediatr Blood Cancer*. 2013;60(9):1431–1436.

48. Song S, Park HJ, Yoon JH, et al. Proton beam therapy reduces the incidence of acute haematological and gastrointestinal toxicities associated with craniospinal irradiation in pediatric brain tumors. *Acta Oncol*. 2014;53(9):1158–1164.

49. McGovern SL, Okcu MF, Munsell MF, et al. Outcomes and acute toxicities of proton therapy for pediatric atypical teratoid/rhabdoid tumor of the central nervous system. *Int J Radiat Oncol Biol Phys*. 2014;90(5):1143–1152.

50. Cox MC, Kusters JM, Gidding CE, et al. Acute toxicity profile of craniospinal irradiation with intensity-modulated radiation therapy in children with medulloblastoma: a prospective analysis. *Radiat Oncol*. 2015;10:241. doi:10.1186/s13014-015-0547-9

51. Ballesteros-Zebadua P, Chavarria A, Celis MA, et al. Radiation-induced neuroinflammation and radiation somnolence syndrome. *CNS Neurol Disord Drug Targets*. 2012;11(7):937–949.

52. Kelsey CR, Marks LB. Somnolence syndrome after focal radiation therapy to the pineal region: case report and review of the literature. *J Neurooncol*. 2006;78(2):153–156.

53. Lal DR, Foroutan HR, Su WT, et al. The management of treatment-related esophageal complications in children and adolescents with cancer. *J Pediatr Surg*. 2006;41(3):495–499.

54. Holmqvist AS, Olsen JH, Andersen KK, et al. Adult life after childhood cancer in Scandinavia: diabetes mellitus following treatment for cancer in childhood. *Eur J Cancer*. 2014;50(6):1169–1175.

55. Mayson SE, Parker VE, Schutta MH, et al. Severe insulin resistance and hypertriglyceridemia after childhood total body irradiation. *Endocr Pract*. 2013;19(1):51–58.

56. Lee SH, Shin CH. Reduced male fertility in childhood cancer survivors. *Ann Pediatr Endocrinol Metab*. 2013;18(4):168–172.

57. Hess CB, Thompson HM, Benedict SH, et al. Exposure risks among children undergoing radiation therapy: considerations in the era of image guided radiation therapy. *Int J Radiat Oncol Biol Phys*. 2016;94(5):978–992.

58. van Nimwegen FA, Schaapveld M, Cutter DJ, et al. Radiation dose-response relationship for risk of coronary heart disease in survivors of hodgkin lymphoma. *J Clin Oncol*. 2016;34(3):235–243.

59. Hancock SL, Tucker MA, Hoppe RT. Factors affecting late mortality from heart disease after treatment of Hodgkin's disease. *JAMA*. 1993;270(16):1949–1955.

60. Darby SC, Ewertz M, McGale P, et al. Risk of ischemic heart disease in women after radiotherapy for breast cancer. *N Engl J Med*. 2013;368(11):987–998.

61. Cheuk DK, Sieswerda E, van Dalen EC, et al. Medical interventions for treating anthracycline-induced symptomatic and asymptomatic cardiotoxicity during and after treatment for childhood cancer. *Cochrane Database Syst Rev*. 2016;8:CD008011. doi:10.1002/14651858.CD008011.pub3

62. Gondi V, Pugh SL, Tome WA, et al. Preservation of memory with conformal avoidance of the hippocampal neural stem-cell compartment during whole-brain radiotherapy for brain metastases (RTOG 0933): a phase II multi-institutional trial. *J Clin Oncol*. 2014;32(34):3810–3816.

63. Gondi V, Tome WA, Mehta MP. Why avoid the hippocampus? A comprehensive review. *Radiother Oncol*. 2010;97(3):370–376.

64. Merchant TE, Sharma S, Xiong X, et al. Effect of cerebellum radiation dosimetry on cognitive outcomes in children with infratentorial ependymoma. *Int J Radiat Oncol Biol Phys*. 2014;90(3):547–553.

65. Zureick AH, Pulsifer M, Niemierko A, et al. Elevated proton radiation therapy dose to left temporal lobe or whole-brain correlates with decline in full-scale iq components for pediatric cns tumor survivors. *Int J Radiat Oncol Biol Phys*. 2016;96(2S):S120.

66. Kazda T, Jancalek R, Pospisil P, et al. Why and how to spare the hippocampus during brain radiotherapy: the developing role of hippocampal avoidance in cranial radiotherapy. *Radiat Oncol*. 2014;9:139. doi:10.1186/1748-717X-9-139

67. Balentova S, Adamkov M. Molecular, cellular and functional effects of radiation-induced brain injury: a review. *Int J Mol Sci*. 2015;16(11):27796–27815.

68. Zeltzer LK, Recklitis C, Buchbinder D, et al. Psychological status in childhood cancer survivors: a report from the Childhood Cancer Survivor Study. *J Clin Oncol*. 2009;27(14):2396–2404.

69. Littley MD, Shalet SM, Beardwell CG, et al. Radiation-induced hypopituitarism is dose-dependent. *Clin Endocrinol (Oxf)*. 1989;31(3):363–373.

70. Vatner RE, Weyman E, Goebel C, et al. Endocrine deficiency as a function of proton radiation dose to the hypothalamus in children with brain tumors. *Int J Radiat Oncol Biol Phys*. 2016;96(2S):S231–S232.

71. Chemaitilly W, Li Z, Huang S, et al. Anterior hypopituitarism in adult survivors of childhood cancers treated with cranial radiotherapy: a report from the St Jude Lifetime Cohort study. *J Clin Oncol*. 2015;33(5):492–500.

72. Lustig RH, Post SR, Srivannaboon K, et al. Risk factors for the development of obesity in children surviving brain tumors. *J Clin Endocrinol Metab*. 2003;88(2):611–616.

73. Saultier P, Auquier P, Bertrand Y, et al. Metabolic syndrome in long-term survivors of childhood acute leukemia treated without hematopoietic stem cell transplantation: an L.E.A. study. *Haematologica*. 2016;101(12):1603–1610.

74. Djogo T, Robins SC, Schneider S, et al. Adult NG2-Glia are required for median eminence-mediated leptin sensing and body weight control. *Cell Metab*. 2016;23(5):797–810.

75. Bretault M, Boillot A, Muzard L, et al. Clinical review: Bariatric surgery following treatment for craniopharyngioma: a systematic review and individual-level data meta-analysis. *J Clin Endocrinol Metab*. 2013;98(6):2239–2246.

76. Weirich A, Ludwig R, Graf N, et al. Survival in nephroblastoma treated according to the trial and study SIOP-9/GPOH with respect to relapse and morbidity. *Ann Oncol*. 2004;15(5):808–820.
77. Levin TL, Roebuck D, Berdon WE. Long-segment narrowing of the abdominal aorta and its branches in a survivor of infantile neuroblastoma treated without radiation therapy. *Pediatr Radiol*. 2011;41(7):933–936.
78. Venkatramani R, Kamath S, Wong K, et al. Correlation of clinical and dosimetric factors with adverse pulmonary outcomes in children after lung irradiation. *Int J Radiat Oncol Biol Phys*. 2013;86(5):942–948.
79. Palma DA, Senan S, Tsujino K, et al. Predicting radiation pneumonitis after chemoradiation therapy for lung cancer: an international individual patient data meta-analysis. *Int J Radiat Oncol Biol Phys*. 2013;85(2):444–450.
80. Abugideiri M, Nanda RH, Butker C, et al. Factors influencing pulmonary toxicity in children undergoing allogeneic hematopoietic stem cell transplantation in the setting of total body irradiation-based myeloablative conditioning. *Int J Radiat Oncol Biol Phys*. 2016;94(2):349–359.
81. Lanier JC, Abrams AN. Posterior fossa syndrome: Review of the behavioral and emotional aspects in pediatric cancer patients. *Cancer*. 2017;123(4):551–559.
82. Korah MP, Esiashvili N, Mazewski CM, et al. Incidence, risks, and sequelae of posterior fossa syndrome in pediatric medulloblastoma. *Int J Radiat Oncol Biol Phys*. 2010;77(1):106–112.
83. Inskip PD, Sigurdson AJ, Veiga L, et al. Radiation-related new primary solid cancers in the childhood cancer survivor study: comparative radiation dose response and modification of treatment effects. *Int J Radiat Oncol Biol Phys*. 2016;94(4):800–807.
84. Morton LM, Onel K, Curtis RE, et al. The rising incidence of second cancers: patterns of occurrence and identification of risk factors for children and adults. *Am Soc Clin Oncol Educ Book*. 2014:e57–e67.
85. Armstrong GT, Chen Y, Yasui Y, et al. Reduction in late mortality among 5-year survivors of childhood cancer. *N Engl J Med*. 2016;374(9):833–842.
86. National Research Council (U.S.). Committee to Assess Health Risks from Exposure to Low Level of Ionizing Radiation. *Health risks from exposure to low levels of ionizing radiation: BEIR VII phase 2*. Washington, DC: National Academies Press; 2006.
87. Armstrong GT, Liu W, Leisenring W, et al. Occurrence of multiple subsequent neoplasms in long-term survivors of childhood cancer: a report from the childhood cancer survivor study. *J Clin Oncol*. 2011;29(22):3056–3064.
88. Zhang J, Walsh MF, Wu G, et al. Germline mutations in predisposition genes in pediatric cancer. *N Engl J Med*. 2015;373(24):2336–2346.
89. Radivoyevitch T, Sachs RK, Gale RP, et al. Defining AML and MDS second cancer risk dynamics after diagnoses of first cancers treated or not with radiation. *Leukemia*. 2016;30(2):285–294.
90. Krasovec M, Trueb RM. Temporary roentgen epilation after embolization of a cerebral arteriovenous malformation. *Hautarzt*. 1998;49(4):307–309.
91. Crossland PM. Therapy of tinea capitis; the value of x-ray epilation. *Calif Med*. 1956;84(5):351–353.
92. Martin NE, Ng AK. Good things come in small packages: low-dose radiation as palliation for indolent non-Hodgkin lymphomas. *Leuk Lymphoma*. 2009;50(11):1765–1772.

93. Lawenda BD, Gagne HM, Gierga DP, et al. Permanent alopecia after cranial irradiation: dose-response relationship. *Int J Radiat Oncol Biol Phys*. 2004;60(3):879–887.

94. Min CH, Paganetti H, Winey BA, et al. Evaluation of permanent alopecia in pediatric medulloblastoma patients treated with proton radiation. *Radiat Oncol*. 2014;9:220. doi:10.1186/s13014-014-0220-8

95. Haas RL, de Klerk G. An illustrated case of doxorubicin-induced radiation recall dermatitis and a review of the literature. *Neth J Med*. 2011;69(2):72–75.

96. Hattangadi J, Esty B, Winey B, et al. Radiation recall myositis in pediatric Ewing sarcoma. *Pediatr Blood Cancer*. 2012;59(3):570–572.

97. Boaventura P, Pereira D, Mendes A, et al. Thyroid and parathyroid tumours in patients submitted to X-ray scalp epilation during the tinea capitis eradication campaign in the north of Portugal (1950–1963). *Virchows Arch*. 2014;465(4): 445–452.

98. Hirsch JF, Renier D, Czernichow P, et al. Medulloblastoma in childhood. Survival and functional results. *Acta Neurochir (Wien)*. 1979;48(1–2):1–15.

99. Nadol'nik LI, Netsetskaia ZV, Kardash NA, et al. [Functional and morphological characterization of rat thyroid gland at remote periods following single high and low dose radiation exposure]. *Radiats Biol Radioecol*. 2004;44(5):535–543.

100. Lin Z, Wang X, Xie W, et al. Evaluation of clinical hypothyroidism risk due to irradiation of thyroid and pituitary glands in radiotherapy of nasopharyngeal cancer patients. *J Med Imaging Radiat Oncol*. 2013;57(6):713–718.

101. Ronjom MF, Brink C, Bentzen SM, et al. Hypothyroidism after primary radiotherapy for head and neck squamous cell carcinoma: normal tissue complication probability modeling with latent time correction. *Radiother Oncol*. 2013;109(2):317–322.

102. Sobol G, Musiol K, Kalina M, et al. The evaluation of function and the ultrasonographic picture of thyroid in children treated for medulloblastoma. *Childs Nerv Syst*. 2012;28(3):399–404.

103. Paulino AC. Hypothyroidism in children with medulloblastoma: a comparison of 3600 and 2340 cGy craniospinal radiotherapy. *Int J Radiat Oncol Biol Phys*. 2002;53(3):543–547.

104. Hancock SL, McDougall IR, Constine LS. Thyroid abnormalities after therapeutic external radiation. *Int J Radiat Oncol Biol Phys*. 1995;31(5):1165–1170.

105. Constine LS, Donaldson SS, McDougall IR, et al. Thyroid dysfunction after radiotherapy in children with Hodgkin's disease. *Cancer*. 1984;53(4):878–883.

106. de Vathaire F, Haddy N, Allodji RS, et al. Thyroid radiation dose and other risk factors of thyroid carcinoma following childhood cancer. *J Clin Endocrinol Metab*. 2015;100(11):4282–4290.

107. Krawczuk-Rybak M, Tomczuk-Ostapczuk M, Panasiuk A, et al. Carotid intima-media thickness in young survivors of childhood cancer. *J Med Imaging Radiat Oncol*. 2017;61(1):85–92.

108. Reynolds MR, Haydon DH, Caird J, Leonard JR. Radiation-induced moyamoya syndrome after proton beam therapy in the pediatric patient: a case series. *Pediatr Neurosurg*. 2016;51(6):297–301.

109. Zwagerman NT, Foster K, Jakacki R, et al. The development of Moyamoya syndrome after proton beam therapy. *Pediatr Blood Cancer*. 2014;61(8):1490–1492.

110. Kim TG, Kim DS, Chung SS, et al. Moyamoya syndrome after radiation therapy: case reports. *Pediatr Neurosurg*. 2011;47(2):138–142.

111. Bitzer M, Topka H. Progressive cerebral occlusive disease after radiation therapy. *Stroke*. 1995;26(1):131–136.

112. Bansal LR, Belair J, Cummings D, et al. Late-onset radiation-induced vasculopathy and stroke in a child with medulloblastoma. *J Child Neurol*. 2015;30(6): 800–802.

113. Mueller S, Sear K, Hills NK, et al. Risk of first and recurrent stroke in childhood cancer survivors treated with cranial and cervical radiation therapy. *Int J Radiat Oncol Biol Phys*. 2013;86(4):643–648.

114. Drezner N, Hardy KK, Wells E, et al. Treatment of pediatric cerebral radiation necrosis: a systematic review. *J Neurooncol*. 2016;130(1):141–148.

115. Zawaski JA, Gaber MW, Sabek OM, et al. Effects of irradiation on brain vasculature using an in situ tumor model. *Int J Radiat Oncol Biol Phys*. 2012;82(3): 1075–1082.

116. Wilson CM, Gaber MW, Sabek OM, et al. Radiation-induced astrogliosis and blood-brain barrier damage can be abrogated using anti-TNF treatment. *Int J Radiat Oncol Biol Phys*. 2009;74(3):934–941.

117. Yuan H, Gaber MW, Boyd K, et al. Effects of fractionated radiation on the brain vasculature in a murine model: blood-brain barrier permeability, astrocyte proliferation, and ultrastructural changes. *Int J Radiat Oncol Biol Phys*. 2006;66(3):860–866.

118. Zheng Q, Yang L, Tan LM, et al. Stroke-like migraine attacks after radiation therapy syndrome. *Chin Med J (Engl)*. 2015;128(15):2097–2101.

119. Black DF, Morris JM, Lindell EP, et al. Stroke-like migraine attacks after radiation therapy (SMART) syndrome is not always completely reversible: a case series. *AJNR Am J Neuroradiol*. 2013;34(12):2298–2303.

120. Armstrong AE, Gillan E, DiMario FJ, Jr. SMART syndrome (stroke-like migraine attacks after radiation therapy) in adult and pediatric patients. *J Child Neurol*. 2014;29(3):336–341.

121. Pereira P, Cerejo A, Cruz J, et al. Intracranial aneurysm and vasculopathy after surgery and radiation therapy for craniopharyngioma: case report. *Neurosurgery*. 2002;50(4):885–887; discussion 7–8.

122. Murakami N, Tsukahara T, Toda H, et al. Radiation-induced cerebral aneurysm successfully treated with endovascular coil embolization. *Acta Neurochir Suppl*. 2002;82:55–58.

123. Ishikawa T, Houkin K, Yoshimoto T, et al. Vasoreconstructive surgery for radiation-induced vasculopathy in childhood. *Surg Neurol*. 1997;48(6):620–626.

124. Scott RM, Smith ER. Moyamoya disease and moyamoya syndrome. *N Engl J Med*. 2009;360(12):1226–1237.

125. Bali L, Silhol F, Kateb A, et al. Renal artery stenosis after abdominal radiotherapy. *Ann Cardiol Angeiol (Paris)*. 2009;58(3):183–186.

126. Marmagkiolis K, Finch W, Tsitlakidou D, et al. Radiation toxicity to the cardiovascular system. *Curr Oncol Rep*. 2016;18(3):15. doi:10.1007/s11912-016-0502-4

127. Wu W, Chaer RA. Nonarteriosclerotic vascular disease. *Surg Clin North Am*. 2013;93(4):833–875, viii.

128. Seregard S, Pelayes DE, Singh AD. Radiation therapy: posterior segment complications. *Dev Ophthalmol*. 2013;52:114–123.

129. Westekemper H, Anastassiou G, Sauerwein W, et al. Analysis of ocular surface alterations following proton beam radiation in eyes with conjunctival malignant melanoma. *Ophthalmologe*. 2006;103(7):588–595.

# 9

# Systemic Effects of Radiation Therapy

*Monica Krishnan and Ron Shiloh*

## OVERVIEW
While radiation side effects are often localized, radiation may also be associated with systemic effects. This chapter focuses on pain, anxiety, fatigue, and anorexia as they specifically relate to radiation therapy (RT). Table 9.1 summarizes management strategies for each of these.

## PAIN
### Definition
- Worsening of pain in the treated site after an intervention, such as external beam radiation therapy (EBRT).
- In some studies, it is specifically defined as a 2-point increase in the pain scale of 0 to 10 compared to baseline, with no decrease in analgesic intake or a 25% increase in analgesic intake (daily oral morphine equivalent), with no decrease in pain score and with a subsequent return to baseline after the transient increase. If increase persists, it is defined as progression rather than a pain flare (1).
- Mechanism of postradiation pain flare is unknown. Hypotheses include edema resulting in nerve compression or release of inflammatory cytokines (2).

### Patient Assessment
- Two-point increase in the pain scale of 0 to 10 compared to baseline, with no decrease in analgesic intake or a 25% increase in analgesic intake employing daily oral morphine equivalent, with no decrease in pain score and with a subsequent return to baseline after the transient increase (1).

### Time Course of Pain Flare
- Usually occurs within 48 hours of first (or single) treatment and lasts 3 days or less.

### Potential Treatments for Pain Flare
- Dexamethasone 8 mg orally at least 1 hour before the start of RT and every day for 4 days after RT.
- Other treatments include those used for management of bone pain in general, including nonsteroidal anti-inflammatory drugs (NSAIDs) and opioids.

Table 9.1 Common Systemic Toxicities Related to Radiation Treatment and Management Strategies

| Ailment | Usual timing | Mild (first step) | Moderate/severe (second steps) | Preventative strategies |
|---|---|---|---|---|
| Pain | Pain flare usually occurs within 48 hours after RT | • OTC analgesics<br>• Acetaminophen<br>• NSAIDs | • Prescription opioids, etc.<br>• Palliative care consultation | • Dexamethasone 8 mg PO 1 hour before RT (for pain flare) and every day for 4 days afterward |
| Anxiety | Pretreatment, may persist long term | • Exercise<br>• Lifestyle modification (reducing caffeine/alcohol, sleep hygiene)<br>• Complementary therapies, including hypnotherapy, music therapy, relaxation training, acupuncture, mindfulness meditation, aromatherapy, massage, and art therapy | • Benzodiazepines (ie, lorazepam 0.25–2 mg PO/SL every 6 h prn) **(not long term)**<br>• Clonazepam<br>• SSRI<br>• SNRI<br>• Psychotherapy, including cognitive behavioral therapy, supportive-expressive group therapy, dignity therapy, and meaning-centered psychotherapy | • Anticipatory guidance regarding what to expect during simulation and treatment |
| Fatigue | At any time | • Exercise<br>• Mind-body techniques, art therapy, sleep therapy | • Methylphenidate<br>• Corticosteroids (dexamethasone 4 mg twice a day) **(not long term)** | • Address comorbidities<br>• Sleep hygiene |
| Anorexia | At any time | • Megestrol | • Corticosteroids<br>• Dronabinol | • Nutritional counseling |

NSAIDs, non-steroidal anti-inflammatory drugs; OTC, over-the-counter; PO, by mouth; RT, radiation therapy; SL, sublingual; SNRI, serotonin-norepinephrine reuptake inhibitor; SSRI, selective serotonin reuptake inhibitor.

Dexamethasone may be effective prophylactically, as evidenced by the National Cancer Institute of Canada (NCIC) Clinical Trials Group Symptom Control 23 Study (3). In that study, all patients were to receive a single dose of 8 Gy to one or two target volumes. Patients were randomized to receive either 8 mg of dexamethasone or placebo to be taken orally at least 1 hour before the start of RT and every day for 4 days after RT. In the sensitivity analysis, 18% of patients in the dexamethasone group versus 29% of patients in the placebo group developed a pain flare with a statistically significant ($P = .01$) difference of 11%. There was no statistically significant difference in the overall pain response, although it trended toward a higher response rate in patients in the dexamethasone group. Patients in the dexamethasone group trended toward having a greater reduction in mean pain scores. Three patients in the dexamethasone group had biochemically identified hyperglycemic episodes, none of which were clinically significant. There were no serious adverse events reported. At day 10, patients in the dexamethasone group also reported significantly reduced nausea and functional interference and improved appetite. However, at day 42, significantly more patients in the dexamethasone group reported high depression scores (8% versus 1%, $P = .04$).

Patients who developed pain flares have reported interference with activities of daily life (ADLs) and anxiety and worry about the success of treatment. Eight-five percent of patients preferred prophylaxis for management of pain flare to an increase in analgesic use when pain flare occurred (4). For patients receiving palliative RT for bone metastases, the incidence of pain flare has been described in several studies. In the Chow study, the incidence of pain flare for patients receiving a single treatment was 14% on day 1 and 2, and for those receiving five daily treatments, the incidence was 15% on day 1 and 21% on day 2 (1). In the Canadian Bone Metastases Trial, the incidence of pain flare was 41%. More specifically, the incidence for patients receiving a single treatment of 8 Gy was 56.5% and for patients receiving 20 Gy in 5 fractions the incidence was 24%. This difference of 32.7% is statistically significant ($P = .04$) (5). Pain flare did not predict for pain relief at 3 months in a statistically significant manner. This result is different from that described for pain flares after radiopharmaceutical administration in patients with metastatic prostate cancer.

Pain flare has also been documented in patients receiving spine stereotactic body radiation therapy (SBRT). In one study, pain flare was observed in 23% of patients (6). Single-fraction SBRT was predictive of pain flare compared to multifraction SBRT with OR 2.48. This suggests that whatever the mechanism of pain flare is, hypofractionation may exacerbate it (6). There was a trend toward a protective effect from prior surgery, suggesting that the surgical stabilization may address a mechanical component of the pain flare (6).

# ANXIETY

## Definition

- Feeling of fear or helplessness, generally associated with a sense of loss of control.
- Anxiety may often be associated with illness, especially if there is possibility of pain or death.

- Common manifestations of anxiety include:
  - Emotional symptoms: edginess or feeling of impending doom
  - Cognitive difficulties: fear, worry, dread
  - Behavioral problems: avoidance or agitation
  - Autonomic symptoms: gastrointestinal distress, dizziness, tachycardia, tachypnea, diaphoresis

## Scope of Problem

- While many patients with cancer express fear or worry about their diagnosis, prognosis, or treatment, not all patients develop anxiety.
- In the Coping with Cancer study, 8% of patients met *DSM-IV* criteria for an anxiety disorder (7).
  - Women, physically impaired patients, and younger patients were more likely to meet criteria for an anxiety disorder.
- In a smaller study specific to patients undergoing RT, 13% of study participants met criteria for clinically relevant anxiety (8).
- It has been posited that patients undergoing RT may develop anxiety specific to the treatment itself due to preconceived notions about the efficacy and safety of radiation. Their anxiety may be heightened by fear of an unfamiliar form of medical treatment (9).

## Patient Assessment

- A short screening tool like the Patient Health Questionnaire for Depression and Anxiety (PHQ-4) may be used to identify patients with anxiety (10).
- If an individual has a positive screen for anxiety on the PHQ-4, it may be reasonable to administer the seven-question Generalized Anxiety Disorder scale (GAD-7) (11).
- It would also be appropriate to refer the patient to a mental health provider or their primary care provider (PCP) for further evaluation.

## Time Course of Anxiety

- Anecdotally, anxiety related to RT appears to develop early in treatment, often before treatment even begins. This is likely related to fear of the unknown.
- Once radiation commences, treatment-related anxiety often diminishes over time.
- For some patients, especially those who are claustrophobic and who are receiving RT that requires more confining immobilization, anxiety may persist.

## Potential Treatments for Anxiety

- Symptoms of anxiety should be addressed when interfering with quality of life (QOL) or with the patient's ability to undergo treatment.
- Current American Society of Clinical Oncology (ASCO) guidelines from 2015 advocate for treatment of moderate to severe symptomatology, defined specifically as a score of 10 or greater on the GAD-7 score (12).

- Psychotherapy, including cognitive behavioral therapy, supportive-expressive group therapy, dignity therapy, and meaning-centered psychotherapy, has been shown to improve symptoms of anxiety.
- Although the data were limited by patient attrition, in the Managing Cancer and Living Meaningfully (CALM) trial, patients who underwent a semistructured individual psychotherapy program experienced improved spiritual well-being and a reduction in depressive symptoms and anxiety (13).
- Complementary therapies, including hypnotherapy, music therapy, relaxation training, acupuncture, mindfulness meditation, aromatherapy, massage, and art therapy, may also be useful adjuncts to help decrease anxiety.
- Exercise may improve emotional well-being and decrease worry and anxiety.
- Lifestyle modification, including reducing caffeine and alcohol intake and improving sleep hygiene, may be helpful.
- Pharmacotherapy with benzodiazepines and/or antidepressants with anxiolytic properties may be useful for some patients.
  - For patients who have direct treatment-related anxiety, a short-acting benzodiazepine may be most effective. Lorazepam is commonly used and may be dosed at 0.25 to 2 mg po/sl every 6 hours prn anxiety.
  - For more generalized anxiety, clonazepam or a selective serotonin reuptake inhibitor (SSRI) or serotonin-norepinephrine reuptake inhibitor (SNRI) may be considered. It is prudent that the patient's PCP or a mental health specialist be involved, as the patient may require longer term monitoring and titration of these medications.

## FATIGUE

### Definition

- Related to cancer or to its treatment.
- Specifically, it is defined as tiredness, weakness, and lack of energy that:
  - Do not correspond with the level of exertion
  - Are not relieved by rest or sleep.

### Patient Assessment

- Start with a full history regarding the fatigue. As fatigue can be multifactorial, you must assess for:
  - Sleep disorders (ie, insomnia): Patients reporting fatigue are 2.5 times more likely to have insomnia than others (14).
  - Depression: While this can be caused by fatigue, it can also be the cause of fatigue. It is therefore important to tease out any history of depression, as well as any other depressive symptoms.
  - Pain: Pain itself can contribute to fatigue due to lack of sleep and anxiety.
  - Anemia: Anemia affects a large proportion of cancer patients and can contribute to fatigue if uncorrected.

- Determine when the fatigue started, that is, prior to radiation or during the radiation course. Fatigue can be related to cancer itself, chemotherapy, or radiation, and establishing a time course can help to identify the etiology.
- Elicit any treatments that a patient has already tried for fatigue.
- Elicit any extraneous stressors in the patient's life that may be contributing to fatigue.
- Data shows that a simple single-question scale can be quite effective at eliciting the scale of a patient's fatigue: "How would you rate your fatigue on a scale of 0 to 10 over the past 7 days?" (15).

## Time Course of Radiation-Induced Fatigue

- Fatigue tends to begin 1 to 2 weeks into treatment course and has been shown to peak 1 to 2 weeks *post*-RT (16).
- It has also been shown to remain higher than baseline for months to years following radiation (16,17).

## Potential Treatments for Fatigue

- First, any correctable, non–radiation related causes of fatigue (ie, anemia) should be addressed and corrected if possible.
- Treatments for radiation-induced fatigue and data assessing these treatments are limited.
- Treatments can be divided into pharmacologic and nonpharmacologic.

### *Nonpharmacologic Treatments*

- Exercise
  - Multiple studies have shown an improvement in fatigue with physical exercise (18–21).
  - These studies have assessed a wide range of exercise modalities, from moderate exercise to strength training to progressive resistance training.
  - There is currently no consensus as to the appropriate type or amount of exercise in the treatment of cancer-related fatigue.
  - Yoga has also shown promising results, although data are limited (22).
  - At our institute, we recommend light to moderate exercise (ie, walking) about 3 to 4 times a week for radiation-induced fatigue.
- Other integrative therapies, such as mindfulness-based stress reduction (23), art therapy (24), and sleep therapy (25) have been shown to improve fatigue, but again, data is limited on these therapies.

### *Pharmacologic Treatments*

- If fatigue is due to underlying depression or a sleep disorder caused by anxiety, these underlying causes should be treated before using one of the following treatments. Please see section on anxiety and depression in this chapter for appropriate treatments.

- Methylphenidate (Ritalin)
  - Psychostimulant: stimulates adrenergic receptors.
  - Results have been mixed: Methylphenidate has been shown in several studies to improve cancer-related fatigue, decrease drowsiness, and increase activity (26,27) but a subsequent study showed no significant improvement when compared to placebo (28).
  - Patients with more severe or advanced fatigue may benefit to a greater extent (29).
  - Side effects may include irritability, anorexia, insomnia, labile mood, nausea, and tachycardia, but no clear increase in adverse events has been found in studies when compared with placebo (30).
  - National Comprehensive Cancer Network (NCCN) guidelines:
    - Psychostimulants are useful for fatigue in advanced disease or those who are receiving active treatment.
    - Limited evidence in reducing fatigue in patients who are disease free after active treatment.
- Corticosteroids
  - Given potential inflammatory etiology of cancer-related fatigue, corticosteroids have been postulated as a potential treatment.
  - Data are limited with respect to specific improvements in cancer-related fatigue
    - One placebo-controlled randomized study of 4 mg dexamethasone twice daily showed a significant improvement in cancer-related fatigue (31).
      - No significant differences in adverse events between placebo and dexamethasone groups.
      - Improvements seen at two timepoints: day 8 and day 15.
  - Corticosteroids may be beneficial in the short term, but given long-term side effects, it should be used cautiously in patients with long-term fatigue.
- Other agents such as modafinil (psychostimulant) (32), paroxetine (SSRI) (33), L-carnitine (34), and bupropion (35) have also been studied, but have limited randomized data to show a benefit.

The etiology of cancer-related fatigue, and radiation-related fatigue specifically, is as of yet still unknown. It is likely multifactorial in nature and related to environmental, genetic, and molecular factors. In one study of breast cancer patients receiving adjuvant RT, age 45 years of less, the presence of psychiatric and pain-related comorbidities and baseline sadness and anxiety were predictive of maximum fatigue scores (4). An immune-mediated etiology has also been postulated (36,37).

Approximately 80% of patients receiving RT for cancer report fatigue as one of the their major side effects (38). Fatigue has been shown to have a significant impact on QOL. Data suggests that fatigue has a higher impact on QOL than other symptoms such as pain and nausea (39,40). Described as one of the most distressing symptoms patients experience while receiving radiation, symptoms of fatigue can persist for months to years, affecting

QOL over a long time span. Radiation-related fatigue occurs across a wide range of cancer types and can contribute to depression, anxiety, concentration difficulties, decreased participation in work and recreational activities, and difficulty with relationships (41).

# ANOREXIA

## Definition

Definition: Loss of appetite/aversion to food due to cancer or cancer-related treatment.

## Patient Assessment

- Start with a full history regarding the anorexia. Anorexia, like fatigue, can be multifactorial and related to:
  - Mechanical difficulties eating, including mucositis, xerostomia, dysphagia
  - Dysgeusia
  - Nausea
  - Constipation
  - Diarrhea—patients may feel as though eating will result in diarrhea and may therefore limit intake
  - Psychological issues such as anxiety and depression
  - Cancer related cachexia-anorexia
    - Characterized by a loss of weight and muscle mass and associated with anorexia
    - Specific etiology is unknown, but thought to represent an interaction of various inflammatory cytokines (42).
- Elicit timeline of symptoms to determine whether the anorexia is related directly to radiation treatment or may be an effect of the cancer in general.
- Elicit any treatments the patient has already tried.
- Elicit any emotional stressors that may be contributing to the patient's anorexia.
- Determine percent weight loss, both from the prior week and from the start of treatment. Doing so can help to determine the extent of the problem.
- Assess vital signs, including heart rate and blood pressure to look for any signs of orthostasis.
- Perform a full physical exam, paying attention to signs of mucositis and thrush, as well as abdominal distention.

## Time Course of Radiation-Induced Anorexia

- The time course of radiation-related anorexia is dependent on the cause of anorexia.
- Time course of mucositis, xerostomia, dysgeusia, esophagitis, nausea, and diarrhea are detailed in their respective chapters.

## Potential Treatments for Anorexia

- Treatment should be tailored to etiology.
- Recommended treatments for mucositis, dysgeusia, esophagitis, nausea, and diarrhea are detailed in their respective chapters.
- This chapter focuses on treatments for generalized anorexia that does not respond to the treatments mentioned previously.
- Nutritional counseling
    - Should focus on dietary modifications, managing specific symptoms that may be causing anorexia, dealing with social/financial burdens that may be affecting caloric intake, and techniques to meet nutritional requirements.
    - Limited data focusing specifically on benefits of nutritional counseling in patients receiving radiation, but smaller studies do show a likely benefit (43,44), and additional studies show a benefit in the general cancer population (45).
    - At our institution, nutritional counseling is offered to all patients with anorexia.
- Megestrol (Megace)
    - Progesterone derivative.
    - Randomized data and a meta-analysis suggest that Megace leads to increased appetite and weight and calorie intake in patients with advanced cancer (46–48).
    - Approved by the U.S. Food and Drug Administration (FDA) for treatment of cachexia-anorexia syndrome.
    - Side effects can include fatigue, diminished libido, and potentially decreased muscle mass.
- Corticosteroids
    - May have benefits for short-term improvements in appetite and weight gain (12).
    - Given long-term side effects, should be used cautiously in those with long-term symptoms.
- Cannabinoids
    - Dronabinol has shown promising results in anorexia caused by noncancer etiologies, such as AIDS (49).
    - Randomized study of 289 patients with advanced cancer showed no significant benefit over placebo (8).
    - FDA approved for chemotherapy-related nausea and for treatment of anorexia in AIDS patients.

Radiation treatment to several different regions (head and neck, gastrointestinal, pelvis, thoracic) can cause anorexia and result in significant weight loss. Anorexia can cause functional limitations, as well as significant emotional distress. Treatment related anorexia may have implications for survival in certain patient populations. In a study of 364 patients receiving preoperative chemoradiation for locally advanced rectal cancer, severe weight loss during chemoradiation was found to impact survival (Overall survival 71.8% versus 88.0%, $P = .030$) (50). Critical weight loss (>10%) was found to be independently associated with worse overall survival in patients with head and neck cancer receiving RT (HR 1.7, $P = .002$) (51).

## REFERENCES

1. Chow E, Ling A, Davis L, et al. Pain flare following external beam radiotherapy and meaningful change in pain scores in the treatment of bone metastases. *Radiother Oncol*. 2005;75(1):64–69.

2. Svendsen KB, Andersen S, Arnason S, et al. Breakthrough pain in malignant and non-malignant diseases: a review of prevalence, characteristics and mechanisms. *Eur J Pain*. 2005;9(2):195–206.

3. Chow E, Meyer RM, Ding K, et al. Dexamethasone in the prophylaxis of radiation-induced pain flare after palliative radiotherapy for bone metastases: a double-blind, randomised placebo-controlled, phase 3 trial. *Lancet Oncol*. 2015;16(15):1463–72.

4. Hird A, Chow E, Zhang L, et al. Determining the incidence of pain flare following palliative radiotherapy for symptomatic bone metastases: results from three canadian cancer centers. *Int J Radiat Oncol Biol Phys*. 2009;75(1):193–197.

5. Loblaw DA, Wu JS, Kirkbride P, et al. Pain flare in patients with bone metastases after palliative radiotherapy—a nested randomized control trial. *Support Care Cancer*. 2007;15(4):451–455.

6. Pan HY, Allen PK, Wang XS, et al. Incidence and predictive factors of pain flare after spine stereotactic body radiation therapy: secondary analysis of phase 1/2 trials. *Int J Radiat Oncol Biol Phys*. 2014;90(4):870–876.

7. Spencer R, Nilsson M, Wright A, et al. Anxiety disorders in advanced cancer patients: correlates and predictors of end-of-life outcomes. *Cancer*. 2010;116(7):1810–1819.

8. Frick E, Tyroller M, Panzer M. Anxiety, depression and quality of life of cancer patients undergoing radiation therapy: a cross-sectional study in a community hospital outpatient centre. *Eur J Cancer Care (Engl)*. 2007;16(2):130–136.

9. Poroch D. The effect of preparatory patient education on the anxiety and satisfaction of cancer patients receiving radiation therapy. *Cancer Nurs*. 1995;18(3):206–214.

10. Kroenke K, Spitzer RL, Williams JB, Löwe B. An ultra-brief screening scale for anxiety and depression: the PHQ-4. *Psychosomatics*. 2009;50(6):613–621.

11. Spitzer RL, Kroenke K, Williams JB, Löwe B. A brief measure for assessing generalized anxiety disorder: the GAD-7. *Arch Intern Med*. 2006;166(10):1092–1097.

12. Andersen BL, DeRubeis RJ, Berman BS, et al. Screening, assessment, and care of anxiety and depressive symptoms in adults with cancer: an American Society of Clinical Oncology guideline adaptation. *J Clin Oncol*. 2014;32(15):1605–1619.

13. Lo C, Hales S, Jung J, et al. Managing Cancer And Living Meaningfully (CALM): phase 2 trial of a brief individual psychotherapy for patients with advanced cancer. *Palliat Med*. 2014;28(3):234–242.

14. Roscoe JA, Kaufman ME, Matteson-Rusby SE, et al., Cancer-related fatigue and sleep disorders. *Oncologist*. 2007;12(Suppl 1):35–42.

15. Morrow GR, Shelke AR, Roscoe JA, et al. Management of cancer-related fatigue. *Cancer Invest*. 2005;23(3):229–239.

16. Spratt DE, et al., Time course and predictors for cancer-related fatigue in a series of oropharyngeal cancer patients treated with chemoradiation therapy. *Oncologist*. 2012;17(4):569–576.

17. Lilleby W, Stensvold A, Dahl AA. Fatigue and other adverse effects in men treated by pelvic radiation and long-term androgen deprivation for locally advanced prostate cancer. *Acta Oncol.* 2016;55(7):807–813.

18. Campbell A, Mutrie N, White F, et al. A pilot study of a supervised group exercise programme as a rehabilitation treatment for women with breast cancer receiving adjuvant treatment. *Eur J Oncol Nurs.* 2005;9(1):56–63.

19. Courneya KS, Friedenreich CM, Quinney HA, et al. A randomized trial of exercise and quality of life in colorectal cancer survivors. *Eur J Cancer Care (Engl).* 2003;12(4):347–357.

20. Courneya KS, Mackey JR, Bell GJ, et al., Randomized controlled trial of exercise training in postmenopausal breast cancer survivors: cardiopulmonary and quality of life outcomes. *J Clin Oncol.* 2003;21(9):1660–1668.

21. Hojan K, Kwiatkowska-Borowczyk E, Leporowska E, et al. Physical exercise for functional capacity, blood immune function, fatigue, and quality of life in high-risk prostate cancer patients during radiotherapy: a prospective, randomized clinical study. *Eur J Phys Rehabil Med.* 2016;52(4):489–501.

22. Cohen L, Warneke C, Fouladi RT, et al. Psychological adjustment and sleep quality in a randomized trial of the effects of a Tibetan yoga intervention in patients with lymphoma. *Cancer.* 2004;100(10):2253–2260.

23. Johns SA, Brown LF, Beck-Coon K, et al. Randomized controlled pilot trial of mindfulness-based stress reduction compared to psychoeducational support for persistently fatigued breast and colorectal cancer survivors. *Support Care Cancer.* 2016;24(10):4085–4096.

24. Koom WS, Choi MY, Lee J, et al. Art therapy using famous painting appreciation maintains fatigue levels during radiotherapy in cancer patients. *Radiat Oncol J.* 2016;34(2):135–144.

25. Berger AM, VonEssen S, Kuhn BR, et al. Adherence, sleep, and fatigue outcomes after adjuvant breast cancer chemotherapy: results of a feasibility intervention study. *Oncol Nurs Forum.* 2003;30(3):513–522.

26. Bruera E, Chadwick S, Brenneis C, et al. Methylphenidate associated with narcotics for the treatment of cancer pain. *Cancer Treat Rep.* 1987;71(1):67–70.

27. Bruera E, Driver L, Barnes EA, et al. Patient-controlled methylphenidate for the management of fatigue in patients with advanced cancer: a preliminary report. *J Clin Oncol.* 2003;21(23):4439–4443.

28. Bruera E, Yennurajalingam S, Palmer JL, et al. Methylphenidate and/or a nursing telephone intervention for fatigue in patients with advanced cancer: a randomized, placebo-controlled, phase II trial. *J Clin Oncol.* 2013;31(19):2421–2427.

29. Moraska AR, Sood A, Dakhil SR, et al. Phase III, randomized, double-blind, placebo-controlled study of long-acting methylphenidate for cancer-related fatigue: North Central Cancer Treatment Group NCCTG-N05C7 trial. *J Clin Oncol.* 2010;28(23):3673–3679.

30. Minton O, Richardson A, Sharpe M, et al. Psychostimulants for the management of cancer-related fatigue: a systematic review and meta-analysis. *J Pain Symptom Manage.* 2011;41(4):761–767.

31. Yennurajalingam S, Frisbee-Hume S, Palmer JL, et al. Reduction of cancer-related fatigue with dexamethasone: a double-blind, randomized, placebo-controlled trial in patients with advanced cancer. *J Clin Oncol.* 2013;31(25):3076–3082.

32. Spathis A, Fife K, Blackhall F, et al, Modafinil for the treatment of fatigue in lung cancer: results of a placebo-controlled, double-blind, randomized trial. *J Clin Oncol.* 2014;32(18):1882–1888.

33. Morrow GR, Hickok JT, Roscoe JA, et al. Differential effects of paroxetine on fatigue and depression: a randomized, double-blind trial from the University of Rochester Cancer Center Community Clinical Oncology Program. *J Clin Oncol*. 2003;21(24):4635–4634.

34. Cruciani RA, Dvorkin E, Homel P, et al. L-carnitine supplementation for the treatment of fatigue and depressed mood in cancer patients with carnitine deficiency: a preliminary analysis. *Ann N Y Acad Sci*. 2004;1033:168–176.

35. Cullum JL, Wojciechowski AE, Pelletier G, Simpson JS. Bupropion sustained release treatment reduces fatigue in cancer patients. *Can J Psychiatry*. 2004;49(2):139–144.

36. Saligan LN, Kim HS. A systematic review of the association between immunogenomic markers and cancer-related fatigue. *Brain Behav Immun*. 2012;26(6):830–848.

37. Xiao C, Beitler JJ, Higgins KA, et al., Fatigue is associated with inflammation in patients with head and neck cancer before and after intensity-modulated radiation therapy. *Brain Behav Immun*. 2016;52:145–152.

38. Hofman M, Ryan JL, Figueroa-Moseley CD, et al. Cancer-related fatigue: the scale of the problem. *Oncologist*. 2007;12(Suppl 1):4–10.

39. Curt GA, Breitbart W, Cella D, et al. Impact of cancer-related fatigue on the lives of patients: new findings from the Fatigue Coalition. *Oncologist*. 2000;5(5):353–360.

40. Jean-Pierre P, Morrow GR, Roscoe JA, et al. A phase 3 randomized, placebo-controlled, double-blind, clinical trial of the effect of modafinil on cancer-related fatigue among 631 patients receiving chemotherapy: a University of Rochester Cancer Center Community Clinical Oncology Program research base study. *Cancer*. 2010;116(14):3513–3520.

41. Mustian KM, Morrow GR, Carroll JK, et al. Integrative nonpharmacologic behavioral interventions for the management of cancer-related fatigue. *Oncologist*. 2007;12(Suppl 1):52–67.

42. Loprinzi CL, Bernath AM, Schaid DJ, et al. Phase III evaluation of 4 doses of megestrol acetate as therapy for patients with cancer anorexia and/or cachexia. *Oncology*. 1994;51(Suppl 1):2–7.

43. Wood L, Palmer M, Hewitt J, et al. Results of a phase III, double-blind, placebo-controlled trial of megestrol acetate modulation of P-glycoprotein-mediated drug resistance in the first-line management of small-cell lung carcinoma. *Br J Cancer*. 1998;77(4):627–631.

44. Bruera E, Macmillan K, Kuehn, et al. A controlled trial of megestrol acetate on appetite, caloric intake, nutritional status, and other symptoms in patients with advanced cancer. *Cancer*. 1990;66(6):1279–1282.

45. Loprinzi CL, Michalak JC, Schaid DJ, et al. Phase III evaluation of four doses of megestrol acetate as therapy for patients with cancer anorexia and/or cachexia. *J Clin Oncol*. 1993;11(4):762–767.

46. Gomez F, Ruiz P, Lopez R, Rivera C. Treatment with megestrol acetate improves human immunodeficiency virus-associated immune thrombocytopenia. *Clin Diagn Lab Immunol*. 2002;9(3):583–587.

47. Beal JE, Olson R, Lefkowitz L, et al. Long-term efficacy and safety of dronabinol for acquired immunodeficiency syndrome-associated anorexia. *J Pain Symptom Manage*. 1997;14(1):7–14.

48. Hansen MV, Andersen LT, Madsen MT, et al. Effect of melatonin on depressive symptoms and anxiety in patients undergoing breast cancer surgery: a randomized, double-blind, placebo-controlled trial. *Breast Cancer Res Treat*. 2014;145(3):683–695.

49. Khan L, Chiang A, Zhang L, et al. Prophylactic dexamethasone effectively reduces the incidence of pain flare following spine stereotactic body radiotherapy (SBRT): a prospective observational study. *Support Care Cancer.* 2015;23(10):2937–2943.
50. Lin J, Peng J, Qdaisat A, et al. Severe weight loss during preoperative chemoradiotherapy compromises survival outcome for patients with locally advanced rectal cancer. *J Cancer Res Clin Oncol.* 2016;142(12):2551–2560.
51. Nelson KA, Walsh D. The cancer anorexia-cachexia syndrome: a survey of the Prognostic Inflammatory and Nutritional Index (PINI) in advanced disease. *J Pain Symptom Manage.* 2002;24(4):424–428.

# 10

# Radioprotection for Radiation Therapy

*Noah S. Kalman, Sherry Zhao, Mitchell S. Anscher, and Alfredo I. Urdaneta*

## OVERVIEW

As cancer screening, diagnosis, and treatment improve, more patients are surviving their illnesses and living longer (1). It has been estimated that there are over 13 million cancer survivors in the United States alone (2,3). Because of these improvements, concern regarding the toxicity of treatment has become a major public health issue.

In the field of radiation oncology, the acute and late toxicities of treatment are well established. The primary option for limiting the risk of toxicity has been to minimize the volume of normal tissue receiving radiation. Advances in radiation delivery technology have enabled radiation oncologists to deliver higher doses to the tumor, while simultaneously improving normal tissue protection. Despite these great technological advances, it is not possible to completely eliminate exposure of normal tissues surrounding the tumor. Thus, the risk of developing normal tissue injury cannot be completely eliminated by dose avoidance alone.

In recent years, much work has been done to better elucidate the underlying molecular mechanisms responsible for the development of both acute and late radiation-related injuries. Building on this accumulating knowledge, researchers have begun to target molecular pathways implicated in these injuries. Three approaches have been taken to address the phenomenon of radiation-related complications. Most commonly, scientists have attempted to prevent injury by administering drugs before and during radiation exposure. Alternatively, drugs have been administered after radiation exposure, but before the development of overt injury, in an attempt to mitigate the development of radiation-related side effects. Finally, others have attempted to treat patients only after radiation injuries have already developed.

In this chapter, we briefly summarize pertinent preclinical studies, but mainly focus on clinical trials designed to prevent, mitigate, or treat radiation injury. Herein we review important aspects of this research and evaluate what therapies have demonstrated benefit.

## CENTRAL NERVOUS SYSTEM

Radiation therapy (RT) aimed at the central nervous system has a multitude of potential side effects. These are most frequently categorized according to the interval from treatment to the onset of symptoms. The earliest effects are termed *acute*. These are reversible, occur during treatment or shortly after completion, and manifest as fatigue, headaches, and dizziness that are thought to be secondary to edema and disruption of the blood-brain barrier (BBB). The second category of side effects are termed *early delayed*. These occur up to 12 weeks after treatment and are thought to be reversible and related to transient demyelination. These effects are expressed as somnolence and generalized weakness. The final category of radiation effects are *late toxicities*, occurring more than 12 weeks after treatment. These events most often manifest as cognitive impairment and symptoms related to radiation-induced necrosis, which may vary depending on the location affected. Preventing, mitigating, and treating the latter has been the area of greatest interest as long-term survivorship rises (4,5).

## Cognitive Impairment

As overall survival increases in patients who undergo whole-brain radiation therapy (WBRT), cognitive impairment induced by RT has been increasingly observed. A proposed mechanism of action suggests a vascular hypothesis where induction of accelerated atherosclerosis and mineralizing microangiopathy cause cognitive decline similar to that seen in small vessel disease–induced vascular dementia (6,7). Interventions to reverse or decrease this process have been tested with mixed results.

### *Memantine (N-Methyl-D-Aspartate [NMDA] Receptor Antagonist)*

Glutamate, the most important excitatory neurotransmitter in the cortical and hippocampal neurons, activates NMDA, which is involved in the processes of learning and memory. Ischemia can induce excessive stimulation of NMDA, potentially creating a toxic effect. Memantine, a NMDA noncompetitive receptor antagonist, blocks this overstimulation and has proven to be effective in patients with vascular dementia, especially in patients whose dementia is related to small vessel disease. Based on these findings, the Radiation Therapy Oncology Group (RTOG) investigated the use of memantine in patients who underwent WBRT. The study, RTOG 0614, examined patients with metastatic disease to the brain with controlled systemic disease for at least 3 months, with no prior history of WBRT, although treatment with stereotactic radiosurgery (SRS) or surgical resection of previous brain metastasis was allowed as long as they had occurred over 2 weeks prior to enrollment. All patients underwent WBRT to a total dose of 37.5 Gy in 15 fractions, with randomization to either placebo or memantine in an escalating dose of 5 mg in the morning for the first week, then 5 mg twice daily for the second, 10 mg in the morning and 5 mg in the evening during the third week, and finally 10 mg BID from week 4 through 24. The primary and secondary endpoints were preservation of cognitive function and time to cognitive failure, respectively, all based on several standardized tests that were given at baseline, weeks 8, 16, 24, and 48. A total of 508 patients were eligible for analysis. The memantine group showed lower decline in delayed recall at 24 weeks compared to the control group, 53.8% versus 64.9% respectively ($P = .059$). First cognitive failure favored the memantine arm with hazard ratio (HR) 0.78 (95% CI 0.62–0.99). Overall grade 3 and grade 4 toxicity occurred in 14% of patients and did not differ between the groups. The authors suggested that statistical significance was not reached due to the fact that 173 patients died before assessment at 24 weeks (8). Although statistical significance was not reached on the primary outcome, this trial did show significant delay in first cognitive failure, a key component of cognitive impairment induced by RT. Easy tolerance and ready availability of this drug supports its use on patients undergoing WBRT with a life expectancy of more than 6 months.

### *Donepezil (Acetyl Cholinesterase Inhibitor)*

Early pathologic and radiographic studies in a murine model suggest that part of the cognitive decline seen in WBRT is similar to that seen in patients with Alzheimer disease (9). Hence, the use of drugs effective in the treatment of Alzheimer disease, such as donepezil, an acetyl cholinesterase inhibitor, have been tested in an attempt to slow or improve WBRT-induced cognitive decline. Shaw et al analyzed the outcome of 24 patients on a phase II open-label study who had undergone partial or WBRT over 6 months prior to enrollment. Patients were given donepezil 5 mg daily for 6 weeks followed by 10 mg for 18 weeks. Improvement in cognitive function was the primary endpoint, with mood and quality of life as secondary endpoints. Scores regarding attention/concentration, verbal memory, and figural memory showed statistical improvement at 24 weeks, and a trend toward significance for verbal fluency. No significant change was seen in global cognitive function or executive function. Quality of life and mood also showed a significant improvement, particularly related to brain-specific concerns (10). Given these positive initial results, a phase III randomized, double-blind, placebo-controlled study of 198 patients led by the same group was published in 2015. Patients with similar clinical characteristics to the prior study were randomized to donepezil versus placebo. The primary endpoint was improvement in cognitive composite score (CCS). The researchers found that both groups had a significant improvement in the CCS, but there was no difference between groups ($P = .59$). While a significant improvement in verbal testing scores was seen in the donepezil group (11), the routine use of donepezil for cognitive decline after WBRT was not supported based on these results.

### *Methylphenidate*

Children who survive primary brain tumors that require radiation are known to suffer from attention deficit disorders (ADD). In 1992, DeLong et al reported the outcomes in 12 childhood survivors of either primary brain tumor or acute lymphoblastic leukemia (ALL) that were treated with methylphenidate (a mixed dopaminergic-noradrenergic agonist) for 6 months to 6 years. The response was rated as good, fair, and poor in 8, 2, and 2 children, respectively (12). Conversely, Torres et al analyzed the outcome in six children with similar clinical scenarios, which showed no benefit to methylphenidate (13). A 32-patient randomized double-blind placebo-controlled study looked at immediate neurocognitive effects of methylphenidate in children suffering from neurocognitive impairment after surviving a brain tumor or ALL. Patients were tested prior to and 90 minutes after the administration of either placebo or methylphenidate. The primary endpoint was improvement in attention ability performance tests. There was a statistically significant improvement on the sustained attention testing scores favoring the methylphenidate group ($P = .015$) (14). Based on these findings, a similar trial examined the long-term effects of methylphenidate use for 12 months versus placebo in this population. The primary endpoint was increased sustained attention with secondary objectives looking at academic, social, and behavioral skills. A total of 122 patients were enrolled, 68 in the methylphenidate group and 54 in the placebo. Overall measures of sustained attention were significantly increased ($P <.05$) in the methylphenidate group as well as measures of social and behavioral skills when compared to the placebo group. There was no difference in the academic skills in both groups (15).

In adults, Butler et al analyzed the rate of fatigue in patients undergoing WBRT pre- and posttreatment. A total of 68 patients were randomly assigned to placebo or methylphenidate. Using the Functional Assessment of Cancer Therapy pre- and posttreatment they did not find any improvement in the rate of fatigue or quality of life in either group (16). Survivors of childhood brain malignancies and ALL with symptoms of ADD seemed to benefit from long-term use of methylphenidate. The use of this drug in adults is not recommended.

## Radiation Necrosis

In the treatment of tumors of the brain and head and neck, high biologically effective doses (120 Gy and 150 Gy) at standard dose per fraction have an incidence of 5% and 10% of radiation necrosis, respectively. For single-fraction radiosurgery, there is a clear correlation of target size and risk of adverse events (17). Studies suggest that white matter necrosis is related to a gradual depletion of vascular endothelial cells forming the BBB, which leads to activation of vascular endothelial growth factor (VEGF), among others. This overstimulation of VEGF leads to worsening vasogenic edema, inflammation, and tissue hypoxia, subsequently leading to white matter necrosis (18). Steroids form the mainstay of treatment, but they are sometimes insufficient or cause significant toxicity.

### *Bevacizumab (VEGF Inhibitor)*

Initial studies in a murine model showed that VEGF antagonism significantly reduced the edema formation and tissue damage after ischemia/reperfusion injury (19). Several years later, Gonzalez et al reported on 8 patients treated with bevacizumab at either 5 mg/kg every 2 weeks or 7.5 mg/kg every 3 weeks. All patients demonstrated reduction on MRI in the T1 postcontrast and fluid attenuation inverse response (FLAIR) imaging at a median of 8.1 weeks postadministration. The average change in the T1 sequence and the FLAIR images was 48% and 60% respectively (20). Wang et al described 17 patients treated with bevacizumab at a dose of 7.5 mg/kg every 2 weeks with a median of four cycles for radiation-induced brain necrosis confirmed by MRI and spectroscopy after poor response to high-dose steroids. MRI was performed before and after bevacizumab and postcontrast T1 sequences, as well as FLAIR sequence were analyzed. There was a 54.9% and 48.4% average reduction based on imaging for both sequences, respectively. Significant neurological improvement was expressed in 10 patients. Dexamethasone dose reduction was achieved on all patients an average of 4 weeks after commencing therapy, and 4 were able to remain off steroids (21). More recently, the group at Memorial Sloan Kettering published the results of 14 episodes of image-diagnosed cerebral radiation necrosis in 11 patients after SRS, who were treated with bevacizumab after a lack of response to high-dose steroids. MRI pre- and posttreatment (mean of 26 days) showed an average reduction of 64.4% and 64.3% on T1 postcontrast and FLAIR, respectively. All patients had reduction in steroid requirements, and all but one reported improvement or stabilization of radiation necrosis–induced symptoms (22). A small randomized double-blind placebo-controlled trial of bevacizumab in the treatment of biopsy or radiological confirmed radiation necrosis was published by Levin et al. Fourteen patients were enrolled and randomized to placebo or bevacizumab at a dose of 7.5 mg/kg every 3 weeks for two cycles. Posttreatment imaging was obtained 3 weeks after last infusion. T1 postcontrast and FLAIR images were compared. None of the patients on the placebo group demonstrated response compared to all patients on the bevacizumab arm with a median decrease in the T1 postcontrast and FLAIR imaging of 63% and 59% respectively (23). These results suggest that bevacizumab has a role in the treatment of radiation-induced necrosis, although steroids remain first-line treatment.

### Summary

For prevention/mitigation of radiation-induced cognitive impairment:

- **Memantine has** evidence of benefit in preventing cognitive impairment from WBRT.
- While improvement in certain domains of cognitive function was seen with **donepezil**, it was **not** found to benefit overall cognitive function.
- Use of **methylphenidate has** demonstrated benefit in children who received WBRT, but its use is **not** recommended in adults.

For treatment of radiation-induced radiation necrosis:

- **Steroids and bevacizumab** are the mainstay of treatment for radiation necrosis.

Recommended reviews are available for who that desire more information (4,5,24,25). Table 10.1 provides a summary of the randomized human prevention/mitigation studies discussed in this section.

### THORAX

In RT for lung cancer, radiation pneumonitis is the primary toxicity of interest. Patients present with cough, fever, shortness of breath, and radiographic lung changes. Once symptoms develop, high-dose steroids are the mainstay of treatment (26). As patients' symptoms improve, steroids are tapered slowly, as abrupt withdrawal of steroids can cause subclinical pneumonitis to be exacerbated (27). Preemptive treatment with steroids to prevent the development of radiation pneumonitis has not proven to be successful (28).

**Table 10.1** CNS: Randomized Human Prevention/Mitigation Studies of Interest

| Agent | Study | Patients | Control Arm | Treatment Arm | Results (Primary endpoint(s) in bold) | Comment |
|---|---|---|---|---|---|---|
| Memantine (8) | RTOG 06-14 | 508 patients with brain metastases | Whole brain radiation at 37.5 Gy in 15 daily fractions of 2.5 Gy | Control arm plus memantine 5 mg PO daily (escalated to 10 mg BID by week 4 if tolerated) for 24 weeks starting with RT | *24 weeks* **HVLT-R delayed recall decline 0.9 vs 0.0 ($P = .059$)** HVLT-R delayed recognition decline 1.0 vs 0.0 ($P = .0149$) MMSE decline 1 vs 0 ($P = .0093$) Cognitive function failure 65% vs 54% ($P = .01$) No difference in late toxicity | 149 evaluable patients at 24 weeks 33% of patients died before 24 weeks |

*(continued)*

Table 10.1 CNS: Randomized Human Prevention/Mitigation Studies of Interest (continued)

| Agent | Study | Patients | Control Arm | Treatment Arm | Results (Primary endpoint(s) in bold) | Comment |
|---|---|---|---|---|---|---|
| Donepezil (11) | Multi-institution, USA | 198 patients with primary or metastatic brain tumors | Cranial (whole or partial) irradiation 30+ Gy in daily fractions | Control arm plus donepezil 5–10 mg PO daily for 24 weeks starting with RT | *24 weeks* **Similar cognitive composite scores ($P = .57$)** HVLT-R delayed recognition and discrimination favor donepezil arm ($P = .03$ and .01 respectively) | Benefit greater with lower baseline scores Results published in abstract form only |
| Methylphenidate (16) | Wake Forest, USA | 68 patients with primary or metastatic brain tumors | Cranial (whole or partial) irradiation 25+ Gy in daily fractions | Control arm plus 5 mg PO BID (escalated to 15 mg BID if tolerated) during RT and for 8 weeks after completion of RT | *8 weeks* **FACIT fatigue subscale 36 vs 34 ($P = .64$)** No difference in cognitive function | 32 evaluable patients at 8 weeks |

BID, twice daily; CNS, central nervous system; FACIT, Functional Assessment of Chronic Illness Therapy; HVLT-R, Hopkins Verbal Learning Test-Revised; MMSE, Mini-Mental Status Exam; PO, by mouth; RT, radiation therapy; RTOG, Radiation Therapy Oncology Group.

Radiation-induced lung injury is mediated by inflammatory processes, which include increased presence of reactive oxygen and nitrogen species, increased cytokine production such as transforming growth factor (TGF) beta and tumor necrosis factor, and increased hypoxia and edema in lung tissue. Multiple classes of medications have been evaluated to prevent this inflammatory cascade and reduce radiation-induced lung injury (29).

## Preclinical Studies

Antioxidants such as taurine, genistein, flaxseed, and cerium oxide nanoparticles, have all demonstrated efficacy in preventing radiation pneumonitis in animal models; one study specifically showed that taurine lowered TGF beta (30–33). Superoxide dismutases have also demonstrated efficacy (34–38). A nitric oxide synthase inhibitor reduced radiation pneumonitis, possibly owing to decreased production of highly reactive nitric oxide byproducts that form in the presence of superoxides (39). Statins reduce the vascular damage that radiation induces and appear to lessen the development of radiation pneumonitis by limiting hypoxia and profibrotic factors such as TGF beta (40–42). Direct inhibition of tumor necrosis factor and other growth factors improves the risk for pneumonitis as well (43,44). Rapamycin, an mTOR inhibitor, was recently shown to reduce pneumonitis in an animal model (45). Natural products such as curcumin, the active ingredient in turmeric, have demonstrated benefit as well (46–49).

## Amifostine

Amifostine, or WR-2721, an inorganic thiophosphate that acts as a free-radical scavenger, was initially developed by the U.S. Army to protect soldiers from a nuclear weapon attack. It has been extensively studied in preventing pulmonary and esophageal toxicity from lung RT (50).

The largest randomized study, RTOG 98-01, examined 243 patients with stage II to IIIB non-small cell lung cancer that received induction chemotherapy (carboplatin and paclitaxel every 3 weeks for 2 cycles) followed by hyperfractionated RT (69.6 Gy at 1.2 Gy BID) with concurrent weekly carboplatin and paclitaxel. Patients were randomly assigned to receive amifostine or not. Results did not show a benefit to amifostine in preventing grade 3 or higher esophagitis, while incidence of nausea, vomiting, and hypotension were increased in the amifostine arm (51). Interestingly, patients reported improved quality of life, more pain reduction, and less dysphagia and weight loss in the amifostine arm, although clinician reported outcomes did not differ between treatment groups (52).

Single institution randomized studies demonstrated benefit to amifostine. A study of 62 patients who received hyperfractionated RT (69.6 Gy at 1.2 Gy BID) with concurrent cisplatin and etoposide found that amifostine reduced acute pneumonitis (0% versus 16%, $P = .020$) and grade 3 or higher esophagitis (16% versus 35%, $P = .021$) (53). Another study with patients undergoing concurrent chemoradiation demonstrated reduced pneumonitis and esophagitis with amifostine (54). A similar effect was seen in patients undergoing RT alone (55). However, other studies showed little or no benefit (56–58). One study showed no benefit to amifostine compared to erythropoietin use in limited stage small cell lung cancer (59).

Despite evidence of some benefit, few providers have adopted amifostine into their practice. Amifostine causes nausea, vomiting, and hypotension. Delivery is either subcutaneous or intravenous, making it inconvenient to administer. Furthermore, there have been concerns that the drug may negatively impact tumor control rates, although a meta-analysis (60) and long-term follow-up of RTOG 98-01 failed to find a decrement in survival with amifostine (61).

### Angiotensin Converting Enzyme Inhibitors and Angiotensin II Receptor Blockers

Angiotensin converting enzyme (ACE) inhibitors and angiotensin II receptor blockers (ARBs) impact the renin-angiotensin-aldosterone system. These classes of medications have also been shown to reduce the presence of TGF beta in animal models (62). TGF beta is a multifunctional protein involved in the pathogenesis of fibrosis (29). RT activates TGF beta (63,64), and higher levels of TGF beta predict the development of pneumonitis in retrospective human studies (65,66). In animal models, inhibition of TGF beta prevents the development of radiation pneumonitis (67,68). Animal studies of ACE inhibitors and ARBs have demonstrated reduction in radiation pneumonitis (62,69–72), with no tumor-protective effects (73).

Retrospective human studies in patients who had undergone thoracic radiation found an association between ACE inhibitors and reduced incidence of radiation pneumonitis. With ACE inhibitor use, grade 2 or higher pneumonitis was lower (2% versus 11%, $P = .032$) (74). In another report, a statistically significant difference was also seen in a subset of patients with mean lung dose of 20 Gy or lower (75). More recently, the association of ACE inhibitors with reduced pneumonitis incidence was also seen in patients undergoing stereotactic body RT for early-stage cancer (76).

A randomized study, RTOG 01-23, was initiated to evaluate the benefit of captopril in reducing radiation pneumonitis in stage II to IIIB non-small cell lung cancer patients undergoing chemoradiation. Captopril has a thiol group that acts as a free-radical scavenger and exhibits superoxide dismutase–like activity (29). Unfortunately, the study accrued poorly and was closed, with insufficient number of patients to perform a meaningful analysis (77). At this time, ACE inhibitors and ARBs have not been proven to reduce radiation pneumonitis, but these classes of drugs remain promising for future investigation.

### Other Human Studies

Pentoxifylline inhibits platelet aggregation and enhances microvascular blood flow. It also exerts an anti-inflammatory effect by inhibiting proinflammatory cytokines such as tumor necrosis factor (78). Alpha-tocopherol (vitamin E), an antioxidant, is often used with pentoxifylline to treat established radiation injury; however, the role of these drugs in prevention of toxicity is less established (79). Two small randomized studies evaluated these drugs in preventing pneumonitis. One study using only pentoxifylline found that its use during lung or breast radiation improved patients' diffusing capacity of carbon monoxide (DLCO) at 3 and 6 months posttreatment relative to control patients ($P = .01$) (80). A follow-up study from the same group found that pentoxifylline and vitamin E reduced acute and subacute (but not late) pulmonary toxicity relative to placebo in patients undergoing thoracic RT (81).

Berberine, another antioxidant, has been evaluated in prevention of radiation pneumonitis in a randomized study. Patients receiving thoracic RT with berberine had lower levels of TGF beta, less radiation-induced lung injury at 6 weeks and 6 months after start of RT, and improved DLCO compared to patients treated with thoracic RT and placebo (all $P$ <.05) (82). No assessments of tumor control rates with berberine or pentoxifylline have been published.

Metformin, an antidiabetic agent, has been evaluated in lung cancer as a therapeutic agent. One retrospective analysis demonstrated that the use of metformin improved progression-free survival and overall survival in patients with metastatic lung cancer (83). The authors hypothesized that the drug sensitized cancer cells to systemic therapy through disruption of tumor glucose metabolism. Animal studies of metformin in non-small cell lung cancer models showed that it enhanced radiation response by activating the ataxia-telangiectasia–mutated (ATM) pathway, reducing angiogenesis, and enhancing apoptotic marker expression (84). Future study will determine if metformin exhibits radioprotective effects on normal tissues.

### Summary

For prevention/mitigation of radiation-induced injury in the chest:

- Despite evidence of benefit in preventing pneumonitis, **amifostine** is **not** recommended due to significant treatment toxicity.
- **ACE inhibitors and ARBs** have shown promise in mitigating the development of pulmonary toxicity but their benefit has **not** been definitively demonstrated.
- **Pentoxifylline and vitamin E**, as well as the antioxidant **berberine, have** randomized evidence documenting their benefit, but the data is limited to single institution studies.

For treatment of radiation-induced injury in the chest:

- **High-dose steroids** are the mainstay of treatment for radiation pneumonitis.

Recommended reviews are available for those who desire more information (29,50,60). Table 10.2 provides a summary of the randomized human prevention/mitigation studies of interest discussed in this section.

## HEAD AND NECK

In RT for head and neck cancer, multiple organs are at risk. During and immediately after treatment, acute mucositis of the oral cavity and pharynx can be severe, as can be acute skin breakdown. Low radiation doses to the parotid glands cause xerostomia. Odynophagia, dysphagia, and infection associated with RT can be life threatening. Disease-associated anemia has been shown to be associated with decreased survival. Following completion of RT, parotid function may not recover, leading to chronic xerostomia. High

**Table 10.2** Thorax: Randomized Human Prevention/Mitigation Studies of Interest

| Agent | Study | Patients | Control Arm | Treatment Arm | Results (Primary endpoint(s) in bold) | Comment |
|---|---|---|---|---|---|---|
| Amifostine (51,52,61) | RTOG 98-01 | 242 patients stage II–IIIB NSCLC | Induction carboplatin-paclitaxel x 2c then concurrent weekly carboplatin-paclitaxel and 69.6 Gy at 1.2 Gy BID (50.4 Gy to larger volume) | Control arm plus amifostine 500 mg IV four times per week during chemoradiation given before afternoon treatment | *Acute* <br> Swallow scores, weight loss, and pain scores during treatment favored amifostine arm ($P = .025, .045$, and $.015$ respectively) <br><br> **Gr 3+ esophagitis 34% vs 30% ($P = .9$)** <br> Gr 2+ CV (hypotension) 7% vs 16% ($P = .0001$) <br> Gr 2+ nausea 21% vs 33% ($P = .03$) <br> Gr 2+ vomiting 14% vs 30% ($P = .007$) <br><br> *Late* <br> Gr 3+ pneumonitis 17% vs 8% (NS) <br> **No OS difference** | 80% patient compliance with amifostine <br> Results consistent with multiple other studies <br> Amifostine can be delivered IV or SQ |

*(continued)*

**Table 10.2** Thorax: Randomized Human Prevention/Mitigation Studies of Interest (*continued*)

| Agent | Study | Patients | Control Arm | Treatment Arm | Results (Primary endpoint(s) in bold) | Comment |
|---|---|---|---|---|---|---|
| Captopril (77) | RTOG 01-23 | 20 patients stage II–IIIB or central stage I NSCLC, or LS-SCLC | Thoracic RT per the treating physician | Control arm plus captopril 12.5 mg PO TID (escalated to 50 mg TID by week 5 if tolerated) starting after completion of RT for 1 year | **Gr 2+ pulmonary toxicity 23% vs 14% (NS)** | 40% discontinued captopril due to side effects Planned accrual 205 patients |
| Pentoxifylline + Vitamin E (81) | Ankara, Turkey | 91 patients localized NSCLC or SCLC | Thoracic RT to 40+ Gy (median 54 Gy) | Control arm plus pentoxifylline 400 mg PO TID and vitamin E 300 mg PO BID during RT followed by 3 months of daily treatment with each drug | Physician assessed radiation induced lung toxicity:<br>– **At 1–2 months post RT 34% vs 16% ($P = .042$)**<br>– **At 12 months post RT 31% vs 16% ($P = .256$)** | 75% received chemotherapy 25% required dose reduction of pentoxifylline due to nausea Only 25 patients were evaluable at 12 months |

(*continued*)

**Table 10.2** Thorax: Randomized Human Prevention/Mitigation Studies of Interest (*continued*)

| Agent | Study | Patients | Control Arm | Treatment Arm | Results (Primary endpoint(s) in bold) | Comment |
|---|---|---|---|---|---|---|
| Berberine (82) | Shandong, China | 85 patients stage III unresectable NSCLC | Thoracic RT 60–70 Gy with concurrent platinum-based chemotherapy | Control arm plus berberine 20 mg/kg PO daily during RT | TGF beta levels at 3 and 6 weeks during RT lower in berberine group ($P$ <.05)<br><br>Physician assessed radiation induced lung injury:<br>– **At 6 weeks post RT Gr 2+ 30% vs 17% ($P$ <.05)**<br>– **At 6 months post RT Gr 2+ 26% vs 12% ($P$ <.05)**<br><br>No OS difference | Mixed results in pulmonary function testing. |

BID, twice daily; LS-SCLC, limited-stage small cell lung cancer; NSCLC, non-small cell lung cancer; OS, overall survival; RT, radiation therapy; RTOG, Radiation Therapy Oncology Group; SCLC, small cell lung cancer; SQ, subcutaneously; TID, three times daily.

radiation doses to the mandible and surrounding tissue can lead to osteoradionecrosis and trismus. Tissue scarring can lead to dysphagia and skin fibrosis. Radioprotective measures have been examined to prevent and/or treat these effects. This section addresses these measures, with the exception of acute dermatitis and late skin fibrosis, which is covered in the Breast/Skin section.

## Oral Mucositis

Interventions to reduce mucositis have aimed to prevent symptoms, given the temporary nature of this toxicity. Meta-analyses have assessed the impact of numerous pharmacologic and nonpharmacologic interventions (85,86). The results of these studies are discussed subsequently.

### *Palifermin (Keratinocyte Growth Factor)*

Multiple randomized studies examined palifermin, a keratinocyte growth factor, in prevention of mucositis. A meta-analysis of seven randomized studies showed a 20% to 30% reduction in the risk of mild, moderate, and severe mucositis ($P$ <.01) (85). However, only one of these studies examined patients undergoing head and neck RT. In this study, in patients receiving chemoradiation for head and neck cancer, palifermin did not show a benefit in reducing mucositis (87). Another randomized study completed after publication of the meta-analysis demonstrated reduction in severe mucositis (54% versus 69%, $P$ = .041) with palifermin use during definitive head and neck chemoradiation relative to the control group (88). Evaluation of palifermin use in the postoperative setting also demonstrated a reduction in severe mucositis (51% versus 67%, $P$ = .027) with the drug. Also, with a 33-month median follow-up, no difference in tumor recurrence was observed between treatment arms (89). Palifermin represents a promising option in reducing the incidence and severity of oral mucositis, although more data is required given conflicting study results in the RT setting and concern for a tumor-protective effect of the drug.

### *Amifostine*

Many randomized studies evaluated the use of amifostine in prevention of mucositis. Certain studies in patients demonstrated reduced mucositis severity without any impact on tumor control rates (56,90–95). Other studies showed no difference in mucositis rates between the amifostine and control arms (96–99). A meta-analysis of 11 chemotherapy and/or RT studies concluded that evidence supporting amifostine's use to prevent mucositis was limited (85). Numerous nonrandomized studies have examined amifostine with various chemoradiation regimens with inconsistent results (100–107). Some of the listed studies have examined endpoints other than mucositis, such as acute xerostomia or candidiasis rates, with no definitive benefit shown with amifostine (108). An earlier meta-analysis with five RT studies determined that amifostine improved oral mucositis rates (50), but a later meta-analysis with these five studies plus an additional 10 studies concluded that amifostine lacked evidence to support its use to prevent mucositis (109). Given the conflicting evidence and associated treatment toxicities, providers have not adopted amifostine for routine use in head and neck RT patients.

## Supportive Measures

A meta-analysis evaluated six randomized studies of cryotherapy (ice chips) against no treatment or a saline control in patients undergoing chemotherapy and found a small but statistically significant benefit in prevention of mucositis (85). However, none of the studies involved patients undergoing RT.

The same meta-analysis evaluated nine randomized studies that investigated chlorhexidine mouthwash, an antibacterial treatment, in prevention of mucositis. Only one study included patients undergoing head and neck RT, which demonstrated inferior outcomes relative to the control group (110). Overall, no benefit to chlorhexidine was seen in the included studies (85).

A total of 12 randomized studies investigated sucralfate mouthwash, a sucrose sulfate-aluminum complex that buffers acidic solutions, in prevention of mucositis. Over half of the studies involved RT. While overall it appeared that sucralfate mouthwash reduced the incidence of moderate and severe mucositis, only one of the studies that included RT demonstrated a reduction in severe mucositis (85,111).

## Other Pharmacologic and Nonpharmacologic Interventions

In addition to the treatments discussed, which have each been evaluated in multiple studies, there have been numerous agents and therapies investigated to prevent mucositis in a smaller number of randomized studies. A list of pharmacologic interventions studied includes allopurinol, benzydamine mouthwash, granulocyte and granulocyte/macrophage-colony stimulating factors, iseganan mouthwash, pilocarpine, prostaglandin, and polymyxin/tobramycin/amphotericin antibiotic lozenges. A list of nonpharmacologic interventions includes aloe vera, glutamine mouthwash, honey, hydrolytic enzymes, laser treatment, oral care protocols, povidone mouthwash, and zinc (85,112–114).

Of these interventions, some had some evidence of efficacy. In a single study, IV glutamine supplementation decreased mucositis rates and severity in patients undergoing chemoradiotherapy with cisplatin and fluorouracil (5-FU) (115). Honey applied to the oral mucosa before and after daily radiation treatments has also been shown to limit mucositis (116,117). Similarly, low-energy laser therapy appeared effective in preventing severe mucositis (118), although most studies of this treatment modality examined patients receiving chemotherapy. Aloe vera use was associated with less severe mucositis versus placebo in one study (119) but did not impact development of overall mucositis in another study (120). Two small trials studied granulocyte-colony stimulating factor use during RT; while a small benefit was observed, neither study met its primary endpoint (121,122). Similarly, polymyxin/tobramycin/amphotericin antibiotic lozenge use did not prevent the development of severe mucositis, although it reduced *Candida* colonization (123).

None of these interventions have been widely adopted, although glutamine, honey, and laser therapy have some documented benefit with minimal associated toxicity. More robust data is required to confirm that these therapies provide benefit.

## Anemia

The presence of anemia is associated with poorer outcomes in head and neck cancer, perhaps mediated through tumor hypoxia and subsequent increased resistance to cytotoxic therapies. Two randomized trials examined whether erythropoietin, a stimulator of hematopoiesis, improved the tolerance and effectiveness of treatment. Both studies demonstrated that erythropoietin increased hemoglobin levels above that of the control group, but there was evidence of poorer survival in patients treated with erythropoietin (124,125). A similar detrimental effect to erythropoietin was seen in patients with metastatic breast cancer (126), and a meta-analysis concluded that erythropoietin worsened patient survival (127). Due to these findings, the routine use of erythropoietin has been abandoned.

## Xerostomia

Xerostomia, or dry mouth, is a severe complication of RT. It can cause pain, dysphagia, and odynophagia, which are lifelong; odynophagia is a major factor in tooth decay. The adoption of intensity-modulated RT for head and neck cancer has reduced the incidence of late xerostomia, but it remains a significant issue. Some studies to address acute oral mucositis have also assessed the impact of various interventions on preventing acute and late xerostomia without definitive success. Many therapies specifically addressing xerostomia have also been evaluated.

### *Pilocarpine*

Pilocarpine is a cholinergic receptor agonist with mild beta adrenergic activity that stimulates saliva production. Its use has been evaluated in both prevention and treatment of xerostomia. Meta-analyses assessed its impact on mitigation of xerostomia when given concomitantly with RT (128,129). The authors concluded that pilocarpine increased unstimulated salivary flow and improved clinician-rated xerostomia scores, but it did not impact stimulated salivary flow rate or patient-rated quality of life (130–138).

Studies also evaluated pilocarpine's role in treating postradiotherapy xerostomia. A prospective single-arm study found that pilocarpine improved symptoms in patients with severe xerostomia, with 67% of patients reporting a significant relief of symptoms of xerostomia at 12 weeks (139). However, 25% of patients stopped treatment due to side effects of sweating, nausea, and vomiting. Providers often offer pilocarpine to patients with clinically significant postradiotherapy xerostomia, but many patients decline it or discontinue its use owing to its side effects.

### *Pilocarpine Alternatives*

Multiple interventions have subsequently been compared to pilocarpine with the goal of obtaining similar improvement in xerostomia symptoms with fewer side effects. One drug, phenylephrine, appears to protect salivary glands during RT in an animal model by upregulating nicotinamide phosphoribosyltransferase (NAMPT), an enzyme that promotes cell survival (140). Submandibular gland transfer (141), in which salivary gland tissue is relocated from an area of the oral cavity planned to receive high-dose radiation to an area to receive lower dose radiation, was compared to pilocarpine in prevention of xerostomia. The study demonstrated improved unstimulated and stimulated salivary flow in the salivary gland transfer group compared to pilocarpine ($P$ = .003) and was closed early (142). While gland transfer was effective in preventing xerostomia, the need for a surgical procedure has limited adoption of this procedure.

RTOG 05-37 evaluated acupuncture-like transcutaneous nerve stimulation compared to pilocarpine in patients with existing xerostomia. The trial was underpowered and did not observe a difference in symptom burden between the treatments, although side effects (mostly grade 1) were higher in the pilocarpine group (143).

Bethanechol, an analogue of acetylcholine, acts as a sialagogue similar to pilocarpine. Similar to results using pilocarpine, a randomized study found that bethanechol given concurrently with RT had improved unstimulated salivary flow after treatment (144). In a crossover trial comparing bethanechol to pilocarpine to treat postradiotherapy xerostomia, no statistically significant differences were found between the two drugs in either efficacy or side effect profile (145). Cevimeline, another acetylcholine derivative, also proved effective in improving posttreatment xerostomia in a single-arm study, although with similar side effects to pilocarpine (146).

### Miscellaneous Interventions

For prevention of xerostomia, a small randomized study demonstrated benefit of adjuvant hyperbaric oxygen treatment in improving dry mouth up to 18 months after RT (147). Another randomized study showed that intensity-modulated RT was superior to conventional RT with amifostine in preserving parotid function (148).

For treatment of postradiotherapy xerostomia, Oral Balance gel (2% hydroxypropyl methyl-cellulose, lactic acid, sorbitol, xylitol, and methyl/propyl parabens) and Biotene (an enzyme-based product containing mutanase, dextranase, lysozyme, lactoperoxidase, and glucose oxidase) toothpaste benefited patients after 2 weeks of use in a randomized study (149). However, xanthan gum did not improve patients' xerostomia (150).

## Osteoradionecrosis and Late Tissue Injury

Late tissue injury in the head and neck region progresses in the weeks to months following RT. In irradiated regions, reduced tissue vascularity, especially regarding small blood vessels, develops. This causes poor tissue perfusion, impaired healing, and increased infection risk given the relative hypoxia in these areas. Furthermore, fibrotic changes decrease the functionality of the treated area. These injuries affect bones, muscles, and nerves. In the case of osteoradionecrosis, the irradiated bone fails to heal after definitive treatment, leading to devitalized tissue, infection, and pain. Patients are at particular risk for poor healing if they require dental procedures in an area that has received high-dose radiation. In the case of trismus, the muscles of mastication become fibrotic, limiting the range of motion required for eating. In the case of peripheral neuropathy, decreased blood supply and injury to neuronal support cells damages neurons and leads to neurologic deficits. Conservative management of these injuries is often ineffective. Given the role of reduced tissue vascularity and subsequent tissue hypoxia in these injuries, treatments have aimed to improve blood flow and tissue oxygenation.

## *Hyperbaric Oxygen*

Patients undergoing hyperbaric oxygen treatment are placed in a pressurized room or suit in which the air pressure is raised above normal atmospheric pressure. The elevated pressure, commonly maintained at approximately 2 to 2.5 times atmospheric pressure, raises the partial pressure of oxygen in the circulating blood, thereby achieving improved oxygenation of previously hypoxic areas. Treatments last 1 to 2 hours delivered 1 to 2 times daily over 30 to 60 sessions (151). Rabbit models have demonstrated increased vascularity in injured tissues after treatment (152).

A meta-analysis demonstrated a mixed effect from hyperbaric oxygen in osteoradionecrosis depending on the primary endpoint and comparator arm (151). In one study of patients with overt mandibular osteoradionecrosis, all patients received 30 hyperbaric oxygen treatments of 90 minutes at 2.4 times atmospheric pressure over 6 weeks followed by surgery; 68 patients were subsequently randomized to receive an additional 10 treatments or not. There was no difference between the two groups, with 19% of hyperbaric oxygen patients recovered at 1 year versus 32% of placebo patients ($P = .23$) (153). Another study randomized patients to prophylactic hyperbaric oxygen or penicillin prior to undergoing dental procedures and found that hyperbaric oxygen reduced the incidence of osteoradionecrosis relative to penicillin (154). Similarly, hyperbaric oxygen given before and after dental implantation at an irradiated site of the mandible improved the implant function at 6 weeks and 1 year after the procedure compared to no treatment (155).

Regarding soft tissue and nerve injury, hyperbaric oxygen demonstrated improved vascular function in irradiated facial skin and gingival mucosa relative to a control arm at 6 months after treatment, although no clinical symptom endpoint was assessed (156). One study examined the effect of hyperbaric oxygen on brachial plexopathy, with no benefit seen (157).

Overall, hyperbaric oxygen may be effective in treating postradiotherapy tissue injury. It appears effective in preventing complications in patients undergoing dental procedures and may improve soft tissue injury, but it does not appear to benefit patients with overt osteoradionecrosis or nerve injury. Availability of treatment varies greatly due to the specialized equipment required to deliver treatment. Furthermore, treatment is relatively expensive, and the sensation of increased atmospheric pressure is often uncomfortable and may require tympanoplasty (ear tubes). However, providers often offer patients treatment because of few alternative options.

## *Pentoxifylline and Vitamin E*

Pentoxifylline improves tissue blood flow and exerts an anti-inflammatory effect that downregulates mediators of fibrogenesis, as described earlier in the chapter. Some researchers have hypothesized that fibrosis plays as large a role in late tissue injury as does reduced tissue vascularity. In this scenario, pentoxifylline and antioxidants, such as vitamin E, may improve tissue function through reduction in established radiation-induced fibrosis. In nonrandomized studies, one group demonstrated that a pentoxifylline–vitamin E combination with clodronate, a bisphosphonate, improved patients' existing osteoradionecrosis (158), including in those patients refractory to hyperbaric oxygen treatment (159). Another single-arm study showed that pentoxifylline alone taken for 8 weeks increased the dental gap in patients with RT-induced trismus from a mean of 12.5 mm to 16.5 mm ($P$ = .023) (160).

For mitigation of skin and soft tissue fibrosis in patients undergoing head and neck RT, one randomized study of 78 patients examined the use of pentoxifylline, with half receiving 400 mg pentoxifylline three times per day during RT. Of the 40 patients randomized to pentoxifylline, 7 patients required dose reduction or discontinuation due to gastrointestinal symptoms and dizziness. Skin and soft tissue changes did not differ during RT. However, at later than 8 weeks postradiotherapy, soft tissue injury (necrosis, pain, and/or fibrosis) was reduced in the pentoxifylline arm (42% versus 71%, $P$ <.05) (161). While the evidence supporting preventative treatment with pentoxifylline is limited, its effectiveness in treating established osteoradionecrosis and other soft tissue injury is well established.

### Summary

For prevention/mitigation of radiation-induced injury in the head and neck:

- **Palifermin has** randomized evidence documenting its benefit in reducing the severity of mucositis, but some studies did not show benefit, and long-term follow-up to rule out a possible tumor-protective effect is lacking.
- The evidence that **amifostine** reduces mucositis and xerostomia is conflicting, and its use is **not** recommended given its significant treatment toxicity.
- Supportive measures such as **ice chips**, **chlorhexidine mouthwash**, and **sucralfate mouthwash** have **not** demonstrated efficacy in preventing mucositis.
- **Glutamine**, **honey**, and **laser therapy have** evidence supporting their use to prevent mucositis, although the literature is limited and requires further study.
- **Erythropoietin** should **not** be used routinely in patients with anemia.
- The use of **pilocarpine** during and after RT improves baseline salivary flow but does **not** improve patient quality of life related to xerostomia.
- **Submandibular gland transfer can** prevent xerostomia by removing salivary tissue from the radiation field, although this may be less important in the era of intensity-modulated RT.
- A small study suggests that **hyperbaric oxygen can** mitigate RT-induced xerostomia, but more data is required to validate this effect.
- A small study suggests that **pentoxifylline can** prevent late soft tissue damage from head and neck RT, but more data is required.

For treatment of radiation-induced injury in the head and neck:

- **Pilocarpine, bethanechol**, and **cevimeline** effectively treat symptomatic xerostomia; **oral enzyme-based solutions** may also improve symptoms.
- **Hyperbaric oxygen** appears to have benefit in treating soft tissue fibrosis and preventing complications of dental procedures, but it may not help patients with overt osteoradionecrosis.
- **Pentoxifylline +/– vitamin E** improves soft tissue damage as well as osteoradionecrosis.

Recommended reviews are available for those who desire more information (50,85,86,109,128,129,151). Table 10.3 provides a summary of the randomized human prevention/mitigation studies of interest discussed in this section.

## ABDOMEN AND PELVIS

In RT for pelvic cancers, multiple organs are at risk. Acute gastrointestinal mucositis can lead to diarrhea, dehydration, and weight loss. Acute genitourinary toxicity can also have significant effects on patient quality of life and compliance with treatment. After RT, vascular and soft tissue damage may develop in pelvic organs. Radiation enteritis, proctitis, and cystitis can be painful, life threatening, and, on rare occasion, require highly morbid surgical interventions to address. Similarly, sexual and reproductive dysfunction can severely decrease patient quality of life.

The mechanism of radiation injury in the pelvis is multifactorial. Inflammatory signals, which include TGF beta, have been discussed earlier. Vascular dysfunction similarly plays a role. Acute and chronic oxidative stress is another contributing mechanism (162). Radiation-generated reactive oxygen and nitrogen species damage intracellular components and cell membranes, creating a proinflammatory environment and predisposing to radiation-induced late effects. Another mechanism of damage is the Rho/Rho-associated protein kinase (ROCK) pathway (163). Activation of this pathway is associated with intestinal radiation–induced fibrosis. In animal models, statins block this pathway and can improve existing radiation enteropathy (164,165). Radioprotective measures that address these mechanisms of injury have been examined to both mitigate RT-induced side effects and treat them.

### Acute Gastrointestinal Mucositis and Other Acute Effects

The gastrointestinal mucosa consists of rapidly dividing cells that constantly slough off in response to normal physiologic stress. RT damages the mucosal lining and disrupts the enteric microflora, leading to pain, ulceration, nausea, vomiting, diarrhea, and/or constipation. A recent systematic review evaluated the role of multiple agents in preventing gastrointestinal mucositis (166).

#### Probiotics

Multiple studies have assessed the use of probiotics in preventing acute gastrointestinal mucositis (167–169). One study with 190 patients examined concurrent probiotic use with multiple strains of probiotics in patients undergoing pelvic RT, and found that probiotic use reduced grade 3 to 4 diarrhea

*(text continues on page 236)*

## Table 10.3 Head and Neck: Randomized Human Prevention/Mitigation Studies of Interest

| Agent | Study | Patients | Control Arm | Treatment Arm | Results (Primary endpoint(s) in bold) | Comment |
|---|---|---|---|---|---|---|
| Palifermin (88) | Multinational | 188 patients stage III-IVB SCCa of oral cavity or pharynx | 70 Gy in 2-Gy fractions 5 days per week with concurrent cisplatin every 3 weeks x 3c | Control arm plus palifermin 180 mcg/kg IV weekly x 8 weeks starting Friday before initiation of RT | **Gr 3–4 oral mucositis 69% vs 54% ($P = .041$)** Duration of severe OM 26 day vs 5 days ($P = .112$) Days to development of severe OM 35 vs 47 ($P = .157$) No OS difference | Negative study with palifermin used 60 mcg/kg weekly (87) Similar benefit seen in postop patients (89) 35% of palifermin patients had drug toxicity but did not stop therapy |
| Amifostine (97) | Multinational | 132 patients with SCCa of the head and neck | 60–70 Gy in 2-Gy fractions 5 days per week with concurrent carboplatin for 5 days every 4 weeks x 2c | Control arm plus amifostine 300 mg/m² IV daily on treatment days prior to treatment | *Acute* **Gr 2+ xerostomia 34% vs 39% ($P = .715$) Gr 3+ mucositis 22% vs 39% ($P = .055$)** Gr 3+ treatment-related adverse events 20% vs 42% ($P = .008$) *Late* **Gr 2+ xerostomia 24% vs 37% ($P = .235$)** 1 year LRF 27% vs 38% ($P = .218$) | Amifostine can be delivered IV or SQ. Numerous studies with conflicting results. |

*(continued)*

Table 10.3 Head and Neck: Randomized Human Prevention/Mitigation Studies of Interest (*continued*)

| Agent | Study | Patients | Control Arm | Treatment Arm | Results (Primary endpoint(s) in bold) | Comment |
|---|---|---|---|---|---|---|
| Glutamine (115) | Buenos Aires, Argentina | 29 patients with SCCa of the head and neck | Induction cisplatin/5-FU every 3 weeks x 2c with RT starting on day 28 consisting of 70 Gy at 1.5 Gy BID (2 Gy daily on chemotherapy days) over 5 weeks with concurrent weekly cisplatin and 5-FU | Control arm plus L-alanyl-L-glutamine 0.4 g/kg IV on chemotherapy days | **Severe objective mucositis 67% vs 14% ($P = .007$) Gr 4 mucositis 33% vs 0% ($P = .042$)** Maximum pain scores 6.3/10 vs 1.3/10 ($P = .008$) Need for feeding tube 60% vs 14% ($P = .020$) | No transfusion reactions noted |
| Honey (116) | Babol, Iran | 40 patients with SCCa of the head and neck | Head and neck RT 50–60 Gy in daily fractions of 1.8–2 Gy with 20 mL normal saline rinse before and after each treatment | Control arm plus 20 mL honey 15 minutes before, 15 minutes after, and 6 hours after each treatment (instead of saline) | *Acute toxicity week 2, 4, 6 of RT* **Mucositis score 28/27/20 vs 13/11/8 ($P <.001$)** Weight loss lower in honey arm ($P <.001$) | Results consistent with other studies |

(*continued*)

**Table 10.3** Head and Neck: Randomized Human Prevention/Mitigation Studies of Interest (*continued*)

| Agent | Study | Patients | Control Arm | Treatment Arm | Results (Primary endpoint(s) in bold) | Comment |
|---|---|---|---|---|---|---|
| Low-energy laser (118) | Nice, France | 30 patients | Head and neck RT 65 Gy with standard daily fractionation without surgery or chemotherapy | Control arm plus low-energy laser 2 J/cm$^2$ applied to the mucosa before each treatment | **Gr 3 mucositis 35% vs 8% ($P$ <.001)** Mean mucositis grade 2.1 vs 1.7 ($P$ = .01) Mean pain intensity 2.0 vs 1.8 ($P$ = .025) | Results consistent with other studies in setting of chemotherapy-induced mucositis |
| Erythropoietin (124) | RTOG 99-03 | 141 patients with SCCa of the head and neck with Hgb ≤12.5 in women (≤13.5 in men) | 66–72 Gy using standard or accelerated concomitant boost fractionation with or without platinum-based chemotherapy | Control arm plus erythropoietin 40,000 units SQ starting 7 to 10 days before RT; given weekly unless Hgb ≥16 in men (≥14 in women) | No difference in acute or late toxicity **2 year LRPFS 58% vs 50% (NS)** 2 year OS 67% vs 60% (NS) | Dose increased to 60,000 units if Hgb rise <1 g/dL after fourth treatment Results confirmed in additional study (125) |

(*continued*)

Table 10.3 Head and Neck: Randomized Human Prevention/Mitigation Studies of Interest (continued)

| Agent | Study | Patients | Control Arm | Treatment Arm | Results (Primary endpoint(s) in bold) | Comment |
|---|---|---|---|---|---|---|
| Pilocarpine (133,134) | RTOG 97-09 | 213 patients with SCCa of the head and neck with ≥50% of major salivary glands receiving 50 Gy | 60-70 Gy using standard or BID fractionation without chemotherapy | Control arm plus pilocarpine 5 mg PO QID starting with radiation for 3 months | **Unstimulated salivary flow improved at end of RT, 3 months, and 6 months ($P$ = .002, .047, .093 respectively)**<br><br>No difference in QoL at 3 or 6 months | All patients received pilocarpine between 3 and 6 months after start of radiation Numerous studies show limited preventative effect |
| Submandibular gland transfer (142) | Multi-institution, Canada | 120 patients with SCCa of head and neck | Chemoradiotherapy 54-70 Gy with or without preceding surgery. Control arm also received pilocarpine 5 mg PO QID starting with radiation and for 3 months after completion of RT | Submandibular gland transfer to submental area prior to RT instead of pilocarpine | 6 months outcomes:<br>- **Unstimulated salivary flow 0.01 vs 0.04 mL/min ($P$ = .001)**<br>- **Stimulated salivary flow 0.05 vs 0.18 mL/min ($P$ = .003)**<br>- QoL saliva amount and consistency favor SGT ($P$ = .017 and .005, respectively) | Study closed early due to better outcome in gland transfer arm 1 submental recurrence occurred 97 patients evaluable at 6 months |

(continued)

Table 10.3 Head and Neck: Randomized Human Prevention/Mitigation Studies of Interest (*continued*)

| Agent | Study | Patients | Control Arm | Treatment Arm | Results (Primary endpoint(s) in bold) | Comment |
|---|---|---|---|---|---|---|
| Hyperbaric oxygen (147) | Rotterdam, The Netherlands | 19 patients with SCCa of oro- or nasopharynx | Head and neck RT 60–70 Gy using standard fractionation with or without chemotherapy | Control arm plus hyperbaric oxygen 2.5 absolute atmospheres for 90 minutes daily for 30 treatments over 6 weeks starting within 2 days of completing radiation | Improved QoL scores at 3 to 18 months:<br>– **EORTC H&N35 Swallowing** ($P = .009$)<br>– **EORTC H&N35 Dry Mouth** ($P = .0001$)<br>– **EORTC H&N35 Sticky Saliva** ($P = .004$)<br>– **PSS Eating in Public** ($P = .009$)<br>– **Mouth pain visual analogue scale** ($P = .0001$) | Patients treated with HBO seemed to have less severe symptoms at baseline |
| Pentoxifylline (161) | Ankara, Turkey | 78 patients with SCCa of head and neck | Postoperative RT 65–75 Gy over 6 weeks in daily 2–2.2 Gy fractions without chemotherapy | Control arm plus pentoxifylline 400 mg PO TID during RT and for 2 weeks after completion of RT | **No difference in acute toxicity**<br><br>At 8+ weeks post-RT, soft tissue injury (necrosis, pain, and/or fibrosis) 71% vs 42% ($P < .05$)<br>No OS difference at 10 months | 18% required dose reduction or discontinuation due to GI symptoms or dizziness |

5-FU, fluorouracil; BID, twice daily; EORTC H&N35, European Organization for Research and Treatment of Cancer Head and Neck quality of life toxicity scale; Hgb, hemoglobin; LRF, locoregional failure; LRPFS, locoregional progression free survival; OM, oral mucositis; OS, overall survival; QID, four times a day; QoL, quality of life; RT, radiation therapy; SCCa, squamous cell carcinoma; SQ, subcutaneously; TID, three times daily.

relative to the control group (7% versus 29%, $P$ <.001) (167). Another randomized study with 206 patients showed that concurrent *Lactobacillus* use during pelvic RT reduced the number of bowel movements ($P$ <.10) and improved feces consistency ($P$ <.05) relative to the control group (168). In light of the minimal toxicity with probiotic use, its use is recommended during pelvic RT.

## Amifostine

Amifostine, a free-radical scavenger, has demonstrated benefit in preventing acute pelvic toxicity in a meta-analysis (50). A randomized study with 71 patients examined the use of amifostine in patients undergoing pelvic RT for rectal cancer. Moderate or severe late effects were reduced in the amifostine arm (0% versus 14%, $P$ = .03) with no difference in tumor control rates (170). Another study of 205 patients randomized to either amifostine or placebo with pelvic RT demonstrated a reduction in acute grade 2 to 3 bladder and lower gastrointestinal toxicity ($P$ <.05) with no difference in tumor response rates 6 weeks after completion of RT (171). A smaller study of 36 patients obtained rectosigmoidoscopy at the completion of pelvic RT to evaluate for acute rectal mucosal toxicity. Rectal mucositis was more severe in the placebo group compared to the amifostine group ($P$ = .003), and incidence of grade 1+ rectal toxicity was higher in the placebo group (89% versus 11%, $P$ = .002) (172). More recently, amifostine was evaluated in a 45-patient study of extended field RT for cervical cancer in RTOG 01-16. Acute grade 3 to 4 toxicity was similar in the amifostine and control groups (87% versus 81%, statistically nonsignificant) (173).

Despite some evidence of benefit with amifostine, providers rarely use this drug owing to difficulty of administration, treatment side effects, and concern for tumor protection. Endorectal administration of amifostine during prostate external beam RT has been investigated in a small, nonrandomized study of 11 patients and found to be well tolerated (174). Another study evaluated subcutaneous amifostine in patients undergoing high dose rate prostate brachytherapy (175). Limiting exposure to amifostine to short time periods and/or limiting systemic exposure may be a path forward that requires more study to validate its effectiveness.

## Immunosuppressive Agents

Drugs that suppress the body's inflammatory response have been examined to reduce acute gastrointestinal toxicity during pelvic RT. Three randomized studies evaluated mesalazine and olsalazine versus control, and all three studies found that diarrhea was worse in the experimental group versus the control group (176–178). This has led to the recommendation against the use of these drugs during pelvic RT.

## Miscellaneous Interventions

Two randomized studies examined the effect of misoprostol suppositories to prevent acute radiation proctitis. Neither study showed a benefit (179,180).

One study of 229 patients examined the effect of timing of pelvic RT on acute toxicity. Compared to patients treated between 8 a.m. and 10 a.m., patients treated between 6 p.m. and 8 p.m. had decreased grade 3 to 4 diarrhea ($P$ <.05) (181). However, these results are yet to be validated.

## Late Pelvic Organ Damage

RT-induced inflammation, vascular dysfunction, and fibrosis all affect pelvic organs, causing end-organ dysfunction and morbidity. Organs at high risk include the bowel, rectum, and bladder. Sexual dysfunction is discussed separately.

### Statins

Statin drugs act as hydroxymethylglutaryl-CoA (HMG-CoA) reductase inhibitors. HMG-CoA reductase is involved in cholesterol synthesis, and these drugs are primarily used to lower cholesterol. As stated earlier, these drugs also appear to improve endothelial function in vasculature and downregulate profibrotic pathways. Animal models demonstrated the importance of endothelial dysfunction in the development of radiation enteropathy (182), and showed that simvastatin administration before and after RT mitigated radiation enteropathy (183). Additional studies with statins in human cells resulted in reduced endothelial dysfunction after RT (184,185). A retrospective study of patients who underwent pelvic RT analyzed the association of statin and ACE inhibitor usage with acute and late gastrointestinal toxicity. In the population, 16% took statins, 16% took ACE inhibitors, and 7.5% took both classes of drugs during RT. Statin use (with or without ACE inhibitor use) was associated with reduced acute and late toxicity relative to patients who did not use statins ($P = .04$) (186).

A prospective single-arm study treated 53 patients with lovastatin for 1 year starting during prostate RT and evaluated its effect on rectal toxicity. At 2 years of follow-up, 38% had developed a grade 2+ rectal toxicity, with 6% having an unresolved grade 2+ rectal toxicity (187). The authors concluded that there did not appear to be a treatment effect. While no randomized evidence exists on the efficacy of statins in preventing gastrointestinal or other pelvic toxicity and human data is conflicting, their low cost, low side effect profile, and ease of administration make statins a promising candidate for further study.

### Pentoxifylline and Vitamin E

Pentoxifylline and vitamin E have demonstrated benefit in treating established postradiotherapy fibrosis at other sites. One study found that overexpression of cell signals associated with radiation enteropathy was suppressed by pentoxifylline and vitamin E (188,189). An additional study showed that the drug combination suppressed TGF beta and improved gastrointestinal symptoms scores in patients with established radiation enteropathy by roughly 50% over 6 to 12 months in 10 patients ($P <.01$) (190). A small study with 10 patients demonstrated that vitamin E and vitamin C use for 1 year improved chronic rectal bleeding and diarrhea but not rectal pain (191). Another small nonrandomized study of 6 patients demonstrated that pentoxifylline and vitamin E use increased endometrial thickness and uterine arterial blood flow in women who had received childhood radiation (192). Overall, pentoxifylline and vitamin E remain an established intervention to treat late toxicity after pelvic RT, given the evidence supporting its use in other treatment sites.

## Hyperbaric Oxygen

Two meta-analyses have evaluated the effect of hyperbaric oxygen in treating RT-induced pelvic toxicity (151,166). Both concluded that hyperbaric oxygen improved postradiotherapy proctitis. In a large randomized crossover study, 120 patients received hyperbaric oxygen to treat chronic radiation proctitis. The group initially randomized to hyperbaric oxygen demonstrated better response in late toxicity scores compared to the control group (89% versus 63%, $P$ <.001); the differences disappeared after treatment crossover (193). Another randomized study of 65 patients examined the effect of hyperbaric oxygen on proctitis in patients who previously received pelvic RT. Hyperbaric oxygen demonstrated a reduction in side effect severity and improved quality of life relative to the control group (194). A multitude of retrospective studies have similarly reported benefit of hyperbaric oxygen in treating established radiation proctitis (195–200).

The data supporting hyperbaric oxygen treatment for bladder and gynecologic toxicity is less robust. One randomized study with 36 patients compared intravesicular hyaluronic acid instillation versus hyperbaric oxygen in treating RT-induced chronic hemorrhagic cystitis. Both groups showed improvement over baseline scores with no difference seen between the two groups (201). A retrospective study with 18 patients demonstrated improvement of established radiation cystitis with hyperbaric oxygen (202). In patients with pelvic toxicity after RT for gynecologic malignancies, two small retrospective series demonstrated improvement in vaginal fistulas, cystitis, and proctitis with hyperbaric oxygen (203,204). Overall, there does appear to be benefits to hyperbaric oxygen in treating pelvic toxicity after RT.

## Miscellaneous Interventions

A meta-analysis on gastrointestinal toxicity concluded that sucralfate enemas improve symptoms of radiation proctitis in patients with rectal bleeding (166). Older retrospective single-arm studies and case reports support this conclusion (205–207). Sucralfate enemas have not been shown to prevent acute symptoms (208).

One randomized study with 21 patients evaluated the use of endoscopic bipolar electrocoagulation to treat rectal bleeding from chronic radiation-induced telangiectasias. At 12 months, severe bleeding episodes occurred in fewer patients treated with electrocoagulation relative to medical management (33% versus 75%) (209).

## Erectile Dysfunction

Sexual dysfunction after pelvic RT is mediated through multiple mechanisms, which include vascular dysfunction, neuronal injury, and psychological changes. Normally, the release of nitric oxide and synthesis of cyclic guanosine monophosphate (cGMP) causes relaxation of smooth muscle in the corpus cavernosum, leading to the increased blood flow necessary for erection. Commonly used nonpharmacologic interventions for erectile dysfunction include vacuum erection devices (210) and penile prostheses (211). Extracorporeal shockwave therapy may benefit some patients as well

(212,213). Numerous pharmacologic interventions have been studied to prevent and treat RT-induced erectile dysfunction.

### Interventions With Preclinical Data

A recent meta-analysis of RT-induced erectile dysfunction examined the effect of multiple drugs on animal models of erectile dysfunction (214). Adipose-derived stem cells have been used to improve erectile dysfunction in animal models. Arginine and glutamine, precursors to nitric oxide, were found to prevent RT-induced injury to corpus cavernosum tissue in animals (215). Gingko biloba and Korean red ginseng, which also induce nitric oxide production, can increase cavernosal smooth muscle cell relaxation in animal models (216,217). These results demonstrate promise but have not yet been validated in human studies.

### Phosphodiesterase 5 Inhibitors

Phosphodiesterase 5 (PDE5) inhibitors prevent the breakdown of cGMP, thereby improving erectile function (218). Multiple studies have examined PDE5 inhibitor use in preventing RT-induced erectile dysfunction, with conflicting results. A small study randomized 27 patients undergoing prostate RT to receive 6 months of daily sildenafil or placebo. At 6 months, patients treated with sildenafil had improved sexual function scores ($P = .02$), but no difference was seen at the 2-year endpoint (219). A similar study design with 279 patients randomized 2:1 to 6 months of daily sildenafil or placebo showed improved sexual function scores at 1 year with sildenafil compared to placebo ($P = .018$); however, scores were similar at 2 years ($P = .172$) (220). Another large randomized study with 242 patients, RTOG 08-31, demonstrated that 6 months of tadalafil did not alter retention of erectile function 1 month after stopping therapy (79% versus 74%, $P = .49$). Sexual function scores were also similar between the two groups at 1 year (221).

Although PDE5 inhibitors failed to prevent RT-induced erectile dysfunction, studies have demonstrated benefit to their use in treating erectile dysfunction. In a randomized crossover study of 406 patients with erectile dysfunction at least 6 months after completion of prostate RT, daily sildenafil for 6 weeks improved sexual function scores (222). A similar randomized study of 358 patients with daily tadalafil for 6 weeks in patients who had completed RT at least 12 months prior to enrollment also showed a benefit (223). Even in patients previously treated with androgen-deprivation therapy and prostate RT, daily sildenafil for 12 weeks was found to be effective in improving sexual function scores in a randomized crossover study, RTOG 02-15 (224). A randomized study in prostatectomy patients demonstrated that on demand PDE5 inhibitor use worked similarly to daily use (225). Intracavernosal injections or urethral suppository administration of PDE5 inhibitors have also been used. As seen in multiple studies, PDE5 inhibitors are a mainstay of erectile dysfunction treatment after pelvic RT.

### Statins

A meta-analysis on the use of statins to treat existing erectile dysfunction concluded that statins may improve erectile dysfunction (226). However, this meta-analysis did not focus on RT-induced erectile dysfunction. A recently published prospective single-arm study suggested that lovastatin may mitigate the risk of erectile dysfunction when given during prostate RT (227). However, this result requires validation in future studies.

## Summary

For prevention/mitigation of radiation-induced injury in the pelvis:

- **Probiotics can** mitigate the development of RT-associated gastrointestinal mucositis and proctitis.
- Treatments such as **immunosuppressive agents** and **misoprostol** do **not** prevent acute radiation proctitis.
- The evidence supports that **amifostine** reduces acute gastrourinary and gastrointestinal toxicity but systemic use is **not** recommended given its significant treatment toxicity; limiting duration of exposure and/or systemic exposure may provide an avenue for its use, especially in prostate RT.
- **Statins** may help prevent late radiation proctitis and erectile dysfunction, but this has **not** been definitively shown.
- The use of **PDE5 inhibitors** does **not** prevent erectile dysfunction in patients undergoing prostate RT.

For treatment of radiation-induced injury in the pelvis:

- Both **hyperbaric oxygen** and **pentoxifylline +/− vitamin E** improve soft tissue damage from pelvic RT.
- **Sucralfate enemas** and **endoscopic electrocoagulation** can be used to treat radiation symptomatic radiation proctitis.
- **PDE5 inhibitors** successfully treat RT-associated erectile dysfunction; multiple nonpharmacologic measures are also effective.
- Studies to support **statin** use for erectile dysfunction do not include patients treated with pelvic RT.

Recommended reviews are available for those who desire more information (50,151,162,163,166,214,226). Table 10.4 provides a summary of the randomized human prevention/mitigation studies of interest.

## BREAST AND SKIN

RT that is directed to the breast and/or the skin has the potential to cause significant dermatologic side effects. In the acute setting, radiation dermatitis is the most common effect and usually manifests during the second or third week of a standard course of treatment, causing discomfort, pain, and potential skin breakdown, and may require up to 4 weeks to heal after the end of treatment (228). Late effects (ie, those occurring or persisting greater than 12 weeks posttreatment) include radiation-induced fibrosis (RIF), which can cause discomfort, pain, and decreased mobility, and the development of telangiectasias. Lymphedema is of particular concern in patients undergoing radiation to the axillary and supraclavicular lymph nodes. Radioprotective study designs have mainly been aimed at preventing or treating acute dermatitis and RIF.

Table 10.4 Abdomen and Pelvis: Randomized Human Prevention/Mitigation Studies of Interest

| Agent | Study | Patients | Control Arm | Treatment Arm | Results (Primary endpoint(s) in bold) | Comment |
|---|---|---|---|---|---|---|
| Probiotic VSL#3 (450 bn/g *Lactobacillus*, *Bifidobacterium*, and *Streptococcus* strains) (167) | Messina, Italy | 190 patients with colorectal or cervical cancer | Postoperative RT per treating physician | Control arm plus 1 sachet VSL#3 PO TID during RT | **Any diarrhea 55% vs 38%** ($P = .001$) **Gr 3–4 diarrhea 29% vs 7%** ($P = .001$) **Gr 1–2 diarrhea 21% vs 30%** (NS) **Mean daily BMs 12 vs 5** ($P < .05$) | Results consistent with other studies |
| Amifostine (171) | Multi-institution, Greece | 205 patients with pelvic malignancies | Pelvic RT 45 Gy in daily fractions of 1.8–2 Gy followed by a boost to 50–70 Gy | Control arm plus amifostine 340 mg/m² IV prior to each radiation treatment | *Acute toxicity week 3, 5, 7 of RT* **Gr 2–3 bladder toxicity** 4%/22%/33% vs 1%/4%/0% ($P = .195, <.001, .003$ respectively) **Gr 2–3 GI toxicity** 22%/43%/40% vs 6%/11%/0% ($P = .001, <.001, .003$ respectively) *Late* **No difference in late toxicity** No difference in tumor response rates | 3% of amifostine patients with drug toxicity Results consistent with multiple other studies |

*(continued)*

Table 10.4 Abdomen and Pelvis: Randomized Human Prevention/Mitigation Studies of Interest (*continued*)

| Agent | Study | Patients | Control Arm | Treatment Arm | Results (Primary endpoint(s) in bold) | Comment |
|---|---|---|---|---|---|---|
| Tadalafil (221) | RTOG 08-31 | 242 patients stage II prostate cancer | Prostate RT 75–79.2 Gy in daily fractions of 1.8–2 Gy or prostate brachytherapy | Control arm plus tadalafil 5 mg PO daily for 24 weeks starting with RT | Retained erectile function:<br>– **At 28–30 weeks 74% vs 79% ($P = .49$)**<br>– At 52 weeks 71% vs 72% ($P = .93$) | 86% tolerated tadalafil Results consistent with multiple other studies |

BM, bowel movements; bn, billion; GI, gastrointestinal; PO, by mouth; RT, radiation therapy; RTOG, Radiation Therapy Oncology Group; TID, three times daily.

## Radiation Dermatitis

Interventions to prevent and/or manage radiation-induced skin toxicity vary widely among practitioners (229); this is most likely due to the difficultly in determining whether different approaches are effective. The more generally accepted interventions include gentle hygiene measures and the use of moisturizing creams and corticosteroid creams.

### Skin Washing

In a randomized study, 99 women undergoing RT to the breast were randomized to no skin washing versus washing with water and a light moisturizing soap. Acute toxicity was recorded based on the RTOG acute skin toxicity scale. Grade 1, 2, and 3 to 4 toxicity were 41%, 57%, 0% versus 64%, 34%, 2% for the washing versus nonwashing group, respectively. Moist desquamation was significantly decreased from 33% to 14% favoring the washing group (230). In general, it is well accepted to recommend skin washing with light moisturizing soaps. This practice might also aid in preventing skin infections.

### Axillary Deodorant Use

General skin care guidelines for patients undergoing radiation to the breast including the axilla often recommend avoiding the use of axillary deodorant, as it is believed that this could potentiate radiation-induced skin toxicity (231). However, a randomized noninferiority trial comparing the use of daily deodorant versus none reported that grade 2 axillary dermatitis and breast dermatitis was 23% versus 30% and 30% versus 34%, respectively, with no significant difference seen between the two groups. In addition, no grade 3 or 4 skin toxicity was seen in either group (232). A second randomized control trial by Watson et al found that women who used daily antiperspirant compared to those who did not had no significant difference in the severity of the skin reaction or self-reported quality of life (233). The use of axillary deodorant, based on these results, does not appear to affect the severity of radiation-induced skin toxicity, and its routine avoidance should be reconsidered (234).

### Steroidal Creams

A meta-analysis examined five clinical trials that evaluated the use of topical corticosteroids in the prevention of skin dermatitis (235). Boström et al reported the outcomes of 49 women treated with whole breast RT who were randomized to mometasone versus an emollient cream. Creams were applied twice weekly from the beginning of RT until fraction 12 and then daily until 3 weeks after the completion of treatment. Radiation dermatitis was significantly reduced in the steroidal cream group ($P$ = .0033) with no significant change in skin pigmentation (236). The North Central Cancer Treatment Group published results on a phase III double-blind randomized trial of daily topical 0.1% mometasone versus placebo in 176 women undergoing radiation to the breast after breast conserving surgery for breast cancer. The primary endpoint, which was grade of radiation dermatitis determined by the health care provider, showed no difference between the two groups; however, patient-reported outcomes were significantly better in the steroid arm, specifically in the rate of pruritus, burning sensation, and annoyance with skin problems (237). Shukla et al showed significant reduction in the rate of moist desquamation, 13.3% versus 36.7% for patients undergoing postoperative locoregional RT for breast cancer who used beclomethasone during radiation compared to no topical intervention, respectively (238). Another group reported on a randomized double-blind trial of topical methylprednisolone versus dexpanthenol in patients undergoing fractionated radiation for breast cancer. Outcomes were compared to a preliminary cohort of untreated patients. Both interventions failed to prevent radiation dermatitis although both delayed the onset of dermatitis by about 2 weeks (239).

More recently Ulff et al published the results of a randomized double-blind trial on patients undergoing breast irradiation who were randomized to betamethasone plus an emollient cream, or an emollient cream alone. The use of the cream started on day 1 of radiation, continued daily and ended 2 weeks after the end of treatment. They showed a statistically significant reduction in acute radiation dermatitis as measured by the RTOG clinical scoring scale for the group that included the steroidal cream ($P = .05$). Patients who benefited the most were those who had undergone a mastectomy or RT to the axilla and supraclavicular region (240).

These studies appear to show the effectiveness of steroidal cream in the prevention, delay, and reduction in severity of radiation dermatitis related to breast radiation. However, its use should be individualized, based on which patients are more likely to develop severe dermatitis, such as those undergoing chest wall and axillary irradiation.

### *Curcumin*

Curcumin, a potent antioxidant and a component of turmeric, has proven useful in the treatment of several skin ailments including eczema, and as an aid in the repair of dermal wounds (241–244). Results from a randomized double-blind, placebo-controlled trial from the University of Rochester reported on 30 women undergoing radiation to the breast who took either 6 g of curcumin orally or placebo. This trial showed a significant reduction in the radiation dermatitis severity score index, 2.6 versus 3.4, favoring curcumin ($P = .008$) (245). Although these findings are encouraging, the use of curcumin as a standard to prevent radiation dermatitis still needs to be addressed in larger clinical trials.

### *Moisturizing Lotions*

The use of different nonsteroidal topical creams such as aloe vera, Biafine, and hyaluronidase-based as well as urea-based creams, in the treatment, prevention, and symptomatic relief of radiation-induced skin dermatitis has been the subject of many randomized trials with ambiguous findings (235).

Aloe vera use was examined in two randomized studies. In a small study, aloe vera use in addition to mild soap was superior to mild soap alone in preventing radiation dermatitis if patients received more than 27 Gy, but the results were not statistically significant (246). Aloe vera was found to be inferior to aqueous creams in reducing dry desquamation in a larger study (247). Similarly, various creams such as Biafine and trolamine creams were not found to be superior to aqueous creams such as Aquaphor in preventing dermatitis in patients undergoing breast (248) or head and neck irradiation (249). Sucralfate-based creams also did not show a benefit compared to aqueous cream (250). It was hypothesized that hyaluronic acid could accelerate skin healing from radiation, but a randomized study found that dermatitis was worse in patients using hyaluronic acid instead of petroleum jelly (251).

Other proprietary products have been developed and tested for efficacy in preventing radiation dermatitis. However, data supporting these products is very limited. Overall, aqueous creams have demonstrated benefit when compared to no intervention in limiting the extent of radiation dermatitis, but there is no evidence that one cream is superior to another.

## Radiation-Induced Fibrosis

Similar to other fibrosis-related sequelae, RIF is characterized by nonspecific changes within the connective tissue, which include elevated deposits of extracellular matrix as well as an increased fibroblastic activity. This can lead to poor cosmesis, restrictions in functionality, as well as pain. Initially thought to be irreversible, there are now several randomized studies showing improvement with combination of pentoxifylline and alpha-tocopherol (vitamin E). Other drugs, such as superoxide dismutase mimetics (252–255) and statins (256), have been tested with limited benefit.

### *Pentoxifylline and Vitamin E*

A methylxanthine derivate, pentoxifylline is a competitive nonselective phosphodiesterase inhibitor known to improve blood viscosity by decreasing platelet aggregation and improving red blood cell deformability (257). Preclinical studies on pig models showed that a combination of this drug with vitamin E, a potent antioxidant located primarily in the cellular membrane that protects it from oxidative stress, provided significant regression of subcutaneous fibrotic scarring induced by gamma rays (258). That same group reported on 43 patients with RIF after radiation to the head and neck or breast around 8 years posttreatment who underwent a course of pentoxifylline at 800 mg/day and vitamin E 1000 IU/day for 6 or more months, showed a striking reduction of RIF by 22%, 35%, and 48% at 3, 6, and 12 months, respectively (259). This led to the conduct of a randomized, placebo-controlled study of 24 women with 29 areas of measurable RIF after radiation for breast cancer. Randomization included pentoxifylline + vitamin E, pentoxifylline + placebo, vitamin E + placebo, or placebo + placebo. The primary endpoint was regression of measurable RIF after 6 months of treatment assessed by ultrasonography and associated symptom measurements. There was a significant mean RIF surface regression of 60% in the pentoxifylline/vitamin E group compared to 46% in the double placebo group. No statistical significance was found when all four groups were compared, although there was a trend toward significance for the pentoxifylline/vitamin E group (260). A phase II clinical trial by Haddad et al using the same regimen on 34 sites of RIF showed significant reduction in the surface area of RIF of 43% and 72% at 3 and 6 months, respectively (261).

While pentoxifylline has proven benefit in treating existing RIF, it is not clear whether its use can prevent the development of fibrosis. A phase II study randomized patients to pentoxifylline 400 mg and vitamin E 100 mg every 8 hours or placebo for 12 months starting 1 to 3 months after breast RT, and examined the rate of passive abduction of the shoulder as primary endpoint and difference in arm volumes as a secondary outcome. These investigators found no significant difference among the groups for shoulder abduction, but a significant decrease in the rate of arm volume increase, 1.04% versus 0.5% in the placebo and pentoxifylline/vitamin E groups, respectively (262). Earlier studies out of the United Kingdom failed to show any benefit of this regimen on the rate of lymphedema (263), and similarly did not find benefit to adjuvant hyperbaric oxygen (264). More recently, the group from the University of Iowa published the results of 53 women undergoing radiation for breast cancer who were randomized to pentoxifylline and vitamin E 400 mg every 8 hours and 400 IU daily, respectively, versus standard follow-up for 6 months after RT. Tissue compliance measurements (TCM) were obtained at 18 months and compared to the nonirradiated breast. The mean difference in TCM was 0.88 mm and 2.10 mm for the pentoxifylline/vitamin E arm and standard follow-up, respectively, with the differences reaching statistical significance (265). In summary, the evidence suggests that pentoxifylline and vitamin E might help improve the severity of RIF once it has been established. However, its role in preventing RIF and other potential side effects such as lymphedema and shoulder abduction is not clear.

## Summary

For prevention/mitigation of radiation-induced dermatitis and fibrosis:

- **Skin washing has** evidence of benefit in preventing acute radiation dermatitis.
- Studies do **not** support avoidance of **axillary deodorants** during breast RT.
- Use of **steroidal creams can** lessen the severity of radiation dermatitis, although its use is most validated in patients at high risk of toxicity.
- **Curcumin** use **has** shown improvement in dermatitis rates, although more data is needed.
- The use of **aqueous creams has** evidence of benefit in limiting the severity of radiation dermatitis, although no product has demonstrated superiority over others.
- **Pentoxifylline** and **vitamin E has** demonstrated benefit in preventing radiation-induced fibrosis, although studies have reported mixed results.

For treatment of radiation-induced fibrosis:

- **Pentoxifylline** and **vitamin E** is the mainstay of treatment for radiation-induced fibrosis.

Recommended reviews are available for those who desire more information (234,235). Table 10.5 provides a summary of the randomized human prevention/mitigation studies of interest discussed in this section.

**Table 10.5 Breast and Skin: Randomized Human Prevention/Mitigation Studies of Interest**

| Agent | Study | Patients | Control Arm | Treatment Arm | Results (Primary endpoint(s) in bold) | Comment |
|---|---|---|---|---|---|---|
| Aluminum-based antiperspirant (233) | Calgary, Canada | 198 patients stage 0–II breast cancer | 42.5–50 Gy in 16–25 daily fractions whole breast radiation | Control arm plus aluminum-based antiperspirant topically applied to the axilla once daily during RT | *Week 3, last RT week, 2 weeks after RT* **Gr 2+ skin toxicity 6%/40%/26% vs 8%/40%/25%** (NS) | No axillary directed RT administered Results consistent with other studies |
| Steroid cream (237) | N06C4 | 176 patients with localized breast cancer | 50+ Gy in daily fractions whole breast/chest wall radiation with or without regional nodal radiation | Control arm plus 3 mL 0.1% mometasone furoate cream applied daily to the breast/chest skin during RT | **Mean maximum grade acute dermatitis 1.3 vs 1.2 ($P = .18$)** Gr 2+ pruritus 23% vs 18% ($P = .005$) Patient-reported outcomes showed less symptoms with mometasone ($P < .05$) | Patients were advised to have at least a 4-hour interval between application of cream and radiation treatment Results consistent with other studies |

*(continued)*

**Table 10.5** Breast and Skin: Randomized Human Prevention/Mitigation Studies of Interest (continued)

| Agent | Study | Patients | Control Arm | Treatment Arm | Results (Primary endpoint(s) in bold) | Comment |
|---|---|---|---|---|---|---|
| Curcumin (245) | New York, USA | 30 patients with localized breast cancer | 42+ Gy in daily fractions whole breast radiation | Control arm plus curcumin 2 g PO TID during RT | **Mean end of treatment grade dermatitis 3.4 vs 2.6 ($P = .008$)** **Moist desquamation 88% vs 29% ($P = .002$)** No difference MPQ-SF (patient reported) | No curcumin-related toxicity reported |
| Aloe vera (246) | Florida, USA | 73 patients receiving RT with expected skin reaction | Gentle soap cleansing to the irradiated area | Control arm plus aloe vera gel applied to the irradiated area 6–8 times per day | *Dose above 27 Gy* Erythema 81% vs 50% ($P = .076$) Texture change 24% vs 20% ($P = .813$) Itch 5% vs 0% ($P = .483$) Tanning 43% vs 40% ($P = .880$) *Dose below 27 Gy* Erythema 69% vs 86% ($P = .189$) Texture change 0% vs 32% ($P = .012$) Itch 0% vs 18% ($P = .071$) Tanning 43% vs 32% ($P = .452$) | Benefit only seen in patients receiving over 27 Gy Other studies do not show a difference between various aqueous creams |

*(continued)*

Table 10.5 Breast and Skin: Randomized Human Prevention/Mitigation Studies of Interest *(continued)*

| Agent | Study | Patients | Control Arm | Treatment Arm | Results (Primary endpoint(s) in bold) | Comment |
|---|---|---|---|---|---|---|
| Pentoxifylline + vitamin E (265) | Iowa, USA | 53 patients with localized breast cancer | 46.8–50.4 Gy in daily fractions of 1.8 Gy whole breast/chest wall radiation followed by a 10 Gy boost | Control arm plus pentoxifylline 400 mg PO TID and vitamin E 400 IU PO daily for 6 months following completion of RT | **Difference in TCM between treated and untreated breast at 18 months 2.4 mm vs 1.0 mm ($P = .0478$)**<br><br>No difference in physician-reported late toxicity | Another study demonstrated improvement in arm circumference with adjuvant treatment (262) |

MPQ-SF, McGill pain questionnaire-short form; PO, by mouth; RT, radiation therapy; TCM, tissue compliance measurements; TID, three times daily.

## PERIPHERAL NEUROPATHY

Much care is taken in RT planning to minimize dose to the spinal cord, given the potentially devastating effects of myelopathy. Peripheral nerves are felt to be more radioresistant, but little is known about the pathophysiology of peripheral nerve injury. A review summarized possible mechanisms, including compression by radiation-induced soft tissue fibrosis, vascular dysfunction, and direct neuronal damage (266). Steroids can be used to limit neuronal damage from inflammatory effects, but few interventions have been tested to treat RT-induced peripheral neuropathy (26).

### Pentoxifylline, Vitamin E, and Clodronate

Pentoxifylline and vitamin E have been shown to improve vascular flow and reduce fibrosis in irradiated tissue. Clodronate, a bisphosphonate, also inhibits macrophagic myelin nerve destruction in animal models (26). In two patients with lumbosacral polyradiculopathy after RT, pentoxifylline, vitamin E, and clodronate improved sensorimotor symptoms (267). Further evaluation of this treatment in a larger patient cohort is planned.

### Other Interventions

Hyperbaric oxygen has been used to treat radiation-induced brachial plexopathy. A randomized study did not show significant improvement in neurologic symptoms relative to the control group (157). Additional series have similarly not demonstrated significant benefit with hyperbaric oxygen (266).

Given the role that vascular damage and subsequent ischemia may play in neuronal injury, anticoagulation has been used. In one case report, treatment with acenocoumarol for 3 months improved nerve conduction in a patient with brachial plexopathy (268).

### Summary

For prevention/mitigation of radiation-induced peripheral neuropathy:

- No intervention has been evaluated in humans to prevent/mitigate peripheral neuropathy.

For treatment of radiation-induced injury peripheral neuropathy:

- The combination of **pentoxifylline**, **vitamin E**, and **clodronate** is a viable treatment option with the largest extent of supporting literature and a favorable side effect profile.
- Use of **hyperbaric oxygen** was not shown to be effective in treating peripheral neuropathy.
- **Anticoagulants** may improve symptoms of peripheral neuropathy, although no randomized studies have evaluated its use.

Recommended reviews are available for those who desire more information (26,266).

## TOTAL BODY IRRADIATION

Since the first nuclear weapons were used in 1945, there has been extensive research in protecting soldiers and civilians from a nuclear attack. Similarly, people involved in radiation accidents can receive total body exposure. There are distinct acute radiation syndromes that develop after total body exposure (269,270). First is the hematopoietic syndrome, in which bone marrow production is temporarily halted by the death of hematopoietic stem cells, causing anemia, neutropenia, and thrombocytopenia; this can be caused by exposures lower than 1 Gy but becomes clinically relevant at doses between 2 and 6 Gy. Second is the gastrointestinal syndrome, in which death of the rapidly dividing gastrointestinal mucosal stem cells leads to fluid and electrolyte imbalances, bleeding, and infection; these effects become relevant at exposures between 6 and 8 Gy. Third is the cerebrovascular syndrome, in which damage to endothelial tissue leads to cerebral edema and inevitably death; this effect predominates at exposure above 8 Gy. The total body radiation dose exposure for humans that causes death at 60 days in half of patients (LD50) is 4.5 Gy (271). Interventions seek to increase the LD50, and improve the chances of surviving total body exposure, through drug administration either before or after radiation exposure (270–273).

### Hematopoietic Growth Factors

The Centers for Disease Control and Prevention (CDC) in the United States stockpiles multiple drugs for treatment of acute radiation syndrome. Filgrastim and pegfilgrastim, both granulocyte colony stimulating factors (G-CSFs), have demonstrated efficacy in animal models. Daily filgrastim reduced 60-day mortality to 7.5 Gy total body exposure compared to the control group (21% versus 59%, $P$ <.004) (274). Pegfilgrastim given at day 1 and day 7 postexposure similarly improved neutrophil recovery relative to controls (275). Based on these results, a World Health Organization consensus statement supported its use as a radiation countermeasure (276). Sargramostim, a granulocyte-macrophage colony stimulating factor (GM-CSF), is also stockpiled. Erythropoietin can also be administered, although the recommendation for its use was not as strong as for filgrastim.

Other growth factors have been examined in animal studies. Myelopoietin, an IL-3 and G-CSF agonist, improved hematopoietic recovery (277), but was not as effective as G-CSF itself in human patients undergoing chemotherapy (278). IL-12, a proinflammatory cytokine, reduced the incidence of severe neutropenia and improved 60-day survival in a randomized animal study (279). Thrombopoietin, a stimulator of platelet production, has been examined alone and in combination with IL-11, another stimulator of thrombopoiesis, and found to promote survival in preclinical models (280,281). Insulin-like growth factor 1 (IGF-1) reduced the severity of hematopoietic damage from radiation in an animal study (282). Fibroblast growth factor mimetics have demonstrated efficacy as well (283). To date, these interventions have not received consensus acceptance in treating the hematopoietic syndrome.

## Repurposed Treatments

Many drugs in common use may mitigate radiation injury. ACE inhibitors administered after total body irradiation prevented multiorgan injury in multiple animal studies (284,285). Studies specifically examining the use of ACE inhibitors for prevention of radiation-induced renal injury similarly showed benefit in animal models (286–288). In a randomized study of 55 patients undergoing total body irradiation as part of stem cell transplant conditioning, captopril use for 1 year after neutrophil engraftment improved glomerular filtration rates and serum creatinine levels (86 and 0.95 versus 77 and 1.10, respectively) (289), although the benefit did not reach statistical significance. Long-term follow-up demonstrated that patients in the captopril arm had lower rates of chronic renal failure, pulmonary mortality, and death from any cause (290), although again the differences did not reach statistical significance.

In addition to ACE inhibitors, statins have been evaluated to mitigate radiation injury. Lovastatin has been evaluated in an animal model of total body irradiation, which demonstrated that the drug did not prevent DNA damage but reduced subsequent activation of proinflammatory and profibrotic pathways (291). Overall, ACE inhibitors have promise as an avenue for mitigating multiorgan radiation injury that can be seen after total body irradiation given their availability, low cost, and favorable side effect profile.

## Gastrointestinal Radiation Syndrome Countermeasures

Palifermin, a keratinocyte growth factor, promoted intestinal mucosal recovery after RT in an animal model (292), and it has proven safe in humans (88,89). Pasireotide, a somatostatin analogue, mitigated RT-induced gastrointestinal damage by preventing release of exocrine pancreatic enzymes into the vulnerable bowel lumen (293,294). Anti-ceramide antibodies, which prevent ceramide-induced endothelial cell apoptosis in the intestinal mucosa, protected animals from the gastrointestinal radiation syndrome (295). Beclomethasone, a corticosteroid, has also shown benefit in an animal model. Although no treatment has definitively demonstrated benefit in gastrointestinal radiation syndrome, these novel treatments warrant further investigation.

## Miscellaneous Radiation Syndrome–Preventing Agents

Once radiation damage has occurred, it can be very difficult to treat. Many agents have been administered prior to radiation injury to evaluate if they can prevent radiation injury or lessen the extent of injury. Amifostine administered prior to radiation exposure protected against radiation injury in animal models (296). One study evaluated whether melanin, a natural pigment that can absorb external radiation, conjugated to silica nanoparticles that honed to bone marrow, could protect against radiation injury. In an animal model, the melanin-coated nanoparticles administered prior to exposure reduced radiation-induced hematologic toxicity (297). Another study examined phenylbutyrate, a histone deacetylase inhibitor, in preventing radiation injury. Animals treated with phenylbutyrate prior to radiation exposure had decreased DNA damage and radiation-induced apoptosis in peripheral leukocytes, as well as increased neutrophil and platelet levels (298). Lastly, a thrombopoietin receptor agonist given prior to radiation exposure improved megakaryocyte development and survival in an animal model (299). While amifostine has largely been abandoned as a radioprotector due to its side effects, these other agents are promising avenues of research in preventing or mitigating radiation injury.

### Miscellaneous Radiation Syndrome–Mitigating Agents

Numerous other measures have been examined. Superoxide dismutases have improved survival after radiation exposure in animal models (300–302). The toll-like receptor (TLR) 5 agonist entolimod/flagellin appears to protect against radiation exposure (303). TLR2 and TLR6 agonists have also been studied. Other interventions with published animal data include 5-androstenedione (a steroid that promotes hematopoietic survival by inducing G-CSF) (304), recilisib (an agent that upregulates the PI3K/AKT pathways) (305), flk2/flt3 ligand (306), ciprofloxacin (a fluoroquinolone antibiotic) (307), melatonin (308,309), and curcumin (310). Other interventions with more limited data include genistein (a soy-derived isoflavone), vitamin E derivatives, ARA 290 (an immune system modulator), and Rx100 (an antiapoptotic agent) (271).

### Endocrine Effects

In addition to the immediate damage of irradiation, heavy particles emitted in a potential nuclear reactor meltdown such as iodine and cesium can be taken up in the body, causing damage. Indeed, thyroid cancer is a major concern after such events (311). Iodine loading with potassium iodide pills can saturate the thyroid gland and limit uptake of radioactive iodine in the thyroid. In addition, methimazole has been shown to reduce DNA damage from external irradiation in thyroid cells (312). In the case of cesium, the body incorporates it into bone similar to calcium. To date, no interventions have proven successful in limiting this process.

### Summary

For prevention/mitigation of total body irradiation–induced toxicity:

- Measures including **G-CSF** and to a lesser extent **erythropoietin have** gained acceptance in mitigating the hematopoietic syndrome in acute radiation injury.
- **Sargramostim**, a GM-CSF, **has** been stockpiled by the CDC to treat acute radiation injury.
- The ACE inhibitor **captopril has** demonstrated benefit in mitigating pulmonary and renal injury after total body irradiation for stem cell transplant, but the benefit did not reach statistical significance and requires further validation.
- **Iodine loading** and **methimazole can** reduce thyroid injury from radioactive iodine exposure or total body irradiation, although data is limited.
- Numerous measures for prevention or mitigation of acute radiation injury remain in different stages of development.

## Table 10.6 Total Body Irradiation: Randomized Human Prevention/Mitigation Studies of Interest

| Agent | Study | Patients | Control Arm | Treatment Arm | Results (Primary endpoint(s) in bold) | Comment |
|---|---|---|---|---|---|---|
| Captopril (289,290) | Milwaukee, USA | 55 patients with a hematologic malignancy undergoing stem cell transplant | Total body irradiation 14 Gy in 9 fractions over 3 days with at least 4 hours between fractions with shielding to limit kidney dose to 9.8 Gy and lung dose to 5–7 Gy | Control arm plus captopril 6.25 mg BID (escalated to 25 mg TID if tolerated) starting after neutrophil engraftment for 1 year | *1 year*<br>**Serum creatinine 1.10 vs 0.95** ($P = .2$)<br>**GFR 77 vs 86 ($P = .07$)**<br>GFR if took drug >2 months 80 vs 92 ($P = .1$)<br><br>*4 year*<br>Chronic renal failure 17% vs 11% ($P > .2$)<br>Pulmonary mortality 26% vs 11% ($P = .15$)<br><br>8 year OS 22% vs 37% ($P = .26$)<br>No difference in relapse rates<br>No difference in PFT values | Average time on drug was 2 months; only 20% of patients took full year of drug |

BID, twice daily; GFR, glomerular filtration rate; OS, overall survival; PFT, pulmonary function testing; TID, three times daily.

For treatment of total body irradiation–induced toxicity:

- **Bone marrow transplant** has been attempted in certain cases of acute radiation injury.

Recommended reviews are available for those who desire more information (270–273). Table 10.6 provides a summary of the randomized human prevention/mitigation studies of interest discussed in this section.

## CONCLUSION

Despite improvements in RT delivery that enable providers to better spare critical normal structures for high-dose RT, radiation-induced normal tissue injury remains a significant issue affecting numerous patients (Figure 10.1). Much has been learned regarding the mechanisms of radiation injury of normal tissue, with radioprotective measures developed to prevent/mitigate these effects (Figure 10.2). However, radiation injury is multifactorial

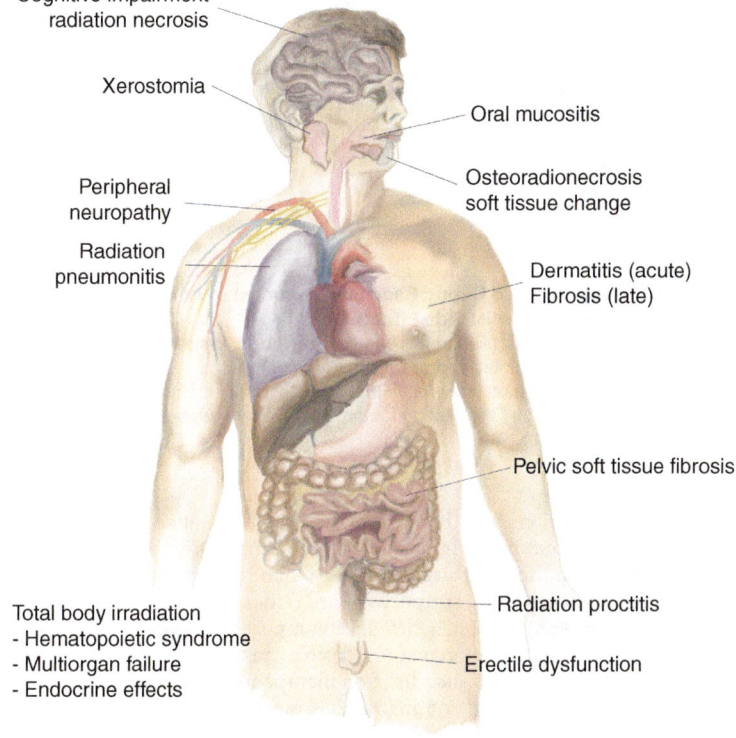

**Figure 10.1** Radiation-Induced Side Effects.

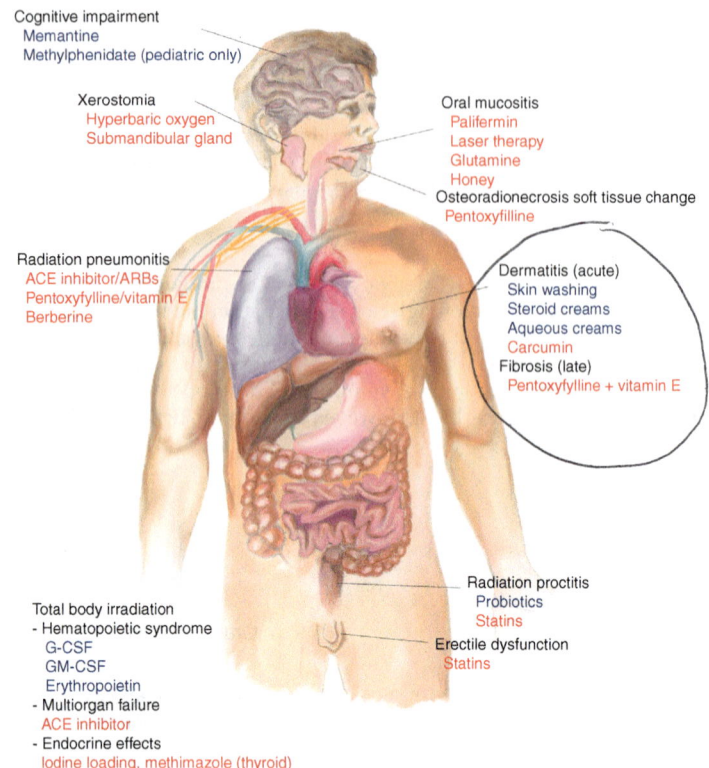

**Figure 10.2 Agents Used During Radiation Treatment or Adjuvantly to Prevent or Mitigate Potential Side Effects.**
*Note:* Blue labels: well-established treatments; Red labels: benefits have been demonstrated in small studies and/or data is conflicting.
ACE, angiotensin-converting enzyme; ARBs, angiotensin II receptor blockers; G-CSF, granulocyte colony stimulating factor; GM-CSF, granulocyte-macrophage colony stimulating factor.

and most interventions have had only a modest, if any, effect on preventing or mitigating normal tissue injury. In addition, many treatments have created concern for a tumor protective effect. Often the most successful treatments have been improved supportive care rather than a targeted therapy. In the case of treating established radiation injury, many options are available, although some toxicity remains refractory to treatment (Figure 10.3).

Additional studies may shed light on therapeutic targets and treatments that prevent/mitigate radiation injury. Existing agents in clinical use, such as ACE inhibitors and statins, represent promising avenues of investigation given their safety profile and ubiquity. In the future, we look forward to seeing further progress in radioprotection.

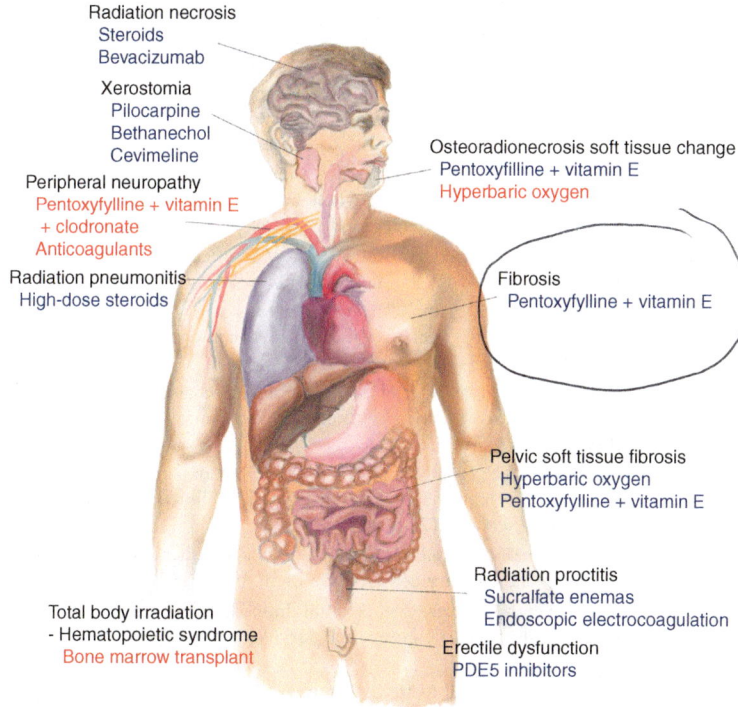

**Figure 10.3 Treatments for Radiation-Induced Side Effects.**
*Note:* Blue labels: well-established treatments; Red labels: benefits have been demonstrated in small studies and/or data is conflicting.
PDE5, phosphodiesterase type 5.

# REFERENCES

1. De Angelis R, Sant M, Coleman MP, et al. Cancer survival in Europe 1999–2007 by country and age: results of EUROCARE-5—a population-based study. *Lancet Oncol.* 2014;15:23–34.

2. de Moor JS, Mariotto AB, Parry C, et al. Cancer survivors in the United States: prevalence across the survivorship trajectory and implications for care. *Cancer Epidemiol Biomarkers Prev.* 2013;22:561–570.`

3. Siegel RL, Miller KD, Jemal A. Cancer statistics, 2016. *CA Cancer J Clin.* 2016;66: 7–30.

4. Belka C, Budach W, Kortmann RD, Bamberg M. Radiation induced CNS toxicity—molecular and cellular mechanisms. *Br J Cancer.* 2001;85: 1233–1239.

5. Kim JH, Brown SL, Jenrow KA, Ryu S. Mechanisms of radiation-induced brain toxicity and implications for future clinical trials. *J Neurooncol.* 2008;87:279–286.

6. Orgogozo JM, Rigaud AS, Stoffler A, et al. Efficacy and safety of memantine in patients with mild to moderate vascular dementia: a randomized, placebo-controlled trial (MMM 300). *Stroke*. 2002;33:1834–1839.

7. Wilcock G, Mobius HJ, Stoffler A. A double-blind, placebo-controlled multicentre study of memantine in mild to moderate vascular dementia (MMM500). *Int Clin Psychopharmacol*. 2002;17:297–305.

8. Brown PD, Pugh S, Laack NN, et al. Memantine for the prevention of cognitive dysfunction in patients receiving whole-brain radiotherapy: a randomized, double-blind, placebo-controlled trial. *Neuro Oncol*. 2013;15:1429–1437.

9. Dimberg Y, Vazquez M, Soderstrom S, Ebendal T. Effects of X-irradiation on nerve growth factor in the developing mouse brain. *Toxicol Lett*. 1997;90:35–43.

10. Shaw EG, Rosdhal R, D'Agostino RB, et al. Phase II study of donepezil in irradiated brain tumor patients: effect on cognitive function, mood, and quality of life. *J Clin Oncol*. 2006;24:1415–1420.

11. Rapp SR, Case LD, Peiffer A, et al. Donepezil for irradiated brain tumor survivors: a phase III randomized placebo-controlled clinical trial. *J Clin Oncol*. 2015;33:1653–1659.

12. DeLong R, Friedman H, Friedman N, et al. Methylphenidate in neuropsychological sequelae of radiotherapy and chemotherapy of childhood brain tumors and leukemia. *J Child Neurol*. 1992;7:462–463.

13. Torres CF, Korones DN, Palumbo D, et al. Effect of methylphenidate in the postradiation attention and memory deficits in children. *Ann Neurol*. 1996;40:331–332.

14. Thompson SJ, Leigh L, Christensen R, et al. Immediate neurocognitive effects of methylphenidate on learning-impaired survivors of childhood cancer. *J Clin Oncol*. 2001;19:1802–1808.

15. Conklin HM, Reddick WE, Ashford J, et al. Long-term efficacy of methylphenidate in enhancing attention regulation, social skills, and academic abilities of childhood cancer survivors. *J Clin Oncol*. 2010;28:4465–4472.

16. Butler JM, Jr, Case LD, Atkins J, et al. A phase III, double-blind, placebo-controlled prospective randomized clinical trial of d-threo-methylphenidate HCl in brain tumor patients receiving radiation therapy. *Int J Radiat Oncol Biol Phys*. 2007;69:1496–1501.

17. Lawrence YR, Li XA, el Naqa I, et al. Radiation dose-volume effects in the brain. *Int J Radiat Oncol Biol Phys*. 2010;76:S20–S27.

18. Liu W, Ahmad SA, Reinmuth N, et al. Endothelial cell survival and apoptosis in the tumor vasculature. *Apoptosis*. 2000;5:323–328.

19. van Bruggen N, Thibodeaux H, Palmer JT, et al. VEGF antagonism reduces edema formation and tissue damage after ischemia/reperfusion injury in the mouse brain. *J Clin Invest*. 1999;104:1613–16120.

20. Gonzalez J, Kumar AJ, Conrad CA, Levin VA. Effect of bevacizumab on radiation necrosis of the brain. *Int J Radiat Oncol Biol Phys*. 2007;67:323–326.

21. Wang Y, Pan L, Sheng X, et al. Reversal of cerebral radiation necrosis with bevacizumab treatment in 17 Chinese patients. *Eur J Med Res*. 2012;17:25. doi:10.1186/2047-783X-17-25

22. Boothe D, Young R, Yamada Y, et al. Bevacizumab as a treatment for radiation necrosis of brain metastases post stereotactic radiosurgery. *Neuro Oncol*. 2013;15:1257–1263.

23. Levin VA, Bidaut L, Hou P, et al. Randomized double-blind placebo-controlled trial of bevacizumab therapy for radiation necrosis of the central nervous system. *Int J Radiat Oncol Biol Phys*. 2011;79:1487–1495.

24. Dye NB, Gondi V, Mehta MP. Strategies for preservation of memory function in patients with brain metastases. *Chin Clin Oncol*. 2015;4:24. doi:10.3978/j.issn.2304-3865.2015.05.05

25. Attia A, Page BR, Lesser GJ, Chan M. Treatment of radiation-induced cognitive decline. *Curr Treat Options Oncol*. 2014;15:539–550.

26. Delanian S, Lefaix J-L. Current management for late normal tissue injury: radiation-induced fibrosis and necrosis. *Semin Radiat Oncol*. 2007;17:99–107.

27. Castellino RA, Glatstein E, Turbow MM, et al. Latent radiation injury of lungs or heart activated by steroid withdrawal. *Ann Intern Med*. 1974;80:593–599.

28. Movsas B, Raffin TA, Epstein AH, Link CJ, Jr. Pulmonary radiation injury. *Chest*. 1997;111:1061–1076.

29. Graves PR, Siddiqui F, Anscher MS, Movsas B. Radiation pulmonary toxicity: from mechanisms to management. *Semin Radiat Oncol*. 2010;20:201–207.

30. Robb WB, Condron C, Moriarty M, et al. Taurine attenuates radiation-induced lung fibrosis in C57/Bl6 fibrosis prone mice. *Ir J Med Sci*. 2010;179:99–105.

31. Para AE, Bezjak A, Yeung IW, et al. Effects of genistein following fractionated lung irradiation in mice. *Radiother Oncol*. 2009;92:500–510.

32. Lee JC, Krochak R, Blouin A, et al. Dietary flaxseed prevents radiation-induced oxidative lung damage, inflammation and fibrosis in a mouse model of thoracic radiation injury. *Cancer Biol Ther*. 2009;8:47–53.

33. Colon J, Herrera L, Smith J, et al. Protection from radiation-induced pneumonitis using cerium oxide nanoparticles. *Nanomedicine*. 2009;5:225–231.

34. Epperly MW, Bray JA, Krager S, et al. Intratracheal injection of adenovirus containing the human MnSOD transgene protects athymic nude mice from irradiation-induced organizing alveolitis. *Int J Radiat Oncol Biol Phys*. 1999;43:169–81.

35. Greenberger JS, Epperly MW, Gretton J, et al. Radioprotective gene therapy. *Curr Gene Ther*. 2003;3:183–195.

36. Gauter-Fleckenstein B, Fleckenstein K, Owzar K, et al. Comparison of two Mn porphyrin-based mimics of superoxide dismutase in pulmonary radioprotection. *Free Radic Biol Med*. 2008;44:982–989.

37. Mahmood J, Jelveh S, Calveley V, et al. Mitigation of radiation-induced lung injury by genistein and EUK-207. *Int J Radiat Biol*. 2011;87:889–901.

38. Antonic V, Rabbani ZN, Jackson IL, Vujaskovic Z. Subcutaneous administration of bovine superoxide dismutase protects lungs from radiation-induced lung injury. *Free Radic Res*. 2015;49:1259–1268.

39. Nozaki Y, Hasegawa Y, Takeuchi A, et al. Nitric oxide as an inflammatory mediator of radiation pneumonitis in rats. *Am J Physiol*. 1997;272:L651–L658.

40. Williams JP, Hernady E, Johnston CJ, et al. Effect of administration of lovastatin on the development of late pulmonary effects after whole-lung irradiation in a murine model. *Radiat Res*. 2004;161:560–567.

41. Bao P, Gao W, Li S, et al. Effect of pretreatment with high-dose ulinastatin in preventing radiation-induced pulmonary injury in rats. *Eur J Pharmacol*. 2009;603:114–119.

42. Fritz G, Henninger C, Huelsenbeck J. Potential use of HMG-CoA reductase inhibitors (statins) as radioprotective agents. *Br Med Bull*. 2011;97:17–26.

43. Zhang M, Qian J, Xing X, et al. Inhibition of the tumor necrosis factor-alpha pathway is radioprotective for the lung. *Clin Cancer Res*. 2008;14:1868–1876.

44. Wang C, Abe S, Matsuda K, et al. Effects of gefitinib on radiation-induced lung injury in mice. *J Nippon Med Sch*. 2008;75:96–105.

45. Chung EJ, Sowers A, Thetford A, et al. Mammalian target of rapamycin inhibition with rapamycin mitigates radiation-induced pulmonary fibrosis in a murine model. *Int J Radiat Oncol Biol Phys*. 2016;96(4):857–866.
46. Shi HS, Gao X, Li D, et al. A systemic administration of liposomal curcumin inhibits radiation pneumonitis and sensitizes lung carcinoma to radiation. *Int J Nanomedicine*. 2012;7:2601–2611.
47. Lee JC, Kinniry PA, Arguiri E, et al. Dietary curcumin increases antioxidant defenses in lung, ameliorates radiation-induced pulmonary fibrosis, and improves survival in mice. *Radiat Res*. 2010;173:590–601.
48. Cho YJ, Lee JD, Jeong YY. Curcumin attenuates pulmonary inflammation in radiation-induced pneumonitis in rat models. *Am J Respir Crit Care Med*. 2012;185:A5731. doi:10.1164/ajrccm-conference.2012.185.1_MeetingAbstracts.A5731
49. Mehta HJ, Patel V, Sadikot RT. Curcumin and lung cancer—a review. *Target Oncol*. 2014;9:295–310.
50. Sasse AD, de Oliveira Clark LG, Sasse EC, Clark OAC. Amifostine reduces side effects and improves complete response rate during radiotherapy: Results of a meta-analysis. *Int J Radiat Oncol Biol Phys*. 2006;64:784–791.
51. Movsas B, Scott C, Langer C, et al. Randomized trial of amifostine in locally advanced non–small-cell lung cancer patients receiving chemotherapy and hyperfractionated radiation: Radiation therapy oncology group trial 98-01. *J Clin Oncol*. 2005;23:2145–2154.
52. Sarna L, Swann S, Langer C, et al. Clinically meaningful differences in patient-reported outcomes with amifostine in combination with chemoradiation for locally advanced non–small-cell lung cancer: an analysis of RTOG 9801. *Int J Radiat Oncol Biol Phys*. 2008;72:1378–1384.
53. Komaki R, Lee JS, Milas L, et al. Effects of amifostine on acute toxicity from concurrent chemotherapy and radiotherapy for inoperable non–small-cell lung cancer: report of a randomized comparative trial. *Int J Radiat Oncol Biol Phys*. 2004;58:1369–1377.
54. Antonadou D, Throuvalas N, Petridis A, et al. Effect of amifostine on toxicities associated with radiochemotherapy in patients with locally advanced non–small-cell lung cancer. *Int J Radiat Oncol Biol Phys*. 2003;57:402–408.
55. Antonadou D, Coliarakis N, Synodinou M, et al. Randomized phase III trial of radiation treatment ± amifostine in patients with advanced-stage lung cancer. *Int J Radiat Oncol Biol Phys*. 2001;51:915–922.
56. Koukourakis MI, Kyrias G, Kakolyris S, et al. Subcutaneous administration of amifostine during fractionated radiotherapy: a randomized phase II study. *J Clin Oncol*. 2000;18:2226–2233.
57. Leong SS, Tan EH, Fong KW, et al. Randomized double-blind trial of combined modality treatment with or without amifostine in unresectable stage III non–small-cell lung cancer. *J Clin Oncol*. 2003;21:1767–1774.
58. Senzer N. A phase III randomized evaluation of amifostine in stage IIIA/IIIB non-small cell lung cancer patients receiving concurrent carboplatin, paclitaxel, and radiation therapy followed by gemcitabine and cisplatin intensification: preliminary findings. *Semin Oncol*. 2002;29:38–41.
59. Han HS, Han JY, Yu SY, et al. Randomized phase 2 study of subcutaneous amifostine versus epoetin-alpha given 3 times weekly during concurrent chemotherapy and hyperfractionated radiotherapy for limited-disease small cell lung cancer. *Cancer*. 2008;113:1623–1631.

60. Mell LK, Malik R, Komaki R, et al. Effect of amifostine on response rates in locally advanced non–small-cell lung cancer patients treated on randomized controlled trials: a meta-analysis. *Int J Radiat Oncol Biol Phys*. 2007;68:111–118.
61. Lawrence YR, Paulus R, Langer C, et al. The addition of amifostine to carboplatin and paclitaxel based chemoradiation in locally advanced non-small cell lung cancer: long-term follow-up of Radiation Therapy Oncology Group (RTOG) randomized trial 9801. *Lung Cancer*. 2013;80:298–305.
62. Molteni A, Wolfe LF, Ward WF, et al. Effect of an angiotensin II receptor blocker and two angiotensin converting enzyme inhibitors on transforming growth factor-beta (TGF-beta) and alpha-actomyosin (alpha SMA), important mediators of radiation-induced pneumopathy and lung fibrosis. *Curr Pharm Des*. 2007;13:1307–1316.
63. Barcellos-Hoff M. How tissues respond to damage at the cellular level: orchestration by transforming growth factor-β (TGF-β). *Br J Radiol*. 2014;27(1). doi:10.1259/bjr/26432956
64. Carl C, Flindt A, Hartmann J, et al. Ionizing radiation induces a motile phenotype in human carcinoma cells in vitro through hyperactivation of the TGF-beta signaling pathway. *Cell Mol Life Sci*. 2016;73:427–443.
65. Fu X-L, Huang H, Bentel G, et al. Predicting the risk of symptomatic radiation-induced lung injury using both the physical and biologic parameters V30 and transforming growth factor β. *Int J Radiat Oncol Biol Phys*. 2001;50:899–908.
66. Anscher MS, Kong F-M, Andrews K, et al. Plasma transforming growth factor β1 as a predictor of radiation pneumonitis. *Int J Radiat Oncol Biol Phys*. 1998;41:1029–1035.
67. Anscher MS, Thrasher B, Rabbani Z, et al. Antitransforming growth factor–β antibody 1D11 ameliorates normal tissue damage caused by high-dose radiation. *Int J Radiat Oncol Biol Phys*. 2006;65:876–8781.
68. Anscher MS, Thrasher B, Zgonjanin L, et al. Small molecular inhibitor of transforming growth factor-beta protects against development of radiation-induced lung injury. *Int J Radiat Oncol Biol Phys*. 2008;71:829–837.
69. Molteni A, Moulder JE, Cohen EF, et al. Control of radiation-induced pneumopathy and lung fibrosis by angiotensin-converting enzyme inhibitors and an angiotensin II type 1 receptor blocker. *Int J Radiat Biol*. 2000;76:523–532.
70. Ward WF, Lin PJ, Wong PS, et al. Radiation pneumonitis in rats and its modification by the angiotensin-converting enzyme inhibitor captopril evaluated by high-resolution computed tomography. *Radiat Res*. 1993;135:81–87.
71. Medhora M, Gao F, Jacobs ER, Moulder JE. Radiation damage to the lung: mitigation by angiotensin-converting enzyme (ACE) inhibitors. *Respirology*. 2012;17:66–71.
72. Ghosh SN, Zhang R, Fish BL, et al. Renin-angiotensin system suppression mitigates experimental radiation pneumonitis. *Int J Radiat Oncol Biol Phys*. 2009;75:1528–1536.
73. Kohl RR, Kolozsvary A, Brown SL, et al. Differential radiation effect in tumor and normal tissue after treatment with ramipril, an angiotensin-converting enzyme inhibitor. *Radiat Res*. 2007;168:440–445.
74. Kharofa J, Cohen EP, Tomic R, et al. Decreased risk of radiation pneumonitis with incidental concurrent use of angiotensin-converting enzyme inhibitors and thoracic radiation therapy. *Int J Radiat Oncol Biol Phys*. 2012;84:238–243.

75. Wang H, Liao Z, Zhuang Y, et al. Do angiotensin-converting enzyme inhibitors reduce the risk of symptomatic radiation pneumonitis in patients with non-small cell lung cancer after definitive radiation therapy? Analysis of a single-institution database. *Int J Radiat Oncol Biol Phys*. 2013;87:1071–1077.

76. Harder EM, Park HS, Nath SK, et al. Angiotensin-converting enzyme inhibitors decrease the risk of radiation pneumonitis after stereotactic body radiation therapy. *Pract Radiat Oncol*. 2015;5:e643–e649.

77. Small W Jr, James JL, Moore TD, et al. Utility of the ACE inhibitor captopril in mitigating radiation-associated pulmonary toxicity in lung cancer: results from NRG Oncology RTOG 0123. *Am J Clin Oncol*. 2016. doi:10.1097/COC.0000000000000289

78. Rübe CE, Wilfert F, Uthe D, et al. Modulation of radiation-induced tumour necrosis factor α (TNF-α) expression in the lung tissue by pentoxifylline. *Radiother Oncol*. 2002;64:177–187.

79. Ward WF, Kim YT, Molteni A, et al. Pentoxifylline does not spare acute radiation reactions in rat lung and skin. *Radiat Res*. 1992;129:107–111.

80. Ozturk B, Egehan I, Atavci S, Kitapci M. Pentoxifylline in prevention of radiation-induced lung toxicity in patients with breast and lung cancer: a double-blind randomized trial. *Int J Radiat Oncol Biol Phys*. 2004;58:213–219.

81. Misirlioglu CH, Demirkasimoglu T, Kucukplakci B, et al. Pentoxifylline and alpha-tocopherol in prevention of radiation-induced lung toxicity in patients with lung cancer. *Med Oncol*. 2007;24:308–311.

82. Liu Y, Yu H, Zhang C, et al. Protective effects of berberine on radiation-induced lung injury via intercellular adhesion molecular-1 and transforming growth factor-beta-1 in patients with lung cancer. *Eur J Cancer*. 2008;44:2425–32.

83. Tan BX, Yao WX, Ge J, et al. Prognostic influence of metformin as first-line chemotherapy for advanced nonsmall cell lung cancer in patients with type 2 diabetes. *Cancer*. 2011;117:5103–5111.

84. Storozhuk Y, Hopmans SN, Sanli T, et al. Metformin inhibits growth and enhances radiation response of non-small cell lung cancer (NSCLC) through ATM and AMPK. *Br J Cancer*. 2013;108:2021–2032.

85. Worthington HV, Clarkson JE, Bryan G, et al. Interventions for preventing oral mucositis for patients with cancer receiving treatment. *Cochrane Database Syst Rev*. 2011:CD000978. doi:10.1002/14651858.CD000978.pub2

86. Stokman MA, Spijkervet FK, Boezen HM, et al. Preventive intervention possibilities in radiotherapy- and chemotherapy-induced oral mucositis: results of meta-analyses. *J Dent Res*. 2006;85:690–700.

87. Brizel DM, Murphy BA, Rosenthal DI, et al. Phase II study of palifermin and concurrent chemoradiation in head and neck squamous cell carcinoma. *J Clin Oncol*. 2008;26:2489–2496.

88. Le QT, Kim HE, Schneider CJ, et al. Palifermin reduces severe mucositis in definitive chemoradiotherapy of locally advanced head and neck cancer: a randomized, placebo-controlled study. *J Clin Oncol*. 2011;29:2808–2814.

89. Henke M, Alfonsi M, Foa P, et al. Palifermin decreases severe oral mucositis of patients undergoing postoperative radiochemotherapy for head and neck cancer: a randomized, placebo-controlled trial. *J Clin Oncol*. 2011;29:2815–2820.

90. Buntzel J, Kuttner K, Frohlich D, Glatzel M. Selective cytoprotection with amifostine in concurrent radiochemotherapy for head and neck cancer. *Ann Oncol*. 1998;9:505–509.

91. Antonadou D, Pepelassi M, Synodinou M, et al. Prophylactic use of amifostine to prevent radiochemotherapy-induced mucositis and xerostomia in head-and-neck cancer. *Int J Radiat Oncol Biol Phys*. 2002;52:739–747.

92. Wasserman TH, Brizel DM, Henke M, et al. Influence of intravenous amifostine on xerostomia, tumor control, and survival after radiotherapy for head-and-neck cancer: 2-year follow-up of a prospective, randomized, phase III trial. *Int J Radiat Oncol Biol Phys*. 2005;63:985–990.

93. Vacha P, Fehlauer F, Mahlmann B, et al. Randomized phase III trial of postoperative radiochemotherapy +/- amifostine in head and neck cancer. Is there evidence for radioprotection? *Strahlenther Onkol*. 2003;179:385–389.

94. Bourhis J, De Crevoisier R, Abdulkarim B, et al. A randomized study of very accelerated radiotherapy with and without amifostine in head and neck squamous cell carcinoma. *Int J Radiat Oncol Biol Phys*. 2000;46:1105–1108.

95. Veerasarn V, Phromratanapongse P, Suntornpong N, et al. Effect of amifostine to prevent radiotherapy-induced acute and late toxicity in head and neck cancer patients who had normal or mild impaired salivary gland function. *J Med Assoc Thai* 2006;89:2056–2067.

96. Brizel DM, Wasserman TH, Henke M, et al. Phase III randomized trial of amifostine as a radioprotector in head and neck cancer. *J Clin Oncol*. 2000;18:3339–3345.

97. Buentzel J, Micke O, Adamietz IA, et al. Intravenous amifostine during chemoradiotherapy for head-and-neck cancer: a randomized placebo-controlled phase III study. *Int J Radiat Oncol Biol Phys*. 2006;64:684–691.

98. Haddad R, Sonis S, Posner M, et al. Randomized phase 2 study of concomitant chemoradiotherapy using weekly carboplatin/paclitaxel with or without daily subcutaneous amifostine in patients with locally advanced head and neck cancer. *Cancer*. 2009;115:4514–4523.

99. Karacetin D, Yucel B, Leblebicioglu B, et al. A randomized trial of amifostine as radioprotector in the radiotherapy of head and neck cancer. *J BUON*. 2004;9:23–26.

100. Suntharalingam M, Jaboin J, Taylor R, et al. The evaluation of amifostine for mucosal protection in patients with advanced loco-regional squamous cell carcinomas of the head and neck (SCCHN) treated with concurrent weekly carboplatin, paclitaxel, and daily radiotherapy (RT). *Semin Oncol*. 2004;31:2–7.

101. Trog D, Bank P, Wendt TG, et al. Daily amifostine given concomitantly to chemoradiation in head and neck cancer. A pilot study. *Strahlenther Onkol*. 1999;175:444–449.

102. Koukourakis MI, Tsoutsou PG, Karpouzis A, et al. Radiochemotherapy with cetuximab, cisplatin, and amifostine for locally advanced head and neck cancer: a feasibility study. *Int J Radiat Oncol Biol Phys*. 2010;77:9–15.

103. Law A, Kennedy T, Pellitteri P, et al. Efficacy and safety of subcutaneous amifostine in minimizing radiation-induced toxicities in patients receiving combined-modality treatment for squamous cell carcinoma of the head and neck. *Int J Radiat Oncol Biol Phys*. 2007;69:1361–1368.

104. Anne PR, Machtay M, Rosenthal DI, et al. A phase II trial of subcutaneous amifostine and radiation therapy in patients with head-and-neck cancer. *Int J Radiat Oncol Biol Phys*. 2007;67:445–4452.

105. Ozsahin M, Betz M, Matzinger O, et al. Feasibility and efficacy of subcutaneous amifostine therapy in patients with head and neck cancer treated with curative accelerated concomitant-boost radiation therapy. *Arch Otolaryngol Head Neck Surg*. 2006;132:141–145.

106. Abitbol A, Abdel-Wahab M, Harvey M, et al. Phase II study of tolerance and efficacy of hyperfractionated radiation therapy and 5-fluorouracil, cisplatin, and paclitaxel (taxol) and amifostine (ethyol) in head and neck squamous cell carcinomas: A-3 protocol. *Am J Clin Oncol*. 2005;28:449–455.

107. Braaksma M, Levendag P. Tools for optimal tissue sparing in concomitant chemoradiation of advanced head and neck cancer: subcutaneous amifostine and computed tomography-based target delineation. *Semin Oncol*. 2002;29:63–70.

108. Nicolatou-Galitis O, Sotiropoulou-Lontou A, Velegraki A, et al. Oral candidiasis in head and neck cancer patients receiving radiotherapy with amifostine cytoprotection. *Oral Oncol*. 2003;39:397–401.

109. Nicolatou-Galitis O, Sarri T, Bowen J, et al. Systematic review of amifostine for the management of oral mucositis in cancer patients. *Support Care Cancer*. 2013;21:357–364.

110. Foote RL, Loprinzi CL, Frank AR, et al. Randomized trial of a chlorhexidine mouthwash for alleviation of radiation-induced mucositis. *J Clin Oncol*. 1994;12:2630–2633.

111. Franzen L, Henriksson R, Littbrand B, Zackrisson B. Effects of sucralfate on mucositis during and following radiotherapy of malignancies in the head and neck region. A double-blind placebo-controlled study. *Acta Oncol*. 1995;34:219–223.

112. Lin LC, Que J, Lin LK, Lin FC. Zinc supplementation to improve mucositis and dermatitis in patients after radiotherapy for head-and-neck cancers: a double-blind, randomized study. *Int J Radiat Oncol Biol Phys*. 2006;65:745–750.

113. Bairati I, Meyer F, Gelinas M, et al. Randomized trial of antioxidant vitamins to prevent acute adverse effects of radiation therapy in head and neck cancer patients. *J Clin Oncol*. 2005;23:5805–5813.

114. Ferreira PR, Fleck JF, Diehl A, et al. Protective effect of alpha-tocopherol in head and neck cancer radiation-induced mucositis: a double-blind randomized trial. *Head Neck*. 2004;26:313–321.

115. Cerchietti LC, Navigante AH, Lutteral MA, et al. Double-blinded, placebo-controlled trial on intravenous L-alanyl-L-glutamine in the incidence of oral mucositis following chemoradiotherapy in patients with head-and-neck cancer. *Int J Radiat Oncol Biol Phys*. 2006;65:1330–1337.

116. Motallebnejad M, Akram S, Moghadamnia A, et al. The effect of topical application of pure honey on radiation-induced mucositis: a randomized clinical trial. *J Contemp Dent Pract*. 2008;9:40–47.

117. Samdariya S, Lewis S, Kauser H, et al. A randomized controlled trial evaluating the role of honey in reducing pain due to radiation induced mucositis in head and neck cancer patients. *Indian J Palliat Care*. 2015;21:268–273.

118. Bensadoun RJ, Franquin JC, Ciais G, et al. Low-energy He/Ne laser in the prevention of radiation-induced mucositis. A multicenter phase III randomized study in patients with head and neck cancer. *Support Care Cancer*. 1999;7:244–252.

119. Su CK, Mehta V, Ravikumar L, et al. Phase II double-blind randomized study comparing oral aloe vera versus placebo to prevent radiation-related mucositis in patients with head-and-neck neoplasms. *Int J Radiat Oncol Biol Phys*. 2004;60:171–177.

120. Puataweepong P, Dhanachai M, Dangprasert S, et al. The efficacy of oral aloe vera juice for radiation induced mucositis in head and neck cancer patients: a double-blind placebo-controlled study. *Asian Biomedicine (Research Reviews and News)*. 2010;3:375–382.

121. Su YB, Vickers AJ, Zelefsky MJ, et al. Double-blind, placebo-controlled, randomized trial of granulocyte-colony stimulating factor during postoperative radiotherapy for squamous head and neck cancer. *Cancer J*. 2006;12: 182–188.

122. Schneider SB, Nishimura RD, Zimmerman RP, et al. Filgrastim (r-metHuG-CSF) and its potential use in the reduction of radiation-induced oropharyngeal mucositis: an interim look at a randomized, double-blind, placebo-controlled trial. *Cytokines Cell Mol Ther*. 1999;5:175–180.

123. Stokman MA, Spijkervet FK, Burlage FR, et al. Oral mucositis and selective elimination of oral flora in head and neck cancer patients receiving radiotherapy: a double-blind randomised clinical trial. *Br J Cancer*. 2003;88:1012–1016.

124. Machtay M, Pajak TF, Suntharalingam M, et al. Radiotherapy with or without erythropoietin for anemic patients with head and neck cancer: a randomized trial of the radiation therapy oncology group (RTOG 99-03). *Int J Radiat Oncol Biol Phys*. 2007;69:1008–1017.

125. Henke M, Laszig R, Rübe C, et al. Erythropoietin to treat head and neck cancer patients with anaemia undergoing radiotherapy: randomised, double-blind, placebo-controlled trial. *Lancet*. 2003;362:1255–1260.

126. Leyland-Jones B. Breast cancer trial with erythropoietin terminated unexpectedly. *Lancet Oncol*. 2003;4:459–460.

127. Bohlius J, Schmidlin K, Brillant C, et al. Recombinant human erythropoiesis-stimulating agents and mortality in patients with cancer: a meta-analysis of randomised trials. *Lancet*. 373:1532–1542.

128. Yang W-f, Liao G-q, Hakim SG, Ouyang D-q, Ringash J, Su Y-x. Is pilocarpine effective in preventing radiation-induced xerostomia? A systematic review and meta-analysis. *Int J Radiat Oncol Biol Phys*. 2016;94:503–511.

129. Cheng C-Q, Xu H, Liu L, et al. Efficacy and safety of pilocarpine for radiation-induced xerostomia in patients with head and neck cancer: A systematic review and meta-analysis. *J Am Dent Assoc*. 2016;147:236–243.

130. Ringash J, Warde P, Lockwood G, et al. Postradiotherapy quality of life for head-and-neck cancer patients is independent of xerostomia. *Int J Radiat Oncol Biol Phys*. 2005;61:1403–1407.

131. Nyarady Z, Nemeth A, Ban A, et al. A randomized study to assess the effectiveness of orally administered pilocarpine during and after radiotherapy of head and neck cancer. *Anticancer Res*. 2006;26:1557–1562.

132. Burlage FR, Roesink JM, Kampinga HH, et al. Protection of salivary function by concomitant pilocarpine during radiotherapy: a double-blind, randomized, placebo-controlled study. *Int J Radiat Oncol Biol Phys*. 2008;70:14–22.

133. Fisher J, Scott C, Scarantino CW, et al. Phase III quality-of-life study results: impact on patients' quality of life to reducing xerostomia after radiotherapy for head-and-neck cancer—RTOG 97-09. *Int J Radiat Oncol Biol Phys*. 2003;56: 832–836.

134. Scarantino C, LeVeque F, Swann RS, et al. Effect of pilocarpine during radiation therapy: results of RTOG 97-09, a phase III randomized study in head and neck cancer patients. *J Support Oncol*. 2006;4:252–258.

135. Gornitsky M, Shenouda G, Sultanem K, et al. Double-blind randomized, placebo-controlled study of pilocarpine to salvage salivary gland function during radiotherapy of patients with head and neck cancer. *Oral Surg Oral Med Oral Pathol Oral Radiol Endod*. 2004;98:45–52.

136. Haddad P, Karimi M. A randomized, double-blind, placebo-controlled trial of concomitant pilocarpine with head and neck irradiation for prevention of radiation-induced xerostomia. *Radiotherapy Oncol*. 2002;64:29–32.

137. Warde P, O'Sullivan B, Aslanidis J, et al. A phase III placebo-controlled trial of oral pilocarpine in patients undergoing radiotherapy for head-and-neck cancer. *Int J Radiat Oncol Biol Phys*. 2002;54:9–13.

138. LeVeque FG, Montgomery M, Potter D, et al. A multicenter, randomized, double-blind, placebo-controlled, dose-titration study of oral pilocarpine for treatment of radiation-induced xerostomia in head and neck cancer patients. *J Clin Oncol*. 1993;11:1124–1131.

139. Horiot J-C, Lipinski F, Schraub S, et al. Post-radiation severe xerostomia relieved by pilocarpine: a prospective French cooperative study. *Radiotherapy Oncol*. 2000;55:233–239.

140. Xiang B, Han L, Wang X, et al. Nicotinamide phosphoribosyltransferase upregulation by phenylephrine reduces X-ray injury in submandibular gland. *Int J Radiat Oncol Biol Phys*. 2016;96(3):538–546.

141. Seikaly H, Jha N, Harris JR, et al. Long-term outcomes of submandibular gland transfer for prevention of postradiation xerostomia. *Arch Otolaryngol Head Neck Surg*. 2004;130:956–961.

142. Jha N, Seikaly H, Harris J, et al. Phase III randomized study: oral pilocarpine versus submandibular salivary gland transfer protocol for the management of radiation-induced xerostomia. *Head Neck*. 2009;31:234–243.

143. Wong RKW, Deshmukh S, Wyatt G, et al. Acupuncture-like transcutaneous electrical nerve stimulation versus pilocarpine in treating radiation-induced xerostomia: results of RTOG 0537 Phase 3 study. *Int J Radiat Oncol Biol Phys*. 2015;92:220–227.

144. Jham BC, Teixeira IV, Aboud CG, et al. A randomized phase III prospective trial of bethanechol to prevent radiotherapy-induced salivary gland damage in patients with head and neck cancer. *Oral Oncology*. 2007;43:137–142.

145. Gorsky M, Epstein JB, Parry J, et al. The efficacy of pilocarpine and bethanechol upon saliva production in cancer patients with hyposalivation following radiation therapy. *Oral Surg Oral Med Oral Pathol Oral Radiol Endod*. 2004;97:190–195.

146. Chambers MS, Jones CU, Biel MA, et al. Open-label, long-term safety study of cevimeline in the treatment of postirradiation xerostomia. *Int J Radiat Oncol Biol Phys*. 2007;69:1369–1376.

147. Teguh DN, Levendag PC, Noever I, et al. Early hyperbaric oxygen therapy for reducing radiotherapy side effects: early results of a randomized trial in oropharyngeal and nasopharyngeal cancer. *Int J Radiat Oncol Biol Phys*. 2009;75:711–716.

148. Rudat V, Münter M, Rades D, et al. The effect of amifostine or IMRT to preserve the parotid function after radiotherapy of the head and neck region measured by quantitative salivary gland scintigraphy. *Radiotherapy Oncol*. 2008;89:71–80.

149. Epstein JB, Emerton S, Le ND, Stevenson-Moore P. A double-blind crossover trial of Oral Balance gel and Biotene® toothpaste versus placebo in patients with xerostomia following radiation therapy. *Oral Oncol*. 1999;35:132–137.

150. Jellema AP, Langendijk H, Bergenhenegouwen L, et al. The efficacy of Xialine® in patients with xerostomia resulting from radiotherapy for head and neck cancer: a pilot-study. *Radiotherapy Oncol*. 2001;59:157–160.

151. Bennett MH, Feldmeier J, Hampson NB, et al. Hyperbaric oxygen therapy for late radiation tissue injury. *Cochrane Database Syst Rev.* 2016;(4):CD005005. doi:10.1002/14651858.CD005005.pub3

152. Marx RE, Ehler WJ, Tayapongsak P, Pierce LW. Relationship of oxygen dose to angiogenesis induction in irradiated tissue. *Am J Surg.* 1990;160:519–524.

153. Annane D, Depondt J, Aubert P, et al. Hyperbaric oxygen therapy for radionecrosis of the jaw: a randomized, placebo-controlled, double-blind trial from the ORN96 study group. *J Clin Oncol.* 2004;22:4893–4900.

154. Marx RE, Johnson RP, Kline SN. Prevention of osteoradionecrosis: a randomized prospective clinical trial of hyperbaric oxygen versus penicillin. *J Am Dent Assoc.* 1985;111:49–54.

155. Schoen PJ, Raghoebar GM, Bouma J, et al. Rehabilitation of oral function in head and neck cancer patients after radiotherapy with implant-retained dentures: effects of hyperbaric oxygen therapy. *Oral Oncol.* 2007;43:379–388.

156. Svalestad J, Thorsen E, Vaagbo G, Hellem S. Effect of hyperbaric oxygen treatment on oxygen tension and vascular capacity in irradiated skin and mucosa. *Int J Oral Maxillofac Surg.* 2014;43:107–112.

157. Yarnold J. Double-blind randomised phase II study of hyperbaric oxygen in patients with radiation-induced brachial plexopathy. *Radiother Oncol.* 2005;77:327.

158. Robard L, Louis MY, Blanchard D, et al. Medical treatment of osteoradionecrosis of the mandible by PENTOCLO: preliminary results. *Eur Ann Otorhinolaryngol Head Neck Dis.* 2014;131:333–338.

159. Delanian S, Chatel C, Porcher R, et al. Complete restoration of refractory mandibular osteoradionecrosis by prolonged treatment with a pentoxifylline-tocopherol-clodronate combination (PENTOCLO): A phase II trial. *Int J Radiat Oncol Biol Phys.* 2011;80:832–839.

160. Chua DT, Lo C, Yuen J, Foo YC. A pilot study of pentoxifylline in the treatment of radiation-induced trismus. *Am J Clin Oncol.* 2001;24:366–369.

161. Aygenc E, Celikkanat S, Kaymakci M, et al. Prophylactic effect of pentoxifylline on radiotherapy complications: a clinical study. *Otolaryngol Head Neck Surg.* 2004;130:351–356.

162. Zhao W, Diz DI, Robbins ME. Oxidative damage pathways in relation to normal tissue injury. *Br J Radiol.* 2007;80:S23–S31.

163. Haydont V, Bourgier C, Vozenin-Brotons MC. Rho/ROCK pathway as a molecular target for modulation of intestinal radiation-induced toxicity. *Br J Radiol.* 2007;80:S32–S40.

164. Haydont V, Bourgier C, Pocard M, et al. Pravastatin inhibits the Rho/CCN2/extracellular matrix cascade in human fibrosis explants and improves radiation-induced intestinal fibrosis in rats. *Clin Cancer Res.* 2007;13:5331–5340.

165. Haydont V, Gilliot O, Rivera S, et al. Successful mitigation of delayed intestinal radiation injury using pravastatin is not associated with acute injury improvement or tumor protection. *Int J Radiat Oncol Biol Phys.* 2007;68:1471–1482.

166. Gibson RJ, Keefe DMK, Lalla RV, et al. Systematic review of agents for the management of gastrointestinal mucositis in cancer patients. *Support Care Cancer.* 2013;21:313–326.

167. Delia P, Sansotta G, Donato V, et al. Prevention of radiation-induced diarrhea with the use of VSL#3, a new high-potency probiotic preparation. *Am J Gastroenterol.* 2002;97:2150–2152.

168. Urbancsek H, Kazar T, Mezes I, Neumann K. Results of a double-blind, randomized study to evaluate the efficacy and safety of antibiophilus in patients with radiation-induced diarrhoea. *Eur J Gastroenterol Hepatol.* 2001;13:391–396.

169. Osterlund P, Ruotsalainen T, Korpela R, et al. Lactobacillus supplementation for diarrhoea related to chemotherapy of colorectal cancer: a randomised study. *Br J Cancer.* 2007;97:1028–1034.

170. Liu T, Liu Y, He S, et al. Use of radiation with or without WR-2721 in advanced rectal cancer. *Cancer.* 1992;69:2820–2825.

171. Athanassiou H, Antonadou D, Coliarakis N, et al. Protective effect of amifostine during fractionated radiotherapy in patients with pelvic carcinomas: results of a randomized trial. *Int J Radiat Oncol Biol Phys.* 2003;56:1154–1160.

172. Kouvaris J, Kouloulias V, Malas E, et al. Amifostine as radioprotective agent for the rectal mucosa during irradiation of pelvic tumors. A phase II randomized study using various toxicity scales and rectosigmoidoscopy. *Strahlenther Onkol.* 2003;179:167–174.

173. Small WJ, Winter K, Levenback C, et al. Extended-field irradiation and intracavitary brachytherapy combined with cisplatin and amifostine for cervical cancer with positive para-aortic or high common iliac lymph nodes: results of Arm II of Radiation Therapy Oncology Group (RTOG) 0116. *Int J Gynecol Cancer.* 2011;21:1266–1275.

174. Menard C, Camphausen K, Muanza T, et al. Clinical trial of endorectal amifostine for radioprotection in patients with prostate cancer: rationale and early results. *Semin Oncol.* 2003;30:63–67.

175. Dziuk T, Senzer N. Feasibility of amifostine administration in conjunction with high-dose rate brachytherapy. *Semin Oncol.* 2003;30:49–57.

176. Baughan CA, Canney PA, Buchanan RB, Pickering RM. A randomized trial to assess the efficacy of 5-aminosalicylic acid for the prevention of radiation enteritis. *Clin Oncol (R Coll Radiol).* 1993;5:19–24.

177. Martenson JA, Jr, Hyland G, Moertel CG, et al. Olsalazine is contraindicated during pelvic radiation therapy: results of a double-blind, randomized clinical trial. *Int J Radiat Oncol Biol Phys.* 1996;35:299–303.

178. Resbeut M, Marteau P, Cowen D, et al. A randomized double blind placebo controlled multicenter study of mesalazine for the prevention of acute radiation enteritis. *Radiother Oncol.* 1997;44:59–63.

179. Hille A, Schmidberger H, Hermann RM, et al. A phase III randomized, placebo-controlled, double-blind study of misoprostol rectal suppositories to prevent acute radiation proctitis in patients with prostate cancer. *Int J Radiat Oncol Biol Phys.* 2005;63:1488–1493.

180. Kertesz T, Herrmann MK, Zapf A, et al. Effect of a prostaglandin--given rectally for prevention of radiation-induced acute proctitis--on late rectal toxicity: results of a phase III randomized, placebo-controlled, double-blind study. *Strahlenther Onkol.* 2009;185:596–602.

181. Shukla P, Gupta D, Bisht SS, et al. Circadian variation in radiation-induced intestinal mucositis in patients with cervical carcinoma. *Cancer.* 2010;116:2031–2035.

182. Wang J, Boerma M, Fu Q, Hauer-Jensen M. Significance of endothelial dysfunction in the pathogenesis of early and delayed radiation enteropathy. *World J Gastroenterol.* 2007;13:3047–3055.

183. Wang J, Boerma M, Fu Q, et al. Simvastatin ameliorates radiation enteropathy development after localized, fractionated irradiation by a protein C-independent mechanism. *Int J Radiat Oncol Biol Phys.* 2007;68:1483–1490.

184. Gaugler MH, Vereycken-Holler V, Squiban C, et al. Pravastatin limits endothelial activation after irradiation and decreases the resulting inflammatory and thrombotic responses. *Radiat Res.* 2005;163:479–487.

185. Nubel T, Damrot J, Roos WP, et al. Lovastatin protects human endothelial cells from killing by ionizing radiation without impairing induction and repair of DNA double-strand breaks. *Clin Cancer Res.* 2006;12:933–939.

186. Wedlake LJ, Silia F, Benton B, et al. Evaluating the efficacy of statins and ACE-inhibitors in reducing gastrointestinal toxicity in patients receiving radiotherapy for pelvic malignancies. *Eur J Cancer.* 2012;48:2117–2124.

187. Anscher MS, Chang MG, Moghanaki D, et al. A phase II study to prevent radiation-induced rectal injury with lovastatin. *Am J Clin Oncol.* 2016. doi:10.1097/COC.0000000000000320

188. Hamama S, Noman MZ, Gervaz P, et al. MiR-210: A potential therapeutic target against radiation-induced enteropathy. *Radiotherapy Oncol.* 2014;111:219–221.

189. Hamama S, Delanian S, Monceau V, Vozenin MC. Therapeutic management of intestinal fibrosis induced by radiation therapy: from molecular profiling to new intervention strategies et vice et versa. *Fibrogenesis Tissue Repair.* 2012;5(Suppl 1):S13.

190. Hamama S, Gilbert-Sirieix M, Vozenin M-C, Delanian S. Radiation-induced enteropathy: molecular basis of pentoxifylline–vitamin E anti-fibrotic effect involved TGF-β1 cascade inhibition. *Radiotherapy Oncol.* 2012;105:305–312.

191. Kennedy M, Bruninga K, Mutlu EA, et al. Successful and sustained treatment of chronic radiation proctitis with antioxidant vitamins E and C. *Am J Gastroenterol.* 2001;96:1080–1084.

192. Letur-Konirsch H, Guis F, Delanian S. Uterine restoration by radiation sequelae regression with combined pentoxifylline-tocopherol: a phase II study. *Fertil Steril.* 2002;77:1219–1226.

193. Clarke RE, Tenorio LM, Hussey JR, et al. Hyperbaric oxygen treatment of chronic refractory radiation proctitis: a randomized and controlled double-blind crossover trial with long-term follow-up. *Int J Radiat Oncol Biol Phys.* 2008;72:134–143.

194. Sidik S, Hardjodisastro D, Setiabudy R, Gondowiardjo S. Does hyperbaric oxygen administration decrease side effect and improve quality of life after pelvic radiation? *Acta Med Indones.* 2007;39:169–173.

195. Jones K, Evans AW, Bristow RG, Levin W. Treatment of radiation proctitis with hyperbaric oxygen. *Radiother Oncol.* 2006;78:91–94.

196. Dall'Era MA, Hampson NB, Hsi RA, et al. Hyperbaric oxygen therapy for radiation induced proctopathy in men treated for prostate cancer. *J Urol.* 2006;176:87–90.

197. Girnius S, Cersonsky N, Gesell L, et al. Treatment of refractory radiation-induced hemorrhagic proctitis with hyperbaric oxygen therapy. *Am J Clin Oncol.* 2006;29:588–592.

198. Woo TC, Joseph D, Oxer H. Hyperbaric oxygen treatment for radiation proctitis. *Int J Radiat Oncol Biol Phys.* 1997;38:619–622.

199. Bui QC, Lieber M, Withers HR, et al. The efficacy of hyperbaric oxygen therapy in the treatment of radiation-induced late side effects. *Int J Radiat Oncol Biol Phys.* 2004;60:871–878.

200. Kitta T, Shinohara N, Shirato H, et al. The treatment of chronic radiation proctitis with hyperbaric oxygen in patients with prostate cancer. *BJU Int.* 2000;85:372–374.

201. Shao Y, Lu GL, Shen ZJ. Comparison of intravesical hyaluronic acid instillation and hyperbaric oxygen in the treatment of radiation-induced hemorrhagic cystitis. *BJU Int.* 2012;109:691–694.
202. Mayer R, Klemen H, Quehenberger F, et al. Hyperbaric oxygen--an effective tool to treat radiation morbidity in prostate cancer. *Radiother Oncol.* 2001;61: 151–156.
203. Fink D, Chetty N, Lehm JP, et al. Hyperbaric oxygen therapy for delayed radiation injuries in gynecological cancers. *Int J Gynecol Cancer.* 2006;16:638–642.
204. Safra T, Gutman G, Fishlev G, et al. Improved quality of life with hyperbaric oxygen therapy in patients with persistent pelvic radiation-induced toxicity. *Clin Oncol (R Coll Radiol).* 2008;20:284–287.
205. Gul YA, Prasannan S, Jabar FM, et al. Pharmacotherapy for chronic hemorrhagic radiation proctitis. *World J Surg.* 2002;26:1499–1502.
206. Kochhar R, Sriram PV, Sharma SC, et al. Natural history of late radiation proctosigmoiditis treated with topical sucralfate suspension. *Dig Dis Sci.* 1999;44:973–978.
207. Melko GP, Turco TF, Phelan TF, Sauers NM. Treatment of radiation-induced proctitis with sucralfate enemas. *Ann Pharmacother.* 1999;33:1274–1276.
208. O'Brien PC, Franklin CI, Dear KB, et al. A phase III double-blind randomised study of rectal sucralfate suspension in the prevention of acute radiation proctitis. *Radiother Oncol.* 1997;45:117–123.
209. Jensen DM, Machicado GA, Cheng S, et al. A randomized prospective study of endoscopic bipolar electrocoagulation and heater probe treatment of chronic rectal bleeding from radiation telangiectasia. *Gastrointest Endosc.* 1997;45:20–25.
210. Pahlajani G, Raina R, Jones S, et al. Vacuum erection devices revisited: its emerging role in the treatment of erectile dysfunction and early penile rehabilitation following prostate cancer therapy. *J Sex Med.* 2012;9:1182–1189.
211. Sherer BA, Levine LA. Current management of erectile dysfunction in prostate cancer survivors. *Curr Opin Urol.* 2014;24:401–406.
212. Chung E, Cartmill R. Evaluation of clinical efficacy, safety and patient satisfaction rate after low-intensity extracorporeal shockwave therapy for the treatment of male erectile dysfunction: an Australian first open-label single-arm prospective clinical trial. *BJU Int.* 2015;115(Suppl 5):46–49.
213. Yee CH, Chan ES, Hou SS, Ng CF. Extracorporeal shockwave therapy in the treatment of erectile dysfunction: a prospective, randomized, double-blinded, placebo controlled study. *Int J Urol.* 2014;21:1041–1045.
214. Mahmood J, Shamah A, Creed TM, et al. Radiation induced erectile dysfunction: recent advances and future directions. *Advan Radiat Oncol.* 2016;1(3):161–169.
215. Medeiros JL, Jr, Costa WS, Felix-Patricio B, et al. Protective effects of nutritional supplementation with arginine and glutamine on the penis of rats submitted to pelvic radiation. *Andrology.* 2014;2:943–950.
216. Cho KS, Park CW, Kim CK, et al. Effects of Korean ginseng berry extract (GB0710) on penile erection: evidence from in vitro and in vivo studies. *Asian J Androl.* 2013;15:503–507.
217. Paick JS, Lee JH. An experimental study of the effect of ginkgo biloba extract on the human and rabbit corpus cavernosum tissue. *J Urol.* 1996;156:1876–1880.
218. Kovanecz I, Rivera S, Nolazco G, et al. Separate or combined treatments with daily sildenafil, molsidomine, or muscle-derived stem cells prevent erectile dysfunction in a rat model of cavernosal nerve damage. *J Sex Med.* 2012;9:2814–2826.

219. Ilic D, Hindson B, Duchesne G, Millar JL. A randomised, double-blind, placebo-controlled trial of nightly sildenafil citrate to preserve erectile function after radiation treatment for prostate cancer. *J Med Imaging Radiat Oncol.* 2013;57:81–88.

220. Zelefsky MJ, Shasha D, Branco RD, et al. Prophylactic sildenafil citrate improves select aspects of sexual function in men treated with radiotherapy for prostate cancer. *J Urol.* 2014;192:868–874.

221. Pisansky TM, Pugh SL, Greenberg RE, et al. Tadalafil for prevention of erectile dysfunction after radiotherapy for prostate cancer: the radiation therapy oncology group [0831] randomized clinical trial. *JAMA.* 2014;311:1300–1307.

222. Incrocci L, Koper PCM, Hop WCJ, Slob AK. Sildenafil citrate (Viagra) and erectile dysfunction following external beam radiotherapy for prostate cancer: a randomized, double-blind, placebo-controlled, cross-over study. *Int J Radiat Oncol Biol Phys.* 2001;51:1190–1195.

223. Incrocci L, Slagter C, Slob AK, Hop WCJ. A randomized, double-blind, placebo-controlled, cross-over study to assess the efficacy of tadalafil (Cialis®) in the treatment of erectile dysfunction following three-dimensional conformal external-beam radiotherapy for prostatic carcinoma. *Int J Radiat Oncol Biol Phys.* 2006;66:439–444.

224. Watkins Bruner D, James JL, Bryan CJ, et al. Randomized, double-blinded, placebo-controlled crossover trial of treating erectile dysfunction with sildenafil after radiotherapy and short-term androgen deprivation therapy: results of RTOG 0215. *J Sex Med.* 2011;8:1228–1238.

225. Montorsi F, Brock G, Lee J, et al. Effect of nightly versus on-demand vardenafil on recovery of erectile function in men following bilateral nerve-sparing radical prostatectomy. *Eur Urol.* 2008;54:924–931.

226. Cui Y, Zong H, Yan H, Zhang Y. The effect of statins on erectile dysfunction: a systematic review and meta-analysis. *J Sex Med.* 2014;11:1367–1375.

227. Anscher MS, Chang MG, Moghanaki D, et al. Lovastatin may reduce the risk of erectile dysfunction following radiation therapy for prostate cancer. *Acta Oncol.* 2016:55(12):1500–1502. doi:10.1080/0284186X.2016.1223882

228. McQuestion M. Evidence-based skin care management in radiation therapy. *Semin Oncol Nurs.* 2006;22:163–173.

229. Lavery BA. Skin care during radiotherapy: a survey of UK practice. *Clin Oncol (R Coll Radiol).* 1995;7:184–187.

230. Roy I, Fortin A, Larochelle M. The impact of skin washing with water and soap during breast irradiation: a randomized study. *Radiother Oncol.* 2001;58:333–339.

231. Bolderston A, Lloyd NS, Wong RK, et al. The prevention and management of acute skin reactions related to radiation therapy: a systematic review and practice guideline. *Support Care Cancer.* 2006;14:802–817.

232. Théberge V, Harel F, Dagnault A. Use of axillary deodorant and effect on acute skin toxicity during radiotherapy for breast cancer: a prospective randomized noninferiority trial. *Int J Radiat Oncol Biol Phys.* 2009;75:1048–1052.

233. Watson LC, Gies D, Thompson E, Thomas B. Randomized control trial: evaluating aluminum-based antiperspirant use, axilla skin toxicity, and reported quality of life in women receiving external beam radiotherapy for treatment of stage 0, I, and II breast cancer. *Int J Radiat Oncol Biol Phys.* 2012;83:e29–e34.

234. Hardefeldt PJ, Edirimanne S, Eslick GD. Deodorant use and the risk of skin toxicity in patients undergoing radiation therapy for breast cancer: a meta-analysis. *Radiothe Oncol.* 2012;105:378–379.

235. Salvo N, Barnes E, van Draanen J, et al. Prophylaxis and management of acute radiation-induced skin reactions: a systematic review of the literature. *Curr Oncol*. 2010;17:94–112.

236. Bostrom A, Lindman H, Swartling C, et al. Potent corticosteroid cream (mometasone furoate) significantly reduces acute radiation dermatitis: results from a double-blind, randomized study. *Radiother Oncol*. 2001;59:257–265.

237. Miller RC, Schwartz DJ, Sloan JA, et al. Mometasone furoate effect on acute skin toxicity in breast cancer patients receiving radiotherapy: a phase III double-blind, randomized trial from the North Central Cancer Treatment Group N06C4. *Int J Radiat Oncol Biol Phys*. 2011;79:1460–1466.

238. Shukla PN, Gairola M, Mohanti BK, Rath GK. Prophylactic beclomethasone spray to the skin during postoperative radiotherapy of carcinoma breast: a prospective randomized study. *Indian J Cancer*. 2006;43:180–184.

239. Schmuth M, Wimmer MA, Hofer S, et al. Topical corticosteroid therapy for acute radiation dermatitis: a prospective, randomized, double-blind study. *Br J Dermatol*. 2002;146:983–991.

240. Ulff E, Maroti M, Serup J, Falkmer U. A potent steroid cream is superior to emollients in reducing acute radiation dermatitis in breast cancer patients treated with adjuvant radiotherapy. A randomised study of betamethasone versus two moisturizing creams. *Radiother Oncol*. 2013;108:287–292.

241. Okunieff P, Xu J, Hu D, et al. Curcumin protects against radiation-induced acute and chronic cutaneous toxicity in mice and decreases mRNA expression of inflammatory and fibrogenic cytokines. *Int J Radiat Oncol Biol Phys*. 2006;65:890–898.

242. Aggarwal BB, Sundaram C, Malani N, Ichikawa H. Curcumin: the Indian solid gold. *Adv Exp Med Biol*. 2007;595:1–75.

243. Gopinath D, Ahmed MR, Gomathi K, et al. Dermal wound healing processes with curcumin incorporated collagen films. *Biomaterials*. 2004;25:1911–1917.

244. Bhagavathula N, Warner RL, DaSilva M, et al. A combination of curcumin and ginger extract improves abrasion wound healing in corticosteroid-impaired hairless rat skin. *Wound Repair Regen*. 2009;17:360–366.

245. Ryan JL, Heckler CE, Ling M, et al. Curcumin for radiation dermatitis: a randomized, double-blind, placebo-controlled clinical trial of thirty breast cancer patients. *Radiat Res*. 2013;180:34–43.

246. Olsen DL, Raub W, Jr, Bradley C, et al. The effect of aloe vera gel/mild soap versus mild soap alone in preventing skin reactions in patients undergoing radiation therapy. *Oncol Nurs Forum*. 2001;28:543–547.

247. Heggie S, Bryant GP, Tripcony L, et al. A phase III study on the efficacy of topical aloe vera gel on irradiated breast tissue. *Cancer Nurs*. 2002;25:442–451.

248. Fisher J, Scott C, Stevens R, et al. Randomized phase III study comparing Best Supportive Care to Biafine as a prophylactic agent for radiation-induced skin toxicity for women undergoing breast irradiation: Radiation Therapy Oncology Group (RTOG) 97-13. *Int J Radiat Oncol Biol Phys*. 2000;48:1307–1310.

249. Elliott EA, Wright JR, Swann RS, et al. Phase III trial of an emulsion containing trolamine for the prevention of radiation dermatitis in patients with advanced squamous cell carcinoma of the head and neck: results of Radiation Therapy Oncology Group Trial 99-13. *J Clin Oncol*. 2006;24:2092–2097.

250. Wells M, Macmillan M, Raab G, et al. Does aqueous or sucralfate cream affect the severity of erythematous radiation skin reactions? A randomised controlled trial. *Radiother Oncol*. 2004;73:153–162.

251. Pinnix C, Perkins GH, Strom EA, et al. Topical hyaluronic acid vs. standard of care for the prevention of radiation dermatitis after adjuvant radiotherapy for breast cancer: single-blind randomized phase III clinical trial. *Int J Radiat Oncol Biol Phys*. 2012;83:1089–1094.

252. Doctrow SR, Lopez A, Schock AM, et al. A synthetic superoxide dismutase/catalase mimetic EUK-207 mitigates radiation dermatitis and promotes wound healing in irradiated rat skin. *J Invest Dermatol*. 2013;133:1088–1096.

253. Delanian S, Baillet F, Huart J, et al. Successful treatment of radiation-induced fibrosis using liposomal Cu/Zn superoxide dismutase: clinical trial. *Radiother Oncol*. 1994;32:12–20.

254. Lefaix JL, Delanian S, Leplat JJ, et al. Successful treatment of radiation-induced fibrosis using Cu/Zn-SOD and Mn-SOD: an experimental study. *Int J Radiat Oncol Biol Phys*. 1996;35:305–312.

255. Campana F, Zervoudis S, Perdereau B, et al. Topical superoxide dismutase reduces post-irradiation breast cancer fibrosis. *J Cell Mol Med*. 2004;8:109–116.

256. Holler V, Buard V, Gaugler MH, et al. Pravastatin limits radiation-induced vascular dysfunction in the skin. *J Invest Dermatol*. 2009;129:1280–1291.

257. Samlaska CP, Winfield EA. Pentoxifylline. *J Am Acad Dermatol*. 1994;30:603–621.

258. Lefaix JL, Delanian S, Vozenin MC, et al. Striking regression of subcutaneous fibrosis induced by high doses of gamma rays using a combination of pentoxifylline and alpha-tocopherol: an experimental study. *Int J Radiat Oncol Biol Phys*. 1999;43:839–847.

259. Delanian S, Balla-Mekias S, Lefaix JL. Striking regression of chronic radiotherapy damage in a clinical trial of combined pentoxifylline and tocopherol. *J Clin Oncol*. 1999;17:3283–3290.

260. Delanian S, Porcher R, Balla-Mekias S, Lefaix JL. Randomized, placebo-controlled trial of combined pentoxifylline and tocopherol for regression of superficial radiation-induced fibrosis. *J Clin Oncol*. 2003;21:2545–2550.

261. Haddad P, Kalaghchi B, Amouzegar-Hashemi F. Pentoxifylline and vitamin E combination for superficial radiation-induced fibrosis: a phase II clinical trial. *Radiother Oncol*. 2005;77:324–326.

262. Magnusson M, Hoglund P, Johansson K, et al. Pentoxifylline and vitamin E treatment for prevention of radiation-induced side-effects in women with breast cancer: a phase two, double-blind, placebo-controlled randomised clinical trial (Ptx-5). *Eur J Cancer*. 2009;45:2488–2495.

263. Gothard L, Cornes P, Earl J, et al. Double-blind placebo-controlled randomised trial of vitamin E and pentoxifylline in patients with chronic arm lymphoedema and fibrosis after surgery and radiotherapy for breast cancer. *Radiother Oncol*. 2004;73:133–139.

264. Gothard L, Haviland J, Bryson P, et al. Randomised phase II trial of hyperbaric oxygen therapy in patients with chronic arm lymphoedema after radiotherapy for cancer. *Radiother Oncol*. 2010;97:101–107.

265. Jacobson G, Bhatia S, Smith BJ, et al. Randomized trial of pentoxifylline and vitamin E vs standard follow-up after breast irradiation to prevent breast fibrosis, evaluated by tissue compliance meter. *Int J Radiat Oncol Biol Phys*. 2013;85:604–608.

266. Pradat P-F, Delanian S. Chapter 43—Late radiation injury to peripheral nerves. In: Gérard S, Christian K, eds. *Handbook of Clinical Neurology*. Amsterdam, The Netherlands: Elsevier; 2013:743–758.

267. Delanian S, Lefaix JL, Maisonobe T, et al. Significant clinical improvement in radiation-induced lumbosacral polyradiculopathy by a treatment combining pentoxifylline, tocopherol, and clodronate (Pentoclo). *J Neurol Sci.* 2008;275:164–166.
268. Soto O. Radiation-induced conduction block: resolution following anticoagulant therapy. *Muscle Nerve.* 2005;31:642–645.
269. Macià i Garau M, Lucas Calduch A, López EC. Radiobiology of the acute radiation syndrome. *Rep Pract Oncol Radiother.* 2011;16:123–130.
270. Singh VK, Ducey EJ, Brown DS, Whitnall MH. A review of radiation countermeasure work ongoing at the Armed Forces Radiobiology Research Institute. *Int J Radiat Biol.* 2012;88:296–310.
271. Sixt KM, Smith FR, Jr, Kim D, Curling CA. *Research and development strategies for the current and future medical treatment of radiation casualties* [DTIC Document; IDA Paper P-5160]. Institute for Defense Analyses, Alexandria, Virginia; 2014:1–108.
272. Singh VK, Romaine PL, Newman VL. Biologics as countermeasures for acute radiation syndrome: where are we now? *Expert Opin Biol Ther.* 2015;15:465–471.
273. Singh VK, Newman VL, Seed TM. Colony-stimulating factors for the treatment of the hematopoietic component of the acute radiation syndrome (H-ARS): A review. *Cytokine.* 2015;71:22–37.
274. Farese AM, Cohen MV, Katz BP, et al. Filgrastim improves survival in lethally irradiated nonhuman primates. *Radiat Res.* 2013;179:89–100.
275. Farese AM, Cohen MV, Stead RB, et al. Pegfilgrastim administered in an abbreviated schedule, significantly improved neutrophil recovery after high-dose radiation-induced myelosuppression in rhesus macaques. *Radiat Res.* 2012;178:403–413.
276. Dainiak N, Gent RN, Carr Z, et al. First global consensus for evidence-based management of the hematopoietic syndrome resulting from exposure to ionizing radiation. *Disaster Med Public Health Prep.* 2011;5:202–212.
277. MacVittie TJ, Farese AM, Smith WG, et al. Myelopoietin, an engineered chimeric IL-3 and G-CSF receptor agonist, stimulates multilineage hematopoietic recovery in a nonhuman primate model of radiation-induced myelosuppression. *Blood.* 2000;95:837–845.
278. Nabholtz JM, Cantin J, Chang J, et al. Phase III trial comparing granulocyte colony-stimulating factor to leridistim in the prevention of neutropenic complications in breast cancer patients treated with docetaxel/doxorubicin/cyclophosphamide: results of the BCIRG 004 trial. *Clin Breast Cancer.* 2002;3:268–275.
279. Gluzman-Poltorak Z, Mendonca SR, Vainstein V, et al. Randomized comparison of single dose of recombinant human IL-12 versus placebo for restoration of hematopoiesis and improved survival in rhesus monkeys exposed to lethal radiation. *J Hematol Oncol.* 2014;7:31. doi:10.1186/1756-8722-7-31
280. Van der Meeren A, Mouthon MA, Gaugler MH, et al. Administration of recombinant human IL11 after supralethal radiation exposure promotes survival in mice: interactive effect with thrombopoietin. *Radiat Res.* 2002;157:642–649.
281. Farese AM, Hunt P, Grab LB, MacVittie TJ. Combined administration of recombinant human megakaryocyte growth and development factor and granulocyte colony-stimulating factor enhances multilineage hematopoietic reconstitution in nonhuman primates after radiation-induced marrow aplasia. *J Clin Invest.* 1996;97:2145–2151.
282. Zhou D, Deoliveira D, Kang Y, et al. Insulin-like growth factor 1 mitigates hematopoietic toxicity after lethal total body irradiation. *Int J Radiat Oncol Biol Phys.* 2013;85:1141–1148.

283. Casey-Sawicki K, Zhang M, Kim S, et al. A basic fibroblast growth factor analog for protection and mitigation against acute radiation syndromes. *Health Phys*. 2014;106:704–712.

284. Cohen EP, Fish BL, Moulder JE. Clinically relevant doses of enalapril mitigate multiple organ radiation injury. *Radiat Res*. 2016;185:313–318.

285. Medhora M, Gao F, Wu Q, et al. Model development and use of ACE inhibitors for preclinical mitigation of radiation-induced injury to multiple organs. *Radiat Res*. 2014;182:545–555.

286. Cohen EP, Molteni A, Hill P, et al. Captopril preserves function and ultrastructure in experimental radiation nephropathy. *Lab Invest*. 1996;75:349–360.

287. Moulder JE, Cohen EP, Fish BL. Captopril and losartan for mitigation of renal injury caused by single-dose total-body irradiation. *Radiat Res*. 2011;175:29–36.

288. Moulder JE, Fish BL, Cohen EP. ACE inhibitors and AII receptor antagonists in the treatment and prevention of bone marrow transplant nephropathy. *Curr Pharm Des*. 2003;9:737–749.

289. Cohen EP, Irving AA, Drobyski WR, et al. Captopril to mitigate chronic renal failure after hematopoietic stem cell transplantation: a randomized controlled trial. *Int J Radiat Oncol Biol Phys*. 2008;70:1546–1551.

290. Cohen EP, Bedi M, Irving AA, et al. Mitigation of late renal and pulmonary injury after hematopoietic stem cell transplantation. *Int J Radiat Oncol Biol Phys*. 2012;83:292–296.

291. Ostrau C, Hülsenbeck J, Herzog M, et al. Lovastatin attenuates ionizing radiation-induced normal tissue damage in vivo. *Radiother Oncol*. 2009;92:492–499.

292. Cai Y, Wang W, Liang H, et al. Keratinocyte growth factor pretreatment prevents radiation-induced intestinal damage in a mouse model. *Scand J Gastroenterol*. 2013;48:419–426.

293. Fu Q, Berbee M, Boerma M, et al. The somatostatin analog SOM230 (pasireotide) ameliorates injury of the intestinal mucosa and increases survival after total-body irradiation by inhibiting exocrine pancreatic secretion. *Radiat Res*. 2009;171:698–707.

294. Fu Q, Berbee M, Wang W, et al. Preclinical evaluation of Som230 as a radiation mitigator in a mouse model: postexposure time window and mechanisms of action. *Radiat Res*. 2011;175:728–735.

295. Rotolo J, Stancevic B, Zhang J, et al. Anti-ceramide antibody prevents the radiation gastrointestinal syndrome in mice. *J Clin Invest*. 2012;122:1786–1790.

296. Rasey JS, Nelson NJ, Mahler P, et al. Radioprotection of normal tissues against gamma rays and cyclotron neutrons with WR-2721: LD50 studies and 35S-WR-2721 biodistribution. *Radiat Res*. 1984;97:598–607.

297. Schweitzer AD, Revskaya E, Chu P, et al. Melanin-covered nanoparticles for protection of bone marrow during radiation therapy of cancer. *Int J Radiat Oncol Biol Phys*. 2010;78:1494–1502.

298. Miller AC, Cohen S, Stewart M, et al. Radioprotection by the histone deacetylase inhibitor phenylbutyrate. *Radiat Environ Biophys*. 2011;50:585–596.

299. Satyamitra M, Lombardini E, Graves J, 3rd, et al. A TPO receptor agonist, ALX-N4100TPO, mitigates radiation-induced lethality and stimulates hematopoiesis in CD2F1 mice. *Radiat Res*. 2011;175:746–758.

300. Gan J, Meng F, Zhou X, et al. Hematopoietic recovery of acute radiation syndrome by human superoxide dismutase–expressing umbilical cord mesenchymal stromal cells. *Cytotherapy*. 2015;17:403–17.

301. Mitchell JB, DeGraff W, Kaufman D, et al. Inhibition of oxygen-dependent radiation-induced damage by the nitroxide superoxide dismutase mimic, tempol. *Arch Biochem Biophys*. 1991;289:62–70.
302. Gao F, Fish BL, Szabo A, et al. Short-term treatment with a SOD/catalase mimetic, EUK-207, mitigates pneumonitis and fibrosis after single-dose total-body or whole-thoracic irradiation. *Radiat Res*. 2012;178:468–480.
303. Burdelya LG, Gleiberman AS, Toshkov I, et al. Toll-like receptor 5 agonist protects mice from dermatitis and oral mucositis caused by local radiation: implications for head-and-neck cancer radiotherapy. *Int J Radiat Oncol Biol Phys*. 2012;83:228–234.
304. Grace MB, Singh VK, Rhee JG, et al. 5-AED enhances survival of irradiated mice in a G-CSF-dependent manner, stimulates innate immune cell function, reduces radiation-induced DNA damage and induces genes that modulate cell cycle progression and apoptosis. *J Radiat Res*. 2012;53:840–853.
305. Kang AD, Cosenza SC, Bonagura M, et al. ON01210.Na (Ex-RAD(R)) mitigates radiation damage through activation of the AKT pathway. *PLOS ONE*. 2013;8:e58355. doi:10.1371/journal.pone.0058355
306. Hudak S, Leach MW, Xu Y, et al. Radioprotective effects of flk2/flt3 ligand. *Exp Hematol*. 1998;26:515–522.
307. Fukumoto R, Burns TM, Kiang JG. Ciprofloxacin enhances stress erythropoiesis in spleen and increases survival after whole-body irradiation combined with skin-wound trauma. *PLOS ONE*. 2014;9:e90448. doi:10.1371/journal.pone.0090448
308. Zetner D, Andersen L, Rosenberg J. Melatonin as protection against radiation injury: a systematic review. *Drug Res (Stuttg)*. 2016;66(6):281–296.
309. Shirazi A, Ghobadi G, Ghazi-Khansari M. A radiobiological review on melatonin: a novel radioprotector. *J Radiat Res*. 2007;48:263–272.
310. Aktas C, Kanter M, Kocak Z. Antiapoptotic and proliferative activity of curcumin on ovarian follicles in mice exposed to whole body ionizing radiation. *Toxicol Ind Health*. 2012;28:852–863.
311. Nagataki S, Takamura N. A review of the Fukushima nuclear reactor accident: radiation effects on the thyroid and strategies for prevention. *Curr Opin Endocrinol Diabetes Obes*. 2014;21:384–393.
312. Kahmann C, Wunderlich G, Freudenberg R, et al. Radioprotection of thyroid cells mediated by methimazole. *Int J Radiat Biol*. 2010;86:811–816.

# 11

# Risk and Prevention of Radiation-Induced Cancers

*Sophia C. Kamran and Akila N. Viswanathan*

## OVERVIEW

- Improvements in cancer prevention, detection, treatment, and survival have greatly contributed to higher survival rates in cancer patients.
- As patients survive for longer periods of time, they are experiencing long-term sequelae associated with cancer treatment, including development of a new secondary malignancy.
- It is estimated that cancer survivors have a 14% increased risk of developing a secondary malignancy as compared to the general population.
- Radiation therapy (RT) has the potential to act as a carcinogen.
- New techniques and therapies may impact secondary-malignancy risk in cancer survivors.

Cancer survivors are living longer as treatment modalities, techniques, and early cancer detection continue to advance. However, treatments are not without long-term consequence. One of the most challenging and serious late effects of treatment is secondary malignant neoplasm (SMN). Cancer survivors included in the National Cancer Institute's (NCI) Surveillance, Epidemiology, and End Results (SEER) database had a 14% increased risk of developing a new malignancy, as compared to the general population (1). The risk of developing an SMN may be multifactorial and may depend on the treatment received, as both chemotherapy and radiation have been linked to SMNs. For an SMN to be considered possibly attributable to radiation, it must fall within the primary or secondary radiation beam, have a different histology than the primary cancer, have a latency period of several years, not have been present at the time of initial cancer diagnosis, and not be in a patient with a cancer-prone syndrome (2).

The carcinogenicity of radiation has long been reported based on data from atomic bomb survivors as well as radiation workers (3). After Roentgen discovered x-rays in 1895, it was quickly discovered that the new technology could harm biologic tissue (3). The recognition that radiation causes malignancies came a few years after Roentgen's discovery, when skin cancers, sarcomas, lung cancers, leukemias, and other cancers were noted in those who conducted early experiments with x-rays, and in workers who had direct contact with the sources. The bombings of Hiroshima and Nagasaki further solidified our understanding of the harmful short-term and long-term effects on humans, especially for those exposed to acute low- to moderate-dose radiation (<2 Gy). However, the risk of secondary malignancy after high-dose therapeutic radiation (>5 Gy) is less well understood.

SMN risk differs across disease subsites, as each have their own inherent risks, either from the disease itself or from treatment. In this chapter, we first discuss the overall radiation biology of SMN along with factors that alter the SMN risk with modern-day radiation. We then review each disease subsite to discuss characteristics and factors unique to it and the related literature. Our goal is to encompass a broad understanding of the SMN risks, and provide guidance as to how radiation oncologists might be able to minimize such risks.

## RADIATION BIOLOGY

- Multiple models have attempted to describe the SMN risk after therapeutic radiation.
- One universal model has not been found to fully describe all observations of effect of radiation on SMN risk.
- SMN risk is altered by multiple factors including patient age, radiation field size, use of chemotherapy, and radiation technique. These factors all play a role in the carcinogenicity of radiation, altering the risk and further muddling the picture.

Multiple studies have attempted to model SMN risk after radiation therapy. In 2013, Berrington de Gonzalez and colleagues conducted a systematic review of epidemiologic studies that evaluated the dose-response relationship after high-dose fractionated RT, and found no clear evidence of nonlinearity in support of a reduction in the risk at high doses, even in doses higher than 60 Gy (4). The only exception applied to patients with thyroid cancer, for whom there was a plateau and then a reduction in risk noted at doses higher than 20 Gy.

Sachs et al suggested a model to explain these observations, which posits significant levels of radiation-induced stem-cell repopulation counteracting comparably large levels of cell killing induced by radiation, so that the response (and risk) remain nearly linear (5). Another theoretical model by Schneider and Schafer (6) analyzed the effects of inflammation and proliferative stress risks from fractionated RT. Tissue injury due to high doses of radiation may be secondary to enhanced cell proliferation, escaping senescence and apoptosis, and reentering the cell cycle, thus triggering enhanced carcinogenesis. An acceleration model parameter, $p$, was introduced and affects the dose-response model at large doses.

In a SEER database analysis of 647,672 cancer patients, 9% of whom developed a second solid cancer, the relative risk (RR) was higher for SMN sites that received higher than 5 Gy than for sites that received 5 Gy or less (excluding intensity-modulated radiation therapy [IMRT] and stereotactic body radiation therapy [SBRT]) (7). It is important to develop a model that predicts for SMN risk in the era of high-dose radiation and newer radiation techniques such as IMRT and SBRT.

### Age and Its Role

- Age plays a large role in carcinogenesis after irradiation. Children and adolescents in puberty are known to be more radiosensitive than adults.

- SMN risk increases indefinitely after radiation exposure, and the cumulative lifetime risks of those treated with radiation are much higher than those of the age-matched population.
- It is, therefore, imperative to focus efforts on limiting radiation dose exposure for children and young adults, for whom radiation carries the greatest long-term risk.

Many tissues are at risk when irradiating a child or a young adult. A study performed by Inskip et al evaluated breast cancer risk in girls relative to doses received in early childhood, when developing breast tissue is of greatest concern. The odds ratio for breast cancer increased linearly with radiation dose, reaching 11-fold for breast doses of approximately 40 Gy, compared to no radiation (8). Other factors modify the risk, including receipt of chemotherapy and hormonal status at time of treatment. A separate study evaluated the SMN risk among patients with Hodgkin lymphoma (HL) treated with radiation, finding that the RR of developing *any SMN* increased with lower age at diagnosis, compared with an age- and gender-matched general population (9). The RR for SMN development was 2.4 for patients diagnosed and treated at age over 50 years, 4.9 for patients aged 20 to 50 years, and 10.7 for patients less than 20 years. However, the absolute excess risk (AR) for those three age groups (youngest to oldest) was 71.0, 88.5, and 211.0 per 10,000 person-years, respectively. This is due to the fact that the elderly have a much greater risk of developing cancers overall. Nevertheless, this, and other studies, demonstrated how crucial continued long-term follow-up is for childhood-cancer survivors.

## Delivery of Radiation

- Radiation techniques have greatly evolved over the years and novel techniques may expose less tissue to high doses compared to older techniques. Some modalities, such as IMRT, can increase the volume of tissue receiving low radiation dose.
- Understanding the SMN risk in the context of these new treatment modalities is difficult as most studies predate this era of new technology.

IMRT creates highly conformal radiation treatment plans that attempt to avoid giving high doses to most normal tissue structures by "conforming" the beam around the tumor. This can allow for dose escalation in many cases. There has been a suggestion that the amount of "low-dose bath" to normal tissues may actually increase with the use of highly conformal radiation and play a role in increased SMNs, but additional studies need to be conducted to further understand this risk.

Given the physical characteristics of the beam, proton therapy has recently become of great interest to treating radiation oncologists. The particles are heavily charged and exhibit rapidly increasing and large energy losses near the end of their ranges, known as the Bragg peak, thereby minimizing radiation exposure to surrounding nontarget tissues (10). Protons are frequently used in the context of pediatric treatment, given the aforementioned risks of unnecessary radiation exposure in children. Because proton treatment has only recently been incorporated into treatments for certain cancers, more studies are needed to truly assess its effects and the risk of SMN in the proton-treated population. Early studies are promising, however. For example, patients treated at the Harvard Cyclotron with proton radiation with passive scattering were matched to photon-treated patients identified in the SEER database (11). After adjusting for gender and age at treatment, proton treatment was not associated with an increased risk of SMN compared to photon therapy (hazard ratio [HR] 0.52, $P$ <.009). There were 6.9 cancers per 1,000 person-years observed in the proton group and 10.3 per 1,000 person-years observed in the photon group. Median follow-up times were 6.0 and 6.7 years in the photon and proton cohorts, respectively, which is considered very short given the normal 10- to 20-year time interval required to assess SMN risk. Future studies with longer follow-up and large patient numbers are needed to determine the true SMN risk.

## Radiation Field Size

- SMN risk increases with increasing radiation field size, as more tissue is irradiated.
- By decreasing radiation field size, SMN risk can be reduced.

It is well known that decreasing radiation field size corresponds to reduced SMN risk. For HL patients, the RR of SMN was estimated to be 2.1 after mantle radiation alone (Figure 11.1), 4.2 for subtotal nodal irradiation, and

**Historical Mantle Field (Dose: 40–44 Gy)**

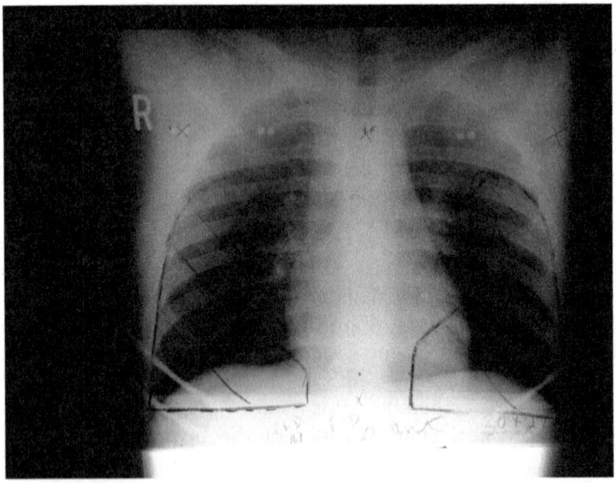

**Figure 11.1 A Depiction of Mantle Radiation Fields on a Patient.** Hand-cut cerrobend blocks were used, and patients were treated AP/PA without subfields. Wedges were used to make up for inhomogeneity. As depicted, radiation was delivered to cover most lymph node stations in the upper half of the body.
AP, anterior–posterior; PA, posterior–anterior.
Photo courtesy of Dr. Andrea Ng.

## 11. RISK AND PREVENTION OF RADIATION-INDUCED CANCERS

5.1 for total nodal irradiation compared to the age- and gender-matched general population (9). Chemotherapy given concurrently with radiation increased the risk in all cases; the same fields had RRs of 4.7, 5.9, and 13.5, respectively ($P = .03$). In a cohort of 1,112 female 5-year HL survivors treated before the age of 51 years, full mantle irradiation was associated with a 2.7-fold increased risk of breast cancer compared with mediastinal irradiation alone (12). The less breast tissue exposed, the lower the risk of breast cancer. This is keeping with the hypothesis that smaller radiation fields will reduce the long-term risk of SMN.

## HEMATOLOGIC MALIGNANCIES

- The literature on late effects of radiation on patients treated for HL is robust, as HL patients are often young, their prognosis for long-term survival is good, and radiation plays an important role in their treatment.
- Lung, stomach, other gastrointestinal (GI) malignancies, and, in particular, breast cancer, are all relatively common SMNs in previously irradiated HL patients.
- A 30-year-old HL patient who received radiation has a 20% risk of SMN by age 60 years.
- Adequate counseling, rigorous follow-up, and appropriate screening tools are important for this population.

Robust data exist on the risk of SMNs among HL survivors. A large study published in 2007 with data from 18,862 5-year HL survivors estimated the RR (compared to the general population) and cumulative incidence for SMN relative to age at HL diagnosis (13). Data are summarized in Table 11.1. For men and women diagnosed with HL at age 30 years, the 30-year cumulative risks of SMN were 18% and 26% respectively, compared to 7% and 9% for age- and gender-matched controls in the general population. The excess cumulative incidence of SMN was highly dependent on age at HL diagnosis, particularly for women. Women diagnosed with HL at age 20 years were estimated to have a 30-year cumulative incidence of SMN that was 20% higher than that of age-matched controls in the general population. These trends have implications for screening recommendations in this population. For example, in the United States, colorectal screening typically commences at age 50 years. However, the absolute risk of colorectal cancer for an HL survivor at age 35 to 40 years has been found to be comparable to that of an average 50- to 54-year-old in the general population. Similarly, breast cancer screening typically begins at age 40 years; however, the absolute risk of breast cancer among young female HL survivors has been shown to be comparable to that of an average 50-year-old woman within 5 to 10 years of HL diagnosis.

Lung cancer after radiation therapy for HL is a major concern given recent growing evidence for and interest in radiation-induced lung tumors. A study by Gilbert et al matched 227 HL survivors with 455 controls, and found an estimated excess RR per Gray received of 0.15 (95% CI: 0.06–0.39) (15).

Stomach cancer is another cause of morbidity and mortality among HL survivors. The risk of stomach cancer after HL treatment was examined in a study by Morton et al in which 89 cases were matched with 190 controls. Stomach cancer risk increased with increasing radiation dose and with

# RADIATION THERAPY TREATMENT EFFECTS

**Table 11.1** Studies Examining the Rates of Secondary Malignancy in Irradiated Populations

| Study | Number of patients | Secondary malignancy | Risk |
|---|---|---|---|
| **Hematologic Malignancy** | | | |
| Hodgson et al (13) | 18,862 5-year survivors | Breast<br>Infradiaphragmatic[b]<br>Supradiaphragmatic[c]<br>Thyroid<br>Soft tissue and bone | 6.1[a]<br>3.7<br>6.0<br>3.1<br>11.7 |
| Travis et al (14) | 3,817 1-year survivors | Breast | [d]1.4%, 11.1%, 29%<br>[e]0.7%, 5.3%, 15% |
| Gilbert et al (15) | 19,046 1-year survivors | Lung | 5.8[a,f] |
| Morton et al (16) | 19,882 ≥5-year survivors | Stomach | 6.8[g] |
| **Breast Malignancy** | | | |
| Berrington de Gonzalz et al (17) | 182,057 5-year survivors | High-dose region[h]<br>Contralateral breast | 1.45[a]<br>1.09 |
| Stovall et al (18) | 2,017 survivors | Contralateral breast | 2.5 and 3.0[a,i] |
| Inskip et al (19) | 8,976 survivors | Lung | 1.8[a] at 10 years |
| Grantzau et al (20) | 23,627 survivors | Lung | 8.5% per Gy[j] |
| Morton et al (21) | 289,748 ≥5-year survivors | Esophagus | 8.3[g,k] |
| **Gynecologic Malignancy** | | | |
| Wright et al (22) | 199,268 6-month survivors with primary tumors of vulva, cervix, uterus, anus, rectum | Leukemia<br>Multiple myeloma | 1.72[l]<br>1.08[m] |
| Onsrud et al (23) | 568 survivors of endometrial cancer | Secondary malignancy, nonspecified | 2.02[l] |
| Wiltink et al (24) | 2,554 patients from TME, PORTEC-1, PORTEC-2 trials | Any secondary malignancy | 2.98[n] |

*(continued)*

## 11. RISK AND PREVENTION OF RADIATION-INDUCED CANCERS 283

**Table 11.1** Studies Examining the Rates of Secondary Malignancy in Irradiated Populations (*continued*)

| Study | Number of patients | Secondary malignancy | Risk |
|---|---|---|---|
| Lonn et al (25) | 60,949 ≥1 year uterine cancer survivors | Any secondary malignancy | 1.26, 1.15, 1.07[o,p] |
| **Genitourinary Malignancy** | | | |
| Travis et al (26) | 40,000 1-year survivors | Secondary solid cancer | 2.0[a] |
| **Pediatric Malignancy** | | | |
| Bowers et al (27) | >150,000 | CNS neoplasms | 8.1–52.3[a] |
| Friedman et al (28) | 14,363 5-year survivors | Meningioma<br>Osteosarcoma<br>Bone cancer<br>Thyroid cancer<br>Head and neck cancer<br>Breast cancer<br>AML | 87.8[n]<br>30<br>19<br>10.9<br>10.8<br>9.8<br>9.3 |

[a]Risk given in relative risk values.
[b]Infradiaphragmatic solid tumors include stomach, colon, rectum and anus, pancreas, urinary bladder, kidney.
[c]Supradiaphragmatic solid tumors include buccal, esophagus, lung, pleura.
[d]Cumulative absolute risk for a female treated with chest irradiation at 25 years of age to a dose of 40 Gy or more without alkylating agents by age 35, 45, and 55 years.
[e]Cumulative absolute risk for a female treated with chest irradiation at 25 years of age to a dose of 40 Gy or more with alkylating agents by age 35, 45, and 55 years.
[f]RR of 5.8 at the median dose of 32 Gy.
[g]Odds ratio.
[h]High-dose region defined as receiving 1 Gy or more, including esophagus, pleura, lung, bone, soft tissue.
[i]Relative risk was 2.5 for women less than 40 years of age who received more than 1.0 Gy of absorbed dose, RR = 3.0 for women less than 40 years of age with follow-up more than 5 years.
[j]Risk increased linearly 8.5% per Gray in patients who developed a primary lung cancer 5 years or longer after breast cancer treatment.
[k]In patients who received 35 Gy or more to the esophagus.
[l]Hazard ratio.
[m]Nonsignificant.
[n]Standardized incidence ratio.
[o]Incidence rate ratios.
[p]1.26 for combined external beam and brachytherapy, 1.16 for external beam alone, 1.07 for brachytherapy alone.
AML, acute myeloid leukemia; CNS, central nervous system; PORTEC, Postoperative Radiation Therapy for Endometrial Cancer; TME, total mesorectal excision.

increasing number of alkylating chemotherapy cycles (16). Another study found that in testicular cancer in HL survivors, mean stomach radiation doses more than 20 Gy were associated with a 9.9-fold increased risk for malignancy, compared with doses under 11 Gy; the risk of gastric cancer increased significantly with increasing estimated stomach dose (29).

Given these risks of lung and stomach cancer, it is especially important for practitioners to counsel HL survivors on the risks of smoking, as well as to evaluate GI symptoms promptly with appropriate work-up, particularly if the patient received infradiaphragmatic radiation therapy along with alkylating chemotherapy.

In 2005, Travis et al sought to estimate the cumulative absolute risk of breast cancer among women diagnosed with HL at age 30 years or less between 1965 and 1994 (Table 11.1) (14). Risks were generated for different cohorts depending on age and the use of alkylating chemotherapy, which has been shown to reduce the risk of breast cancer (Table 11.2). Of note, the study did not account for competing breast cancer risk factors, and the data may not be applicable to modern women treated with smaller radiation fields. Long-term survivors of HL who develop subsequent new breast primary cancers have been shown to have different presentations, clinical characteristics, treatment, and outcomes than women in the general population who develop primary breast cancer (Table 11.3).

A variety of factors play a role in subsequent breast cancer development after radiation treatment for HL. van Leeuwen et al examined the role of radiation dose, chemotherapy use, and hormonal status in breast cancer development (33). Using historical datasets, it was found that increasing radiation dose led to an increased risk for breast cancer (RR of 4.47 for doses

**Table 11.2** Factors That May Reduce the Risk of SMN in Irradiated Populations

| Secondary malignancy by primary site | Factors that have been shown to reduce risk |
|---|---|
| **Hematologic Primary** | |
| Breast<br>Lung<br>Stomach<br>Thyroid<br>Soft tissue and bone<br>Others | Alkylating chemotherapy, menopause (12)<br>Reduced radiation field size for all others (9) |
| **Breast Primary** | |
| Lung<br>Esophagus | Smoking cessation (20)<br>Reduced use of supraclavicular and internal mammary nodal irradiation (21) |
| **Pediatric Primary** | |
| Any SMN | Proton therapy (30) |
| SMN, secondary malignant neoplasm. | |

## 11. RISK AND PREVENTION OF RADIATION-INDUCED CANCERS 285

**Table 11.3** Characteristics of Subsequent New Breast Primary in HL Survivors Compared to General Population With New Breast Primary

| Diagnosis | Characteristics of tumor | Treatment | Outcomes |
|---|---|---|---|
| • Younger at diagnosis (45 years compared to 63) (31)<br>• Diagnosed by mammography (40% versus 33%) (32)<br>• Diagnosed at an earlier stage (DCIS or stage I, 61% versus 42%) (32)<br>• Present with bilateral disease (6% versus 2%) (32)<br>• Metachronous contralateral tumors were four times greater (32) | • More likely to have estrogen- and progesterone-receptor-negative status (31) | • More likely to undergo complete mastectomy (31)<br>• 35% of those who underwent partial mastectomy did not receive radiation (31) | • Lower 15-year overall survival rates than the general population with first primary breast cancer (48% versus 58% for localized breast cancer, $P < .0001$) (31)<br>• Mortality from heart disease also higher than general population (31) |

DCIS, ductal carcinoma in situ; HL, Hodgkin lymphoma.

between 38.5 and 56 Gy compared to referent group doses between 0.26 and 3.9 Gy). The use of alkylating chemotherapy was found to be protective, as it often puts patients into menopause, decreasing breast tissue hormonal exposure (RR of 0.33 for patients receiving <6 cycles of alkylating chemotherapy and 0.28 for ≥6 cycles, compared to a referent group receiving no chemotherapy). Early menopause (age 19–30 years) was associated with a decreased RR for breast cancer after radiation. Volume treated was also important (Table 11.2).

Screening this young population may be difficult, as mammography has been suggested to be less sensitive in patients under age 40 years. Breast MRI has emerged as the preferred technology for screening high-risk women (eg, *BRCA* carriers). Ng et al performed a prospective analysis using breast MRI and mammography to screen female HL survivors who had chest radiation for HL at age less than 35 years and were at least 8 years out from diagnosis (34). Sensitivity was 68% for mammography and 67% for MRI; however, the combined sensitivity of both modalities was 94%. Hence, it was concluded that using both modalities would be more beneficial in the HL survivor population than either alone.

Overall, historically treated female HL survivors are at increased risk of breast cancer, particularly if treated at a young age. Breast cancer after HL appears to differ from de novo breast cancer, with younger age at presentation and poorer biologic characteristics. Overall and cause-specific survival rates are worse in the HL survivors, hence it is important to develop rigorous screening and educational awareness programs in order to detect cancers earlier.

## BREAST CANCER

- Improvements in diagnosis and treatment of primary breast cancer has allowed over 90% of survivors to live 5 or more years. The development of an SMN is of great concern to this healthy population. Radiation also plays an important role in the treatment of breast cancers.
- The risk of radiation-induced SMN is not clear in *BRCA1/2* carriers, as data are conflicting.
- Breast cancer survivors have been found to have an 18% increased risk of SMN compared to the general population (35).

Berrington de Gonzalez and colleagues evaluated long-term cancer risks of breast cancer survivors between 1973 and 2000 using the SEER database (17). Among 182,057 breast cancer survivors, 15,498 SMN had occurred. The RR for SMN in a high-dose site ($\geq$1 Gy) was 1.45 (95% CI: 1.33–1.58) compared to the age- and gender-matched general population. There was no excess risk for sites that received less than 1 Gy. Risks were lower for modern treatment periods (1993 or more recent) and higher for younger age at time of treatment. SMNs that were greatly increased (>2-fold standard incidence ratios) included esophageal, pleural, bone, soft tissue, and contralateral breast. The RR of lung cancer was also significantly increased, and was higher for ipsilateral than for contralateral lung cancer (1.54 versus 1.18). For patients diagnosed with breast cancer in 1983 or later, the lung cancer risk was higher after mastectomy than after breast-conserving therapy. The RR for esophageal cancers was 1.99, and the risk for soft-tissue cancers was 2.52; the risk for angiosarcomas was especially elevated (RR = 13.7). Rubino et al demonstrated a dose-response relation between breast irradiation and soft-tissue or bone sarcoma (36). All sarcomas were relatively rare in that cohort, with a 15-year incidence estimate of 0.3%. Women who received more than 14 Gy had a higher risk than women who received less than 14 Gy; the odds ratios were 1.6 and 30.6 for women who received 14 to 44 Gy and 45 Gy or more at the site of sarcoma, respectively.

Stovall et al addressed the risk of contralateral breast cancer after RT for a first breast cancer using information from the Women's Environmental, Cancer, and Radiation Epidemiology (WECARE) study, with 708 cases of bilateral breast cancer (asynchronous) and 1,399 controls (women with unilateral breast cancer) (18). Dose estimates to the contralateral breast were measured with a thermoluminescent dosimeter in tissue-equivalent phantoms. Mean radiation dose to the specific quadrant of the contralateral breast cancer was 1.1 Gy. Younger women (<40 years) who received more than 1.0 Gy of absorbed dose to the quadrant of contralateral breast cancer had a 2.5-fold greater risk of cancer than unexposed women. Women less than 40 years old with follow-up more than 5 years had an RR of 3.0 (95% CI: 1.1–8.1) with a significant dose dependence (an excess RR per Gy of 1.0). However, no excess risk was observed in women treated at age more than 45 years, which is typically when women experience their first breast cancer.

Risks for lung and esophageal cancers have been studied and are summarized in Table 11.1. A history of smoking increases the risk for lung cancer, while tamoxifen appeared to have a protective effect against the development of esophageal cancer (21).

One interesting question regarding SMN risk after primary breast cancer treatment is how the risk translates to *BRCA1/2* carriers. These patients may have more sensitivity to the carcinogenic effect of RT due to their impaired DNA repair capacity. A review by Drooger et al. examined this risk based on the current literature (37). Data were scarce for patients who developed breast cancer after age 30 years who opted for breast-conserving therapy and there was no hard data indicating an increased risk for a second primary breast cancer, either ipsilateral or contralateral (37). An analysis of the WECARE study, which examined the risk of contralateral breast cancer based on dose to the contralateral breast, also did not find different risks based on germline *BRCA1/2* mutations, but numbers were small (38). However, low-dose radiation exposure from diagnostic procedures has been found to increase the risk of primary breast cancer in young *BRCA1/2* carriers (<30 years) (39). Caution is thus necessary in this group when using radiation as part of primary treatment for breast cancer. Further research is needed on the long-term effects of therapeutic radiation on *BRCA* carriers.

## GYNECOLOGIC MALIGNANCIES

- Pelvic radiation is commonly used for gynecologic malignancies. There is a concern for potential secondary malignancies after pelvic irradiation.
- Studies have shown that the cumulative incidence of any SMN ranges between 9% and 17% following radiation for cervical, vaginal, vulvar, uterine, or ovarian cancer.

Pelvic RT is often employed to ensure local control of gynecologic cancers. Data on SMN due to pelvic irradiation have been conflicting. SEER studies have found an increased risk of SMN among women who received pelvic RT (22,40–45), but as radiation dose and treatment fields are not included in the SEER registry, it is difficult to ascertain whether a relationship exists between radiation dose and treatment fields used. A SEER-based study evaluating survivors 1 year or more after uterine cancer diagnosis found that combined brachytherapy and external beam radiation therapy (EBRT) had an SMN incident rate ratio (IRR) of 1.26 (95% CI: 1.16–1.36), whereas EBRT alone had an IRR of 1.15 (95% CI: 1.08–1.22) and brachytherapy alone had an IRR of 1.07 (95% CI: 1.00–1.16) (25).

However, in a pooled analysis by Wiltink et al (24), which included endometrial cancer patients from the Postoperative Radiation Therapy for Endometrial Cancer (PORTEC)-1 (46) and PORTEC-2 (47) trials and rectal cancer patients from the total mesorectal excision (TME) trial (48), for a total of over 2,500 patients with a median follow-up time of 13 years, there was no difference in the probability of developing an SMN between those who received pelvic irradiation and those who did not (15-year rates: no radiation 26.5%; EBRT 25.6%, $P = .94$). The standardized incidence ratio (SIR) for all included patients for all types of SMN (compared to a matched general population) was 2.98 (95% CI: 2.82–3.14). Practitioners should nevertheless be aware that rectal and endometrial cancer survivors have a three times greater risk of developing an SMN than those in the general population.

## GASTROINTESTINAL MALIGNANCIES

- Many rectal cancer patients present at an early age, and the concern for SMN is therefore greater than it would be for cancers that typically present in an older population. However, data on degree of increased risk are sparse.

Data are conflicting regarding SMN risk after pelvic irradiation. A study in 2007 by Kendal et al demonstrated an increased risk of second primary cancer of the uterus or cervix in females who received radiation for a GI malignancy (48). Using the SEER database, 20,910 individuals with pathologically confirmed rectal cancer were analyzed; rates of second primary cancer were evaluated comparing patients who did not receive radiation to those who did. Pelvic irradiation was found to be associated with an elevated risk of second primary gynecologic cancer (uterus and cervix; HR = 2.5, 95% CI: 1.6–2.4, $P$ <.001). However, as shown earlier, in the Wiltink pooled analysis, the individual TME trial showed no difference in risk of SMN at 10 years by treatment (15.3% in patients who received no radiation versus 14.8% in patients who received EBRT) (24).

## GENITOURINARY MALIGNANCIES

- Testicular cancer is a disease of young men with an estimated 10-year survival of 95%; late manifestations of treatment, including SMN development, are therefore a growing concern.
- For men diagnosed with either seminoma or nonseminoma at age 35 years, cumulative risk of SMN is 35% after 40 years of follow-up, compared with 23% for the general population.
- Prostate cancer patients have multiple options for treatment, including radiation. Within this, there are different modalities (brachytherapy, EBRT, or a combination of both), each with different implications for SMN development.

Management of testicular cancer includes orchiectomy, with or without adjuvant regional radiation or retroperitoneal lymph node dissection, for early stage seminomas or nonseminomatous germ cell tumors. However, since the 1970s, nonseminoma patients have been managed with retroperitoneal lymph node dissection and chemotherapy in place of RT. Adjuvant radiation, in the past, included para-aortic and pelvic lymph nodes, with larger doses given for nonseminomas (45–55 Gy) than for seminomas (25–35 Gy). Hence, it is important to characterize SMN risk within a historical context, as radiation for testicular cancer has substantially changed over the past decades, and to factor in the excellent survival rates achieved (49). Travis et al sought to estimate the long-term site-specific absolute and relative risks of secondary cancers, by analyzing records of 40,000 1-year survivors of testicular cancer (26). The population included patients treated between 1943 and 2001, adequately spanning both the historical treatment cohorts as well as more modern day cohorts. Excess relative risk (ERR) and excess absolute risk (EAR) were evaluated using Poisson regression analysis, and average follow-up time was 11.3 years. Among testicular cancer patients who survived at least 10 years, an increased risk for secondary solid cancer was found for those who received RT alone as compared to chemotherapy alone (RR = 2.0, 95% CI: 1.9–2.2 versus RR = 1.8, 95% CI: 1.9–4.2, respectively). Risk from RT alone increased with increasing time from diagnosis (RR = 1.1 [95% CI: <1–1.6] in follow-up period 1 to 4 years versus RR = 2.0 [95 CI: 1.9–2.2] in follow-up period 10+ years). Among seminoma patients, the relative risk of solid cancers was higher for those diagnosed in 1975 and later than for those diagnosed before (RR difference 0.5, 95% CI: 0.05–0.9, $P$ = .03). This pattern was reversed for nonseminoma patients (RR difference −2.6, 95% CI: <−3 to −0.7, $P$ = .01). The decrease in risk after 1975 may be related to the decreased use of RT; the fact that RT continued to be used for seminoma patients may account for why a similar decrease in this group was not observed.

For testicular cancer patients treated with radiation, SMN sites included the stomach, colon, rectum, pancreas, lung, pleura, prostate, kidney, bladder, connective tissue, and thyroid. For men diagnosed with either seminoma or nonseminoma at age 35 years, cumulative risks were 36% and 31%, respectively, after 40 years of follow-up, compared with 23% for the general population (26). Careful follow-up of these patients is necessary, and additional long-term studies are necessary to further quantify the SMN risk, particularly for those treated in the modern era.

Murray et al sought to describe the SMN risk in prostate cancer patients previously treated with radiation, with particular attention to whether different radiation modalities affect the second cancer risk. Multiple studies were assessed, with heterogeneity between studies and small numbers studied in many. In general, the SMN risk appeared small, in the range of 1 in 220 to 1 in 290 (50). This risk increased up to 1 in 70 for patients followed for more than 10 years; however, because those patients had older radiation techniques and treatments used, their risk may not accurately reflect that of patients treated in the modern era. It is premature for studies involving modern techniques, such as IMRT or protons, to draw firm conclusions, but when comparing EBRT to brachytherapy, there appears to be a lower SMN risk with the utility of brachytherapy or brachytherapy combined with EBRT.

## PEDIATRICS

- Treatment of pediatric malignancies has greatly changed, resulting in improved overall survival.
- Radiation therapy is associated with a risk for SMN development, and this risk may be greater in patients with a germline mutation that contributes to malignancies. These patients may be more sensitive to ionizing radiation.

- Newer techniques have been introduced to decrease the SMN risk in pediatric patients.

The Childhood Cancer Survival Study (CCSS) reported an RR for SMN development of 2.7 (95% CI: 2.2–2.3) among pediatric patients who received RT (28). Patients with germline mutations, such as *TP53* or *RB1*, may have a higher risk (51). New secondary CNS malignancies are common among childhood cancer survivors who received prior radiation for a CNS cancer, which is a common pediatric primary malignancy. This risk is dose related, as identified among atomic bomb survivors (52). A study using the SEER database reported 10-year survival of 13.6% for secondary CNS tumors in childhood cancer survivors, and another study (53) reported that secondary CNS tumors were the second leading cause of death among childhood CNS cancer survivors, behind primary tumor recurrence (54). In a review by Bowers et al examining the recent literature on patients who developed subsequent CNS neoplasms after primary treatment for childhood CNS cancer, survivors had an 8.1 to 52.3 times higher incidence of secondary CNS neoplasms as compared to the general population, with high-grade glioma and meningioma being the two most common. Five-year survival rates ranged from 0 to 19.5% for high-grade gliomas, and overall survival from 6% to 15% (27). Neglia et al analyzed CNS SMN risk using the CCSS data (55), finding a statistically significant relationship between radiation dose and risk of CNS neoplasms, including glioma and meningioma. The excess RR was 0.33 per Gray for glioma, 1.06 per Gray for meningioma, and 0.69 per Gray for all CNS neoplasms, compared with controls matched by age at initial cancer diagnosis and sex.

Thyroid cancer is a common SMN in childhood cancer survivors. Bhatti et al, using data from 12,547 5-year childhood cancer survivors in the CCSS, analyzed radiation dose received (56). Thyroid cancer risk increased linearly with radiation dose up to 20 Gy (RR at 20 Gy = 14.6); however, for doses exceeding 20 Gy, a downturn was observed, similar to that found in the Berrington de Gonzalez study (4). This suggests that thyroid tissue is exceptionally sensitive to radiation.

Because of the increased incidence and concern for SMN in childhood cancer survivors, many radiation oncologists are turning to newer technologies to attempt to reduce this risk, most notably, proton beam therapy. In a study by Brodin et al, risks were modeled for pediatric patients with medulloblastoma treated with either three-dimensional conformal radiation therapy, inversely optimized rapid arc (RA) therapy, or intensity-modulated proton therapy (IMPT) (30). Estimates of SMN were higher for the RA plans, and the IMPT plans fared better than the photon techniques, even when taking secondary neutron irradiation into account (Table 11.2).

## CONCLUSIONS

- Secondary malignancies may be serious long-term consequences of primary cancer treatment.
- Modern radiation techniques and modalities (including IMRT and proton therapy), age at primary treatment, environmental factors, use of chemotherapy, and genetic predisposition can all alter SMN risk.

- Practitioners should be aware of potential SMN development, depending on primary malignancy treatment, and provide appropriate follow-up.
- Due to limited data on the effects of frequent diagnostic whole-body radiation exposure, as used for follow-up scans, the use of nonionizing radiation imaging techniques or biomarkers where available should be considered.
- Ongoing studies that incorporate modern techniques and control for confounders are important to truly assess the incidence and biology of radiation-induced SMN, and to predict those at increased risk in the present era.

## REFERENCES

1. Fraumeni JJ, Curtis R, Edwards B, Tucker M. Introduction. In: Curtis R, Freedman D, Ron E, et al, eds. *New Malignancies Among Cancer Survivors: SEER Cancer Registries, 1973–2000*. Bethesda, MD: National Cancer Institute; 2006:1–7.
2. Travis L, Bhatia S, Allan J, et al. Second primary cancers. In: DeVita VJ, Lawrence T, Rosenberg S, eds. *Cancer: Principles and Practice of Oncology*. 9th ed. Philadelphia, PA: Lippincott Williams and Wilkins; 2011:2393.
3. Doll R. Hazards of ionising radiation: 100 years of observations on man. *Br J Cancer*. 1995;72:1339–1349.
4. Berrington de Gonzalez A, Gilbert E, Curtis R, et al. Second solid cancers after radiation therapy: a systematic review of the epidemiologic studies of the radiation dose-response relationship. *Int J Radiat Oncol Biol Phys*. 2013;86:224–233.
5. Sachs RK, Brenner DJ. Solid tumor risks after high doses of ionizing radiation. *Proc Natl Acad Sci USA*. 2005;102:13040–13045.
6. Schneider U, Schafer B. Model of accelerated carcinogenesis based on proliferative stress and inflammation for doses relevant to radiotherapy. *Radiat Environ Biophys*. 2012;51:451–456.
7. Berrington de Gonzalez A, Curtis RE, Kry SF, et al. Proportion of second cancers attributable to radiotherapy treatment in adults: a cohort study in the US SEER cancer registries. *Lancet Oncol*. 2011;12:353–360.
8. Inskip PD, Robison LL, Stovall M, et al. Radiation dose and breast cancer risk in the childhood cancer survivor study. *J Clin Oncol*. 2009;27:3901–3907.
9. Ng AK, Bernardo MV, Weller E, et al. Second malignancy after Hodgkin disease treated with radiation therapy with or without chemotherapy: long-term risks and risk factors. *Blood*. 2002;100:1989–1996.
10. Bourland J. Radiation oncology physics. In: Gunderson LL, Tepper JE, eds. *Clinical Radiation Oncology*. 3rd ed. Philadelphia, PA: Saunders; 2012:95–153.
11. Chung CS, Yock TI, Nelson K, et al. Incidence of second malignancies among patients treated with proton versus photon radiation. *Int J Radiat Oncol Biol Phys*. 2013;87:46–52.
12. De Bruin ML, Sparidans J, van't Veer MB, et al. Breast cancer risk in female survivors of Hodgkin's lymphoma: lower risk after smaller radiation volumes. *J Clin Oncol*. 2009;27:4239–4246.
13. Hodgson DC, Gilbert ES, Dores GM, et al. Long-term solid cancer risk among 5-year survivors of hodgkin's lymphoma. *J Clin Oncol*. 2007;25:1489–1497.
14. Travis LB, Hill D, Dores GM, et al. Cumulative absolute breast cancer risk for young women treated for Hodgkin lymphoma. *J Natl Cancer Inst*. 2005;97:1428–1437.

15. Gilbert ES, Stovall M, Gospodarowicz M, et al. Lung cancer after treatment for Hodgkin's disease: focus on radiation effects. *Radiat Res.* 2003;159:161–173.
16. Morton LM, Dores GM, Curtis RE, et al. Stomach cancer risk after treatment for Hodgkin lymphoma. *J Clin Oncol.* 2013;31:3369–3377.
17. Berrington de Gonzalez A, Curtis RE, Gilbert E, et al. Second solid cancers after radiotherapy for breast cancer in SEER cancer registries. *Br J Cancer.* 2010;102:220–226.
18. Stovall M, Smith SA, Langholz BM, et al. Dose to the contralateral breast from radiotherapy and risk of second primary breast cancer in the WECARE study. *Int J Radiat Oncol Biol Phys.* 2008;72:1021–1030.
19. Inskip PD, Stovall M, Flannery JT. Lung cancer risk and radiation dose among women treated for breast cancer. *J Natl Cancer Inst.* 1994;86:983–988.
20. Grantzau T, Thomsen MS, Vaeth M, Overgaard J. Risk of second primary lung cancer in women after radiotherapy for breast cancer. *Radiother Oncol.* 2014;111:366–373.
21. Morton LM, Gilbert ES, Hall P, et al. Risk of treatment-related esophageal cancer among breast cancer survivors. *Ann Oncol.* 2012;23:3081–3091.
22. Wright JD, St Clair CM, Deutsch I, et al. Pelvic radiotherapy and the risk of secondary leukemia and multiple myeloma. *Cancer.* 2010;116:2486–2492.
23. Onsrud M, Cvancarova M, Hellebust TP, et al. Long-term outcomes after pelvic radiation for early-stage endometrial cancer. *J Clin Oncol.* 2013;31:3951–3956.
24. Wiltink LM, Nout RA, Fiocco M, et al. No increased risk of second cancer after radiotherapy in patients treated for rectal or endometrial cancer in the randomized TME, PORTEC-1, and PORTEC-2 trials. *J Clin Oncol.* 2015;33(15):1640–1646.
25. Lonn S, Gilbert ES, Ron E, et al. Comparison of second cancer risks from brachytherapy and external beam therapy after uterine corpus cancer. *Cancer Epidemiol Biomarkers Prev.* 2010;19: 464–474.
26. Travis LB, Fossa SD, Schonfeld SJ, et al. Second cancers among 40,576 testicular cancer patients: focus on long-term survivors. *J Natl Cancer Inst.* 2005;97:1354–1365.
27. Bowers DC, Nathan PC, Constine L, et al. Subsequent neoplasms of the CNS among survivors of childhood cancer: A systematic review. *Lancet Oncol.* 2013;14:e321–e328.
28. Friedman DL, Whitton J, Leisenring W, et al. Subsequent neoplasms in 5-year survivors of childhood cancer: the childhood cancer survivor study. *J Natl Cancer Inst.* 2010;102:1083–1095.
29. van den Belt-Dusebout AW, Aleman BM, Besseling G, et al. Roles of radiation dose and chemotherapy in the etiology of stomach cancer as a second malignancy. *Int J Radiat Oncol Biol Phys.* 2009;75:1420–1429.
30. Brodin NP, Munck Af Rosenschold P, Aznar MC, et al. Radiobiological risk estimates of adverse events and secondary cancer for proton and photon radiation therapy of pediatric medulloblastoma. *Acta Oncol.* 2011;50:806–816.
31. Milano MT, Li H, Gail MH, et al. Long-term survival among patients with Hodgkin's lymphoma who developed breast cancer: a population-based study. *J Clin Oncol.* 2010;28:5088–5096.
32. Elkin EB, Klem ML, Gonzales AM, et al. Characteristics and outcomes of breast cancer in women with and without a history of radiation for Hodgkin's lymphoma: a multi-institutional, matched cohort study. *J Clin Oncol.* 2011;29: 2466–2473.

33. van Leeuwen FE, Klokman WJ, Stovall M, et al. Roles of radiation dose, chemotherapy, and hormonal factors in breast cancer following Hodgkin's disease. *J Natl Cancer Inst*. 2003;95:971–980.

34. Ng AK, Garber JE, Diller LR, et al. Prospective study of the efficacy of breast magnetic resonance imaging and mammographic screening in survivors of Hodgkin lymphoma. *J Clin Oncol*. 2013;31:2282–2288.

35. Curtis RE, Ron E, Hankey B, Hoover R. New malignancies following breast cancer. In: Curtis R, Freedman D, Ron E, et al, eds. *New Malignancies among Cancer Survivors: SEER Cancer Registries, 1973–2000*. Bethesda, MD: National Cancer Institute; 2006:181–205.

36. Rubino C, Shamsaldin A, Le MG, et al. Radiation dose and risk of soft tissue and bone sarcoma after breast cancer treatment. *Breast Cancer Res Treat*. 2005;89:277–288.

37. Drooger JC, Hooning MJ, Seynaeve CM, et al. Diagnostic and therapeutic ionizing radiation and the risk of a first and second breast cancer, with special attention for BRCA1 and BRCA2 mutation carriers: a critical review of the literature. *Cancer Treat Rev*. 2015;41:187–196.

38. Bernstein JL, Thomas DC, Shore RE, et al. Contralateral breast cancer after radiotherapy among BRCA1 and BRCA2 mutation carriers: A WECARE study report. *Eur J Cancer*. 2013;49:2979–2985.

39. Pijpe A, Andrieu N, Easton DF, et al. Exposure to diagnostic radiation and risk of breast cancer among carriers of BRCA1/2 mutations: retrospective cohort study (GENE-RAD-RISK). *BMJ*. 2012;345:e5660.

40. Curtis RE, Ron E, Hankey B, Hoover R. New malignancies following cancer of the cervix uteri, vagina, and vulva. In: Curtis R, Freedman D, Ron E, et al, eds. *New Malignancies among Cancer Survivors: SEER Cancer Registries, 1973–2000*. Bethesda, MD: National Cancer Institute; 2006:207–209.

41. Boice JD Jr, Blettner M, Kleinerman RA, et al. Radiation dose and leukemia risk in patients treated for cancer of the cervix. *J Natl Cancer Inst*. 1987;79:1295–1311.

42. Travis LB, Andersson M, Gospodarowicz M, et al. Treatment-associated leukemia following testicular cancer. *J Natl Cancer Inst*. 2000;92:1165–1171.

43. Travis LB, Curtis RE, Stovall M, et al. Risk of leukemia following treatment for non-Hodgkin's lymphoma. *J Natl Cancer Inst*. 1994;86:1450–1457.

44. Boice JD Jr, Engholm G, Kleinerman RA, et al. Radiation dose and second cancer risk in patients treated for cancer of the cervix. *Radiat Res*. 1988;116:3–55.

45. Curtis RE, Boice JD Jr, Stovall M, et al. Relationship of leukemia risk to radiation dose following cancer of the uterine corpus. *J Natl Cancer Inst*. 1994;86:1315–1324.

46. Creutzberg CL, van Putten WL, Koper PC, et al. Surgery and postoperative radiotherapy versus surgery alone for patients with stage-1 endometrial carcinoma: multicentre randomised trial. PORTEC Study Group. Post operative radiation therapy in endometrial carcinoma. *Lancet*. 2000;355(9213):1404–1411.

47. Nout RA, Smit VT, Putter H, et al. Vaginal brachytherapy versus pelvic external beam radiotherapy for patients with endometrial cancer of high-intermediate risk (PORTEC-2): an open-label, non-inferiority, randomised trial. *Lancet*. 2010;375(9717):816–823.

48. Kendal WS, Nicholas G. A population-based analysis of second primary cancers after irradiation for rectal cancer. *Am J Clin Oncol*. 2007;30:333–339.

49. Howlader N, Noone A, Krapcho M, et al. SEER cancer statistics review. 1975–2012. http://seer.cancer.gov/csr/1975_2012/sections.html

50. Murray L, Henry A, Hoskin P, et al. PROBATE group of GEC ESTRO. Second primary cancers after radiation for prostate cancer: a systematic review of the clinical data and impact of treatment technique. *Radiother Oncol*. 2014;110:213–228.
51. Choi DK, Helenowski I, Hijiya N. Secondary malignancies in pediatric cancer survivors: perspectives and review of the literature. *Int J Cancer*. 2014;135:1764–1773.
52. Preston DL, Ron E, Yonehara S, et al. Tumors of the nervous system and pituitary gland associated with atomic bomb radiation exposure. *J Natl Cancer Inst*. 2002;94:1555–1563.
53. Vasudevan V, Cheung MC, Yang R, et al. Pediatric solid tumors and second malignancies: characteristics and survival outcomes. *J Surg Res*. 2010;160:184–189.
54. Morris EB, Gajjar A, Okuma JO, et al. Survival and late mortality in long-term survivors of pediatric CNS tumors. *J Clin Oncol*. 2007;25: 1532–1538.
55. Neglia JP, Robison LL, Stovall M, et al. New primary neoplasms of the central nervous system in survivors of childhood cancer: a report from the childhood cancer survivor study. *J Natl Cancer Inst*. 2006;98:1528–1537.
56. Bhatti P, Veiga LH, Ronckers CM, et al. Risk of second primary thyroid cancer after radiotherapy for a childhood cancer in a large cohort study: an update from the childhood cancer survivor study. *Radiat Res*. 2010;174:741–752.

# 12

# Cancer Survivorship: Approaches and Challenges

*Sophia K. Smith*

## EPIDEMIOLOGY OF SURVIVORSHIP

- "The term **cancer survivor** includes anyone who has been diagnosed with cancer, from the time of diagnosis through the rest of his or her life." (1)
- Long-term survivors are considered those who have *completed active treatment and are at least 5 years postdiagnosis.*
- The number of Americans living with cancer has risen steadily since the mid-1970s, attributed to better treatments, early detection, and aging of the population.
- As of January 2016, 15.5 million cancer survivors are living, or about 5% of the U.S. population.
- Cancer disproportionately affects the elderly; 60% of survivors are 65 years old or older

The term *cancer survivor* has been debated for years. The most commonly used definition is from the National Coalition of Cancer Survivorship, "The term *cancer survivor* includes anyone who has been diagnosed with cancer, from the time of diagnosis through the rest of his or her life." Other definitions have been in place, including one that includes those affected by the diagnosis, such as caregivers. However, for the purposes of this chapter we focus on the subset of long-term survivors who have completed active cancer treatment and are at least 5 years postdiagnosis.

This group of cancer survivors has been increasing steadily in numbers since the mid-1970s—largely attributed to better treatments, early detection, and the aging of our population (see Figures 12.1 and 12.2). Currently, there are about 15.5 million cancer survivors who are living, or about 5% of the U.S. population. This number is expected to increase greatly over the next decade to about 20 million by 2026 (Figure 12.3). This represents an increase by 31%, or 4 million survivors, within the next 10 years. And, cancer disproportionately impacts the elderly population who are already likely to be dealing with a multitude of comorbidities (see Figure 12.4). These factors continue to add stress to the cancer care system.

## TRANSITIONS

- The end of primary treatment is often one of significant emotions and a source of confusion.

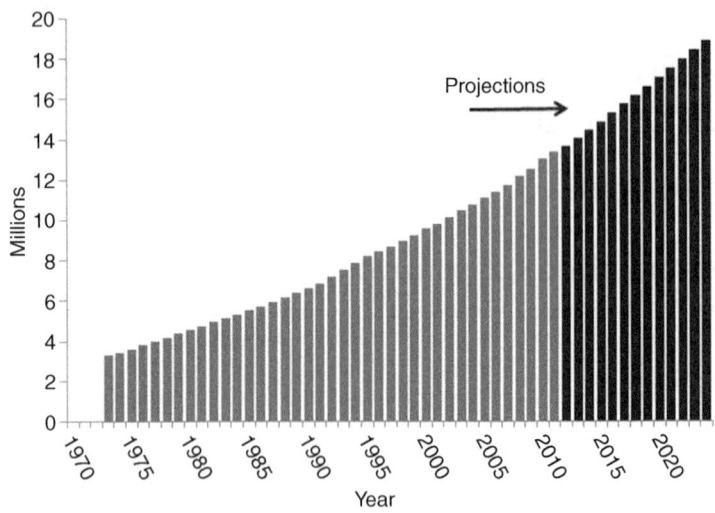

**Figure 12.1 Estimated Number of Cancer Survivors in the United States.**
*Source:* From Ref. (2). DeSantis CE, Lin CC, Mariotto AB, et al. Cancer treatment and survivorship statistics. *CA Cancer J Clin.* 2014;64(4):252–271.

- In addition to celebration, survivors may feel fear that the cancer will come back, sorrow/loss, grief, survivor guilt, uncertainty, anger, numbness, and spiritual distress.

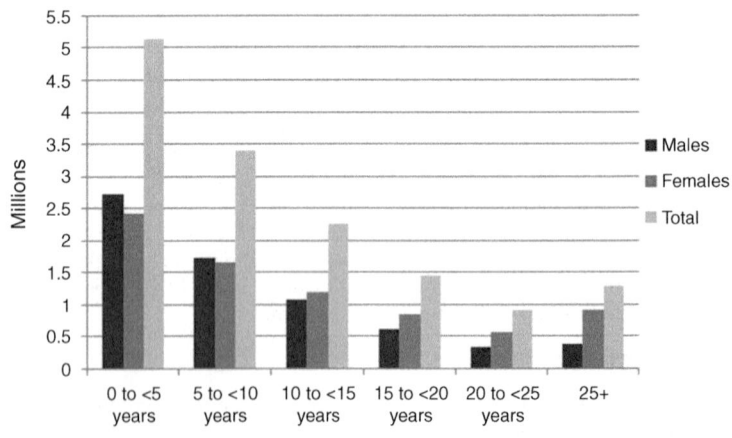

**Figure 12.2 Cancer Survivors in the United States by Years Since Diagnosis.**
*Source:* From Ref. (2). DeSantis CE, Lin CC, Mariotto AB, et al. Cancer treatment and survivorship statistics. *CA Cancer J Clin.* 2014;64(4):252–271.

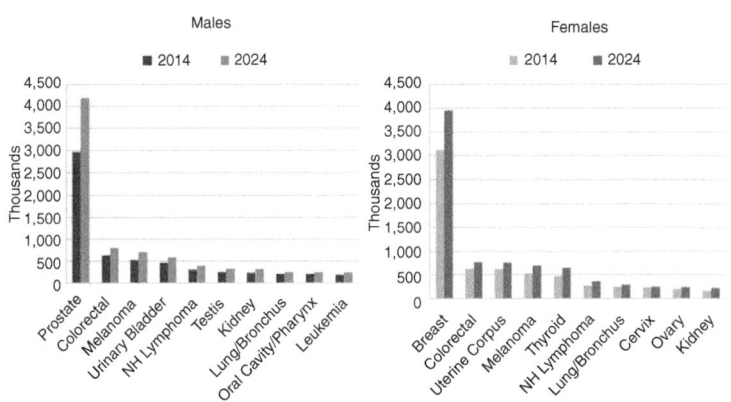

**Figure 12.3** Incidence of Cancer Survivors in the United States by Diagnoses.
NH, non-Hodgkin
*Source:* From Ref. (3). Curigliano G, Cardinale D, Dent S, et al. *CA: A Cancer Journal for Clinicians.* 2016;66(4):265–351. Republished with permission of John Wiley and Sons Inc. Permission conveyed through Copyright Clearance Center, Inc.

- Adjusting to these emotions takes time—survivors should not simply be told to "return to normal" and assume that they are immediately ready to return to activities such as jobs and school.
- Acknowledge that while health care providers are a primary source of support during the treatment phase, they are not as available once treatment ends. This may contribute to anxiety given the reduced surveillance and attention to physical and emotional issues.

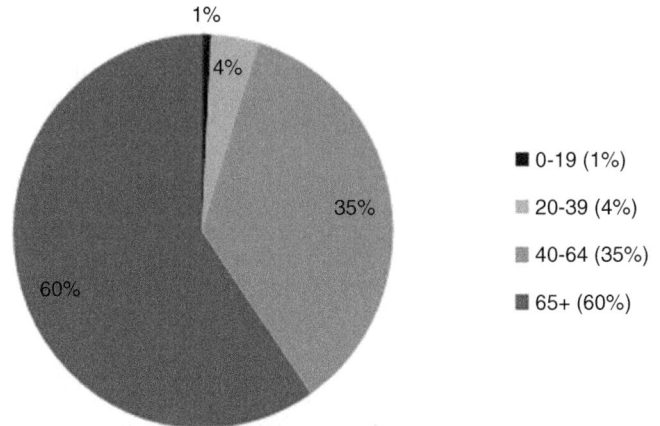

**Figure 12.4** Cancer Survivors in the United States by Age.
*Source:* From Ref. (2). DeSantis CE, Lin CC, Mariotto AB, et al. Cancer treatment and survivorship statistics. *CA Cancer J Clin.* 2014;64(4):252–271.

While the completion of curative treatment is often a time for celebration for the cancer survivor and loved ones, many survivors experience an increase in stress. For example, treatment cessation is also associated with less frequent visits to a health care provider—who was likely to be one of the primary sources of support and encouragement to the survivor and family. Survivors often report increased anxiety that is contributed by surveillance scans and tests and worry that the cancer has returned. Also, survivors are often required to transition back to a full-time job or school while they are still dealing with treatment-related symptoms, such as fatigue, pain, or emotional effects. It is important to recognize that emotional adjustment takes time—and each survivor experiences the transition to posttreatment differently. Normalizing these emotional reactions by assuring the survivor and family members that these emotional reactions often take time to resolve, and providing referrals to social workers or therapists who work with this population is very helpful. In addition, a referral to a career counselor might be beneficial to the survivor who is rethinking their return to "how things were" before cancer due to a reprioritization of life goals or inability to meet the demands of their job due to cancer- or treatment-related effects.

## HEALTH STATUS AND NEEDS OF CANCER SURVIVORS

- Cancer survivors are at increased risk for a second primary cancer and other long-term and late effects related to their physical and mental health.
- The cancer experience can impact the survivors' social life as well, including personal relationships, work or school, and financial well-being.
- While the cancer experience is traumatic, many survivors report positive outcomes (ie, posttraumatic growth) that often coexist with negative impacts.

Many cancer survivors experience impacts to their overall quality of life for up to many years following the diagnosis and treatment phase. Long-term effects such as fatigue and depression often surface early during treatment and may not resolve into survivorship. And late-term effects such as a second primary cancer and treatment-induced cardiomyopathy emerge posttreatment and require ongoing surveillance by the health care providers. The social and financial impacts of the cancer experience often linger well into survivorship; the survivorship phase may encompass efforts to repair family relationships, resolve social isolation, and rebuild personal savings and retirement accounts. Also, many survivors are able to "find the silver lining" and incorporate positive behavioral and existential changes in their lives that will hopefully lead to better health outcomes.

### Physical Effects

- Treatment for cancer is often toxic. Significant symptoms resulting from chemotherapy, radiation, and surgical treatments often impact the survivors' quality of life and well-being.
- Long-term effects are initiated during the cancer diagnosis and treatment phase and extend into survivorship.

- Late-term effects emerge following completion of the primary cancer treatment.

The long- and late-term side effects of cancer treatment are largely associated with the type of treatment received and organ involvement (Table 12.1). Long-term effects are those that are initiated during the treatment phase and do not resolve into survivorship. Certain chemotherapy drugs are likely to cause significant symptoms such as fatigue, premature menopause, sexual dysfunction, and "chemo-brain" (ie, cognitive impairment). Radiation therapy may also contribute to fatigue and cause skin sensitivity and lymphedema. Furthermore, surgery may cause sexual dysfunction, incontinence, and pain.

Importantly, late effects following the completion of primary cancer treatment can arise and may go undetected owing to a decrease in surveillance during the survivorship phase. Chemotherapy can later contribute to significant, and sometimes life-threatening, issues such as infertility, osteoporosis, liver and lung disease, and second primary cancers. Radiation-induced late effects also include second primary cancers, infertility, and lung disease in addition to cardiovascular disease and hypothyroidism. Surgery can later interfere with body image and functional disability while also impacting fertility.

These physical long- and late-term effects may impact and contribute to a wide array of psychosocial issues. For example, a young woman who undergoes premature menopause and is unable to achieve a pregnancy may experience significant sense of loss and grief. Cognitive impairment

**Table 12.1** Long-Term and Late Effects of Cancer Treatment

| Treatment | Long-term side effects | Late side effects |
| --- | --- | --- |
| Chemotherapy | Fatigue<br>Premature menopause<br>Sexual dysfunction<br>Neuropathy<br>"Chemo brain"<br>Kidney failure | Vision/cataracts<br>Infertility<br>Liver problems<br>Lung disease<br>Osteoporosis<br>Reduced lung capacity<br>Secondary primary cancers |
| Radiation therapy | Fatigue<br>Skin sensitivity<br>Lymphedema | Cataracts<br>Cavities and tooth decay<br>Cardiovascular disease<br>Hypothyroidism<br>Infertility<br>Lung disease<br>Intestinal problems<br>Second primary cancers |
| Surgery | Sexual dysfunction<br>Incontinence<br>Pain | Body image disturbance<br>Functional disability<br>Infertility |

*Source:* From Refs. (4,5). George Washington University. Cancer survivorship care. https://smhs.gwu.edu/gwci/sites/gwci/files/NCSRC%20Slides%20FINAL.pdf?src=GWCIwebsite

(ie, chemo-brain) may translate to reduced performance on the job or at school, and ultimately impact emotional and financial well-being.

## Emotional Effects

- Many survivors struggle in their transition from treatment to a new way of life. Fear of recurrence or the cancer coming back is very common, and may take many years to resolve. For some, the fear can be debilitating and impact many areas of life and can be triggered by follow-up visits and tests, anniversary events (eg, date of diagnosis), personal reminders such as smells and locations, and symptoms similar to those experienced at diagnosis.
- Depression, anxiety, and posttraumatic stress disorder (PTSD) symptoms may persist into survivorship. Related feelings of anger, sadness, worry, guilt, numbness, and hopelessness are significant in about one in four cancer survivors. Therapists who are experts in cancer should be consulted.
- Many survivors report positive outcomes (ie, posttraumatic growth) such as the emergence of new opportunities and reprioritization of goals, a greater appreciation for each day, closer relationships with others, a deeper sense of spirituality, and recognition of one's own strength.

Fear of recurrence or the cancer returning is one of the most prevalent emotional side effects experienced by cancer survivors. Survivors often report that the cessation of treatment is a difficult time as they are no longer actively attacking the cancer—and have difficulty transitioning from a "fight" mentality. This is compounded by the reduction in provider visits and reduced surveillance, thereby leading to increased feelings of anxiety and isolation. It is estimated that about one in four survivors has significant symptoms related to depression, anxiety, and PTSD. While emotional effects can be debilitating, many survivors report positive outcomes (ie, posttraumatic growth) such as the emergence of new opportunities and reprioritization of goals, a greater appreciation for each day, closer relationships with others, a deeper sense of spirituality, and recognition of one's own strength. It is not uncommon to hear a survivor express gratitude for each new day.

## Social and Financial Effects

- Family members are often unprepared for the reality that recovery from cancer treatment takes time. Feelings of disappointment, worry, and frustration are experienced by the entire family.
- Survivors may experience greater social isolation due to changes in their physical functioning and vocational situation; this can impact their emotional well-being.
- Cancer and its management can have direct and indirect effects on physical and psychological factors that negatively impact sexual functioning and body image.
- The financial toxicity of cancer is becoming increasingly common and largely attributed to high out-of-pocket costs and lost work productivity.

Family members often express feelings of disappointment, worry, and frustration shortly after the end of treatment. It is common for those around the survivor to underestimate the recovery time and expect that as treatment is over, the survivor should immediately return to where they were before the diagnosis. However, this is often not the case—and the weary caregiver may be experiencing many of the same emotional effects such as depression, anxiety, and posttraumatic stress. In addition, the caregiver is also experiencing greater social isolation and vocational impacts due to accompanying the loved one to appointments and caring for them at home. Therefore, it is not unusual for the caregiver to report significant impacts to quality of life that transition to the survivorship phase. The physical and psychological issues resulting from the cancer experience can negatively impact sexual functioning and body image, creating an additional strain on the survivor's relationships, particularly those with his or her partner or spouse. Furthermore, the increasing cost of cancer treatment and associated high out-of-pocket costs (eg, copayments, medications) and lost work productivity may have drained savings and retirement accounts, thereby often delaying retirement or forcing the return to work by the previously retired survivor or caregiver.

## FOLLOW-UP CARE

- Given the increased risk to survivors' physical and emotional health, regular coordinated surveillance and follow-up care is strongly recommended (GWU).
- Clinical practice guidelines that include screening tools are readily available online from several oncology organizations.
- Survivorship care plans (SCPs) are used to enhance posttreatment care by facilitating communication between the oncology and primary care providers and encouraging healthy survivor behaviors such as nutrition and physical activity.
- Many evidence-based treatments exist to address the physical (eg, rehabilitation) and mental (eg, cognitive behavioral therapy) health needs of cancer survivors.

Given the increased risk to survivors' physical and emotional health, regular coordinated surveillance and follow-up care is strongly recommended. Clinical practice guidelines have been developed by several oncology organizations, such as the American Cancer Society, National Comprehensive Cancer Network, and the American Society of Clinical Oncology (ASCO) (Figure 12.5). These guidelines also include screening tools to assist with late- and long-term side effect surveillance.

In addition, SCPs have been recommended by several prestigious organizations to facilitate communication between oncology and primary care providers and encourage healthy behaviors. ASCO is one of these organizations and has defined minimum data elements (eg, treatment details, follow-up plan) that must be included in an SCP. To facilitate the delivery of SCPs into practice, the Commission on Cancer requires that member organizations achieve 75% coverage by 2018 to maintain their accreditation. In addition, several organizations have published templates and made them available online.

## Cancer Survivorship Clinical Practice Guidelines

| National Comprehensive Cancer Network (NCCN) | American Society of Clinical Oncology (ASCO) | American Cancer Society (ACS) Survivorship Care Guidelines for Primary Care Providers |
|---|---|---|
| • **By Topic:**<br>• Anthracycline-induced cardiac toxicity<br>• Anxiety and depression<br>• Cognitive function<br>• Exercise<br>• Fatigue<br>• Healthy lifestyles<br>• Immunizations and infections<br>• Menopause-related symptoms<br>• Pain<br>• Sexual function (female/male)<br>• Sleep disorders | • **By Topic:**<br>• Anxiety and depression<br>• Cardiac dysfunction<br>• Chronic pain<br>• Fatigue<br>• Fertility preservation<br>• Neuropathy<br>• Palliative care<br>• **By Cancer Site:**<br>• Breast (ASCO/ACS) | • **By Topic:**<br>• Holistic<br>• Care coordination<br>• Health promotion<br>• Long-term and late effects<br>• Nutrition and physical activity<br>• Screening<br>• Surveillance<br>• **By Cancer Site:**<br>• Breast (ACS/ASCO)<br>• Colorectal<br>• Head and neck<br>• Prostate |

THE GEORGE WASHINGTON UNIVERSITY
WASHINGTON, DC

 Cancer Center

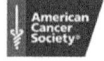

**Figure 12.5 National Cancer Survivorship Guidelines.** In recent years, the National Comprehensive Cancer Network (NCCN), the American Society of Clinical Oncology (ASCO), and the American Cancer Society have been hard at work developing clinical care guidelines to help guide practitioners who care for cancer survivors. NCCN and ASCO have developed many symptom-based guidelines and ACS developed four holistic guidelines for breast, colorectal, head and neck, and prostate cancer as part of the National Cancer Survivorship Resource Center. ASCO jointly released the breast care guideline with ACS.
*Source:* From Refs. (4–7). George Washington University. Cancer survivorship care. https://smhs.gwu.edu/gwci/sites/gwci/files/NCSRC%20Slides%20FINAL.pdf?src=GWCIwebsite.

Consideration for referral and inclusion in the follow-up plan section of the SCP are many evidence-based treatments that exist to address the physical (eg, rehabilitation) and mental health (eg, cognitive behavioral therapy, mindfulness practice) needs of cancer survivors. The survivorship care guidelines are a tremendous resource in identifying effective screening tools and treatments for the symptomatic cancer survivor.

## SPECIAL POPULATIONS

- Racial and ethnic minority survivors are more likely to experience barriers to follow-up care and surveillance, indicate poorer patient-provider communication, indicate not being prepared for side effects after treatment, report more unmet needs, not have access to culturally and linguistically appropriate resources, and report lower quality of life.

- Cancer survivors who live in rural areas report difficulty accessing health providers, face transportation issues, and are more likely to adopt poor health behaviors (eg, smoke, inactivity).
- Individuals who identify as lesbian, gay, bisexual, transgender, or queer (LGBTQ) experience health disparities, including cancer. However, little data exists about their needs posttreatment.
- Survivors of adolescent and young adult (AYA) cancer often have many unique and unmet needs, such as infertility, increased risk of a second primary cancer, chronic medical conditions, and higher financial burden.

Health disparities persist in posttreatment survivorship—and the unmet needs of those within the underserved and vulnerable populations are significant. Racial and ethnic minority survivors are more likely to experience poor outcomes due to poor access to follow-up care, and therefore less likely to receive screening and identification of late- and long-term side effects. In addition, these individuals have expressed more difficulty when engaging with health care providers and being surprised by posttreatment side effects. Furthermore, much of the survivorship resource documentation lacks cultural and linguistic (eg, Spanish) sensitivity. Those survivors living in rural areas experience more difficulty in securing health providers including therapists to address their psychosocial needs. In addition, barriers to care including transportation issues are common. Rural survivors are more likely to smoke, be physically less active, and have health-related unemployment.

However, less is known about the needs of individuals who identify as LGBTQ despite a higher prevalence of health disparities, including cancer. More research is needed to understand the unique challenges and needs facing these posttreatment survivors. AYAs also experience many unique and unmet needs including infertility and increased risks of a second primary cancer and heart damage. In addition, they are more likely to engage in risky behavior, have difficulty securing medical and life insurance policies, and face higher economic burden. Furthermore, a significant number of AYAs do not receive cancer-related follow-up care regularly.

## REFERENCES

1. The National Coalition for Cancer Survivorship. https://www.canceradvocacy.org/about-us/our-history
2. DeSantis CE, Lin CC, Mariotto AB, et al. Cancer treatment and survivorship statistics. *CA Cancer J Clin*. 2014;64(4):252–271.
3. Curigliano G, Cardinale D, Dent S, et al. *CA: A Cancer Journal for Clinicians*. 2016;66(4):265–351. Republished with permission of John Wiley and Sons Inc. Permission conveyed through Copyright Clearance Center, Inc.
4. American Cancer Society, 2016. http://www.cancer.org/treatment/survivorshipduringandaftertreatment/nationalcancersurvivorshipresourcecenter/toolsforhealthcareprofessionals/index
5. George Washington University. Cancer survivorship care. https://smhs.gwu.edu/gwci/sites/gwci/files/NCSRC%20Slides%20FINAL.pdf?src=GWCIwebsite
6. American Society of Clinical Oncology. Guidelines, tools, & resources. http://www.asco.org/practice-guidelines/quality-guidelines/guidelines
7. National Comprehensive Cancer Network. Home page. https://www.nccn.org

## RECOMMENDED READING

American College of Surgeons. Cancer program standards: ensuring patient-centered care: 2016 edition. https://www.facs.org/~/media/files/quality%20programs/cancer/coc/2016%20coc%20standards%20manual_interactive%20pdf.ashx. Published 2015.

Association of Oncology Social Work. Welcome to AOSW. http://www.aosw.org

Cancer*Care*. Our mission. http://www.cancercare.org/mission

Cancer Support Community. Mission & vision and history. http://www.cancersupportcommunity.org/mission-vision-and-history

George Washington University. Supporting cancer survivors through comprehensive cancer control programs. https://smhs.gwu.edu/gwci/survivorship/ncsrc

Institute of Medicine. *Cancer Care for the Whole Patient: Meeting Psychosocial Health Needs*. Washington, DC: National Academies Press; 2008.

Livestrong Foundation. Our mission. https://www.livestrong.org/who-we-are/our-mission

National Cancer Institute. Adolescents and young adults with cancer. http://www.cancer.gov/types/aya. Published 2015.

National Cancer Institute. Research-tested intervention programs (RTIPs). http://rtips.cancer.gov/rtips/index.do

National Coalition for Cancer Survivorship. Our mission. https://www.canceradvocacy.org/about-us/our-mission

National LGBT Cancer Network. About us. Retrieved from http://www.cancer-network.org/about

Oncology Nursing Society. Survivorship care standards for accreditation. https://www.ons.org/practice-resources/standards-reports/survivorship

Stupid Cancer. I'm too young for this! http://www.stupidcancer.org

# 13

# Maximizing the Health and Wellness of Cancer Survivors Through Healthy Lifestyle Behaviors

*Denise Spector*

## OVERVIEW

- Patients must manage cancer treatment effects on the body long after therapy ends. Behavioral approaches can maximize quality of life and reduce comorbidity.
- Physical activity can improve both physical and emotional health.
- Approximately 32% of cancer survivors are obese.
- A healthy diet plays an important role not only for weight management, but also for immune and hematologic support, bone health, as well as risk reduction for comorbid illnesses and potentially secondary malignancies.
- Alcohol may be associated with increased mortality in head and neck, prostate, and breast cancer survivors.
- Smoking is associated with higher rates of mortality, secondary cancers, and recurrence among cancer survivors.
- Use the 5 As (Ask, Advise, Assess, Assist, Arrange) to counsel for behavior change.

## WHY HEALTHY LIFESTYLE BEHAVIORS MATTER

There are over 15.5 million cancer survivors currently living in the United States and the overall 5-year survival rate approaches 70% (1). However, many individuals face a multitude of physical as well as psychosocial, adverse effects following a cancer diagnosis and treatment, such as fatigue, weight gain, and cardiac dysfunction to name a few (2,3). Additionally, some cancer survivors may be at higher risk for recurrence, secondary cancers, and other comorbidities (2). As a result of the unique needs of cancer survivors, significant emphasis has been placed on the optimization of the health and well-being of this population through healthy lifestyle behavior change. Over the past 10 years, the American Cancer Society (ACS) has published guidelines on nutrition and physical activity for cancer survivors, most recently in 2012 (4). There are three broad categories of recommendations, which focus on weight management, physical activity, and diet. The general recommendations also include statements about tobacco cessation and alcohol intake. Subsequent to the release of the ACS healthy lifestyle recommendations, the National Comprehensive Cancer Network (NCCN) has included the recommendations as a component of their clinical practice guidelines for survivorship, and the American Society of Clinical Oncology (ASCO) has developed a toolkit on obesity and cancer for clinicians (5,6). Also, the Institute of Medicine (IOM) report, *Implementing Survivorship Care Planning*, discusses the inclusion of healthy lifestyle recommendations as a standard part of survivorship care plans, with the aim to maximize both the short- and long-term health outcomes of cancer survivors following cancer treatments (7).

Unfortunately, many cancer survivors are either overweight or obese and are not engaging in health-promoting behaviors. Greenlee et al found that among a large sample of cancer survivors, rates of obesity, as defined by a body mass index (BMI) of greater than 30 kg/m$^2$, were higher than among the general population, approximately 32% versus 30%, and about one-third of cancer survivors were overweight (8). Additionally, these cancer survivors were less likely than noncancer controls to be meeting the current exercise guidelines, 36% compared to 38%, respectively. Approximately 27% of cancer survivors reported heavy drinking (ie, at least one day with five or more drinks during the past year) which is only slightly lower than that reported by noncancer patients (28%) (8). Over the past several years, data on prevalence estimates for smoking among cancer survivors have ranged from 9% to 18%, with a recent report revealing a 17% smoking rate, which is comparable to the general population (8,9). While many behavioral researchers and clinicians talk about the diagnosis of cancer as a "teachable moment," there is a significant amount of work that must be done to help decrease rates of unhealthy behaviors among cancer survivors.

To achieve optimal wellness, survivors should be counseled on the importance of diet, physical activity, and the avoidance of harmful behaviors. Many cancer survivors seek this type of information and feel empowered when they are provided with the tools to help enhance their overall health and well-being. Ultimately it is the patient who must engage in healthy lifestyle behaviors, but often the conversation must be initiated by health care providers. With the many resources now available to guide oncology clinicians in counseling their patients about healthy lifestyle promotion, it is hoped that many more survivors will thrive well into the future.

## Physical Activity

There is an ever-growing body of evidence revealing the many benefits of regular physical activity for cancer survivors on both physical and emotional health. The basic physical activity guidelines for cancer survivors, endorsed by both the ACS and the American College of Sports Medicine (ACSM) (4,10), include the following:

- Avoid inactivity and return to normal daily activities as soon as possible following diagnosis.
- Engage in moderate aerobic activity at least 150 minutes per week or 75 minutes of vigorous activity per week.
- Include strength training of all major muscle groups at least twice a week.

While not all cancer survivors will be capable of adhering to all of these recommendations owing to mobility limitations or other special circumstances, such as anemia or bone metastasis, they should still be advised to safely exercise to their ability with the guidance of a qualified exercise specialist, preferably an ACSM-certified oncology exercise trainer.

Data through observational studies has shown that physical inactivity is a risk factor for both breast and colorectal cancers, while physical activity has been associated with a decreased risk for cancer recurrence and cancer-related mortality in some cancer populations, most notably among breast, prostate, and colorectal cancer survivors (11–14). Overall, studies have revealed many positive effects on physical functioning, cardiorespiratory fitness, fatigue, sleep, depression, self-esteem, and overall health-related quality of life (HRQoL) (15).

## *Breast Cancer*

Lack of regular physical activity is a known risk factor for postmenopausal breast cancer (11), but there also appears to be a relationship between breast cancer survival and physical activity. In a review by Schmid and Leitzman, there was a 28% reduction in mortality (95% CI, 0.60–0.85) among breast cancer survivors who were the most active, as well as a 48% decrease in all-cause mortality (13). Preliminary evidence from reviews on breast cancer and physical activity suggest that improved outcomes may be related to biological mechanisms such as enhanced immunity, decreased inflammation, and beneficial effects in circulating insulin levels and insulin-mediated pathways (12).

## *Prostate Cancer*

A growing body of evidence indicates that regular exercise is positively associated with improved outcomes among men with prostate cancer. A recent meta-analysis that included 1,574 men with stage I to IV disease found strong evidence for improvements in cancer-specific quality of life, fatigue, lower-body strength, and aerobic fitness (16). Most of the studies were conducted in men on androgen deprivation therapy, who are known to be at increased risk for loss of muscle strength, bone loss, fatigue, metabolic syndrome, and cardiovascular disease (16). One retrospective study among 470 men treated with radiation therapy (RT) found that men who reported higher levels of physical activity experienced significantly less erectile dysfunction (ED), urinary incontinence, and rectal bleeding than their inactive counterparts (17).

## *Colon Cancer*

Inactivity increases the risk of colon cancer, and it also raises the risk for mortality in colorectal cancer survivors (13). Schmid et al found a statistically significant 39% (95% CI, 0.40–0.92) reduction in the rate of colorectal cancer mortality, and a 42% (95% CI, 0.48–0.70) lower rate of all other causes in the most active survivors of colorectal cancer (13). Colorectal cancer survivors meeting the recommended aerobic physical activity guidelines of at least 150 minutes per week of moderate physical activity, or 75 minutes of vigorous activity, have reported better scores on measures of HRQoL, fatigue, and, in some cases, colorectal cancer symptoms, than those not meeting the guidelines (18). While the body of evidence is small at this time, there is a trend for positive outcomes among colorectal cancer survivors who engage in regular physical activity.

*Other Cancers*

While the number of exercise studies addressing outcomes among survivors of other cancers have been relatively small, there is increasing interest in exploring associations. Among ovarian cancer survivors and endometrial cancer survivors, physical activity has been found to be related to higher HRQoL scores compared to sedentary behavior (19,20). In a recent review of 15 studies of non–small cell lung cancer patients, both presurgical and postsurgical exercise training significantly improved exercise capacity ($P = .02$ and $P = <.00001$, respectively) and physical health, as measured by HRQoL scales (21). A study of a resistance-training exercise program for head and neck cancer patients found significant reductions in postsurgical pain ($P = .01$) and disability ($P < .001$), as well as improvements in fatigue and HRQoL, although these were nonsignificant (22). Improvements in fatigue, physical functioning, and on emotional outcomes have also been found in a recent review among patients with hematologic malignancies, including those who have had a stem cell transplant (23). The number of exercise studies among other cancer populations is steadily growing, and it is expected that many of the outcomes, especially on fatigue, physical functioning, and self-reported HRQoL, will be similar.

## Overweight/Obesity: The Importance of Weight Management

Due to the fact that being overweight and obesity are closely tied with poorer outcomes among cancer patients, there are initiatives through large cancer organizations, such as the ACS, NCCN, and ASCO, to help both oncology providers and cancer survivors toward the goal of obtaining a healthy weight (ie, BMI 18.5–24.9 kg/m$^2$). As previously mentioned, ASCO has developed an obesity and cancer toolkit that includes a guide for oncology providers (6). This guide offers a practical approach for discussing weight with patients with a focus on three main elements:

- Assess—evaluate BMI and discuss as part of the review of systems during survivorship follow-up visits.
- Advise—encourage healthy eating and regular exercise.
- Refer—know what resources are available for weight loss in your community, such as dieticians, health coaches, psychologists, exercise trainers, as well as online resources.

A team effort is typically required to help overweight/obese patients achieve a healthy weight following a cancer diagnosis, and it is through ongoing assessment and encouragement during follow-up visits that sustained healthy lifestyle changes often occur.

Obesity is a known risk factor for the development of several cancers, such as postmenopausal breast cancer, colon, gastric, pancreatic, endometrial, and kidney cancer; there is also strong evidence linking obesity with cancer of the gallbladder and ovaries (24). Additionally, obesity is associated with higher rates of recurrence and lower rates of survival for some common cancers such as breast, colon, and prostate cancers (25–27). Results from a review by Arem and Irwin suggest that obesity among women with endometrial cancer leads to higher rates of recurrence and decreased survival (28). Obesity has been implicated in approximately 15% to 20% of all cancer mortality (6). Of great concern is that rates of obesity among cancer survivors have been trending upward at a higher rate than among noncancer patients over the same period of time (8).

Obesity (ie, BMI $\geq 30$ kg/m$^2$) is one of the most common chronic comorbid conditions among cancer survivors and is related to additional comorbidities such as cardiovascular disease, cerebral vascular disease, diabetes mellitus, metabolic syndrome, as well as some musculoskeletal diseases (29). It also increases an individual's risk for secondary malignancies (30) and can have a negative impact on the delivery of therapeutic strategies. Lin and colleagues (31) found an increased setup error rate among obese endometrial cancer patients receiving daily imagery-guided RT, and Cho et al (32) reported increased challenges for delivering ultrasound-guided RT for obese patients with abdominal cancers. Obesity is also linked with higher rates of thromboembolism in patients receiving chemotherapy, impaired healing following oncologic surgery, and an increased incidence of lymphedema in cancer survivors (6).

Weight gain can be a significant issue for some cancer patients as a result of chemotherapy or surgery that induces premature menopause, especially in women with breast or gynecologic cancers. Also, steroids and some other hormonal therapies are related to a high incidence of weight gain, which is often seen among breast cancer patients on antiestrogen therapy and in men with prostate cancer who are on androgen-deprivation therapy (ADT). Some of these therapies, especially ADT, can lead to body composition changes with increased adipose tissue and decreased lean muscle mass, known as sarcopenic obesity (33). Weight gain while on continued treatment can be particularly challenging to manage and can cause great distress for many cancer patients.

There have been a number of lifestyle behavioral studies addressing weight loss among cancer patients, most of which have been conducted in the breast cancer population. Considering that both diet and exercise are important for weight loss, most studies included multicomponent interventions. Through a combination of dietary modifications that include caloric reduction and regular exercise, it has been shown that lifestyle changes can lead to weight loss of 5% to 7% of body weight (34). Even this small degree of weight loss has been found to decrease the incidence of diabetes in the general population, which would likely be the case for cancer survivors as well. This is of great significance as diabetes mellitus is associated with an increased risk for several cancers, including breast, colorectal cancer, liver cancer, pancreatic cancer, and endometrial cancer (35). While obesity is closely tied with many of these cancers, it appears that the relationship between diabetes and cancer is also directly linked by biological pathways involving insulin and insulin-like growth factors (35). Therefore, combined dietary and exercise interventions are not only important for weight loss and weight maintenance—they are also significant for reducing rates of comorbid conditions in cancer patients.

## Diet/Nutrition

Probably one of the most frequently asked questions from cancer survivors relates to how they can improve their diets. A healthy diet plays an important role not only for weight management, but also for immune and hematologic support, bone health, as well as risk reduction for comorbid illnesses and potentially secondary malignancies. The ACS updated the nutrition and physical activities guidelines in 2012 specifically for cancer survivors (4). The recommendations emphasize that individuals should aim for a diet that is high in fruits, vegetables, and whole grains and specifically states the following:

- Limit consumption of processed meat and red meat;
- eat at least 2.5 cups of vegetables and fruits each day;
- choose whole grains instead of refined grain products;
- and if you drink alcoholic beverages, limit consumption to no more than one drink per day for women or two drinks per day for men.

There are a number of observational and intervention studies that provide evidence for making these recommendations to cancer survivors, although it is unknown at this time if there are any specific dietary changes that will affect long-term survival.

Epidemiologic cohort studies that have evaluated diet and primary cancer prevention reveal a risk reduction for individuals who adhere to dietary guidelines. In fact, in a meta-analysis, Balter et al found a 22% lower cancer-specific mortality rate among adults adhering to dietary guidelines (36). This is of utmost importance to cancer survivors as many are at elevated risk for developing secondary cancers. With regard to data on disease-free survival among cancer survivors, there are several studies that support the consumption of a healthy diet (ie, prudent diet) consistent with the guidelines compared to a typical "Western" diet that is high in meats, processed foods, sweets, and dietary fats. Most of the studies have been conducted among breast cancer survivors and have found reduced risks, from 15% to 43%, for overall mortality among those adhering to a "prudent" diet in comparison to increased rates of mortality for those consuming a "Western" diet. George et al conducted a study among early stage breast cancer survivors that included diet quality and found that women who consumed higher quality diets compared to those with low-quality diets had an 88% (95% CI 0.02–0.99) reduction in breast cancer–specific mortality (37). A prospective study among colon cancer survivors did not find a protective association with a "prudent" diet on either overall survival or disease-specific survival, although higher rates of mortality from other cancers and overall mortality were found among those following a "Western" diet.

Few large randomized clinical trials have assessed dietary factors in relation to risk for recurrence and cancer mortality; however, results from two such studies among breast cancer survivors have been widely recognized in the oncology literature. The first was the Women's Intervention Nutrition Study (WINS) that enrolled 2,437 women with early stage breast cancer. All women were provided with dietary education and counseling and half were randomized to receive a nutritionally adequate diet and the other half received a low-fat diet (ie, no more than 15% of energy from dietary fat).

Among those who received the low-fat diet, breast cancer recurrence was reduced by 24% (HR, 0.76; 95% CI, 0.60–0.98) compared to the control group (38). The Women's Healthy Eating and Living (WHEL) study was also conducted among a large group of early stage breast cancer survivors (39). One intervention arm promoted five servings of fruits and vegetables per day, whereas the other arm promoted 10 servings per day along with a low-fat diet (ie, 15%–20% of energy from fat). While many women improved their diets over the course of the study, there was a high percentage who were already consuming more than five servings of fruits and vegetables per day at baseline. After a mean follow-up of 7.3 years, there was no difference in weight loss or on cancer recurrence between the groups. Smaller intervention studies focused on adding specific dietary components (eg, flaxseed, curcumin) have been conducted among other groups of cancer survivors (ie, prostate and colorectal cancer); however, results have been inconsistent. Further dietary intervention trials are needed.

## Alcohol Intake

As previously stated, the ACS and NCCN recommend that women have no more than one alcoholic drink per day and men no more than two. This general recommendation is supported by evidence indicating cardioprotective effects from alcohol, but it appears that higher alcohol intake does not incur greater benefits and, in fact, can cause more harm (4). While it is well known that alcohol is associated with the risk for several primary cancers, there is also evidence that reveals poorer outcomes among head and neck cancer patients, and possibly among some prostate and breast cancer survivors who consume alcohol (4,40). Additionally, alcohol intake can increase the risk for the development of new primary cancers (41). The discussion about alcohol needs to be tailored to the individual's risk factors and other comorbid conditions (eg, cardiac disease, liver dysfunction). It is important when counseling patients about alcohol intake that they be informed about serving sizes, which are as follows: 150 mL (5 fl oz) of wine, 360 mL (12 fl oz) of beer, and 45 mL (1.5 fl oz) of 80-proof spirits. Providers should also remember that alcohol contributes to weight gain, and overweight/obesity raises risk for many cancers as discussed earlier.

## Tobacco Use

Substantial evidence exists for the association between cigarette smoking and the incidence of many cancers, including liver, colorectal, and breast cancers, in addition to the more commonly associated smoking-related cancers. Evidence also reveals higher rates of mortality, secondary cancers, and recurrence among cancer survivors who smoke or are former smokers. Of 62 studies in cancer patients, 77% found a positive association between higher mortality and smoking, 42% of which were significant (41). There also appears to be a synergistic effect between smoking status and prior RT treatments leading to higher rates of secondary cancers (42). Considering that the prevalence rate of smoking among cancer survivors is approximately 16% compared to 18% in the general population (43), there is a considerable amount of work that needs to be done to help support patients to quit smoking, as well as avoid the use of other tobacco products. Many

| Table 13.1 The 5As for Counseling on Behavior Change | |
|---|---|
| Ask | For example, "On average, how many minutes per week do you do aerobic exercise?" |
| Advise | If not, advise on the exercise recommendations. |
| Assess | For example, "Regular exercise is important, are you willing to begin some form of exercise?" |
| Assist | Have them set a start date and discuss incremental change—start with 10 minutes of walking a day. |
| Arrange | Refer them to a local free LIVESTRONG at the YMCA program for cancer survivors. |

resources are available for clinicians and patients to aid in smoking cessation. Evidence supports the use of combined pharmacologic therapy and behavioral therapy for the highest rates of long-term success at smoking cessation (43).

### Strategies to Improve Healthy Lifestyle Behaviors

Oncologists play a vital role in helping patients lead healthier lives both during and following treatments. Providers often underestimate the impact that healthy lifestyle behaviors can have on enhancing both quality of life and longevity of cancer survivors. Counseling survivors about behavior change can seem like a daunting task, but there are some strategies that have been shown to be effective, such as the 5As approach as outlined in Table 13.1 (15). Realistic goal setting and periodic monitoring during clinic visits will also be important to help patients sustain health behavior change (15). Many health behavior resources are now available for clinicians, and all oncology providers have a responsibility to patients to help them achieve optimal long-term health and well-being.

## REFERENCES

1. Miller KD, Siegel RL, Lin CC, et al. Cancer treatment and survivorship statistics, 2016. *CA Cancer J Clin*. 2016;66(4):271–289.
2. American Cancer Society. *Cancer Treatment and Survivorship Facts & Figures 2012–2013*. Atlanta, GA: American Cancer Society; 2012.
3. Curigliano G, Cardinale D, Dent S, et al. Cardiotoxicity of anticancer treatments: Epidemiology, detection, and management. *CA Cancer J Clin*. 2016;66(4): 309–325.
4. Rock CL, Doyle C, Demark-Wahnefried W, et al. Nutrition and physical activity guidelines for cancer survivors. *CA Cancer J Clin*. 2012;62(4):243–274.
5. National Comprehensive Cancer Network. NCCN clinical practice guidelines in oncology: survivorship—preventive health; https://www.nccn.org/professionals/physician_gls/f_guidelines_nojava.asp#supportive. Published 2016.
6. American Society of Clinical Oncology. *Obesity and Cancer: A Guide for Oncology Providers*. Alexandria, VA: American Society of Clinical Oncology; 2014.

7. Institute of Medicine. *Implementing Cancer Survivorship Care Planning*. Washington, DC: National Academies Press; 2007.

8. Greenlee H, Shi Z, Sardo-Molmenti CL, et al. Trends in obesity prevalence in adults with a history of cancer: Results from the US National Health Interview Survey, 1997 to 2014. *Journal of Clinical Oncology*; 2016; 34:3133–3140.doi:10.1200/JCO.2016.66.4391

9. Shoemaker ML, White MC, Hawkins NA, et al. Prevalence of smoking and obesity among U.S. cancer survivors: estimates from the National Health Interview Survey, 2008–2012. *Oncology Nursing Forum*. 2016;43(4):436–441.

10. Schmitz KH, Courneya KS, Matthews C, et al. American College of Sports Medicine roundtable on exercise guidelines for cancer survivors. *Med Sci Sports Exerc*. 2010;42(7):1409–1426.

11. Kushi LH, Doyle C, McCullough M, et al. American Cancer Society Guidelines on nutrition and physical activity for cancer prevention: reducing the risk of cancer with healthy food choices and physical activity. *CA Cancer J Clin*. 2012;62(1):30–67.

12. Ballard-Barbash R, Friedenreich C, Courneya K, et al. Physical activity, biomarkers, and disease outcomes in cancer survivors: a systematic review. *J Natl Cancer Inst*. 2012;104(11):815–840.

13. Schmid D, Leitzmann MF. Association between physical activity and mortality among breast cancer and colorectal cancer survivors: a systematic review and meta-analysis. *Ann Oncol*. 2014;25(7):1293–1311.

14. Friedenreich CM, Wang Q, Neilson HK, et al. Physical activity and survival after prostate cancer. *Eur Urol*. 2016;70:576–585. doi:10.1016/j.eururo.2015.12.032

15. Demark-Wahnefried W, Rogers LQ, Alfano CH, et al. Practical clinical interventions for diet, physical activity, and weight control in cancer survivors. *CA Cancer J Clin*. 2015;65(3):167–189.

16. Bourke L, Smith D, Steed L, et al. Exercise for men with prostate cancer: a systematic review and meta-analysis. *Eur Urol*. 2016;69(4):693–703.

17. Thomas RJ, Holm M, Williams M, et al. Lifestyle factors correlate with the risk of late pelvic symptoms after prostatic radiotherapy. *Clin Oncol*. 2013;25(4):246–251.

18. Vallance JK, Boyle T, Courneya KS, et al. Associations of objectively assessed physical activity and sedentary time with health-related quality of life among colon cancer survivors. *Cancer*. 2014;120(18):2919–2926.

19. Courneya KS, Karvinen KH, Campbell KL, et al. Associations among exercise, body weight, and quality of life in a population-based sample of endometrial cancer survivors. *Gynecol Oncol*. 2005;97(2):422–430.

20. Smits A, Smits E, Lopes A, et al. Body mass index, physical activity and quality of life of ovarian cancer survivors: time to get moving? *Gynecol Oncol*. 2015;139(1):148–154.

21. Ni H, Pudasaini B, Yuan X, et al. Exercise training for patients pre- and post-surgically treated for non–small cell lung cancer: a systematic review and meta-analysis. *Integr Cancer Ther*. 2016. doi:10.1177/1534735416645180

22. McNeely ML, Parliament MB, Seikaly H, et al. Effect of exercise on upper extremity pain and dysfunction in head and neck cancer survivors: a randomized controlled trial. *Cancer*. 2008;113(1):214–222.

23. Bergenthal N, Will A, Streckmann F, et al. Aerobic physical exercise for adult patients with haematological malignancies. *Cochrane Database Sys Rev.* 2014;(11):CD009075. doi:10.1002/14651858.CD009075.pub2

24. Dobbins M, Decorby K, Choi BC. The association between obesity and cancer risk: a meta-analysis of observational studies from 1985 to 2011. *ISRN Prev Med.* 2013;2013:1–6. doi:10.5402/2013/680536

25. Chan DS, Vieira AR, Aune D, et al. Body mass index and survival in women with breast cancer: systematic literature review and meta-analysis of 82 follow-up studies. *Ann Oncol.* 2014;25(10):1901–1914.

26. Cao Y, Ma J. Body mass index, prostate cancer-specific mortality, and biochemical recurrence: a systematic review and meta-analysis. *Cancer Prev Res.* 2011;4(4):486–501.

27. Wu S, Liu J, Wang X, et al. Association of obesity and overweight with overall survival in colorectal cancer patients: a meta-analysis of 29 studies. *Cancer Causes Control.* 2014;25(11):1489–1502.

28. Arem H, Irwin ML. Obesity and endometrial cancer survival: a systematic review. *Int J Obes.* 2013;37(5):634–639.

29. Sarfati D, Koczwara B, Jackson C. et al. The impact of comorbidity of cancer and its treatment. *CA Cancer J Clin.* 2016;66(4):337–350.

30. Travis LB, Demark-Wahnefried W, Allan JM, et al. Aetiology, genetics and prevention of secondary neoplasms in adult cancer survivors. *Nat Rev Clin Oncol.* 2013;10(5):289–301.

31. Lin LL, Hertan L, Rengan R, et al. Effect of body mass index on magnitude of setup errors in patients treated with adjuvant radiotherapy for endometrial cancer with daily image guidance. *Int J Radiat Oncol Biol Phys.* 2012;83(2):670–675.

32. Choi M, Fuller CD, Wang SJ, et al. Effect of body mass index on shifts in ultrasound-based image-guided intensity-modulated radiation therapy for abdominal malignancies. *Radiother Oncol.* 2009;91(1):114–119.

33. Smith MR, Finkelstein JS, McGovern FJ, et al. Changes in body composition during androgen deprivation therapy for prostate cancer. *J Clin Endocrinol Metab.* 2002;87(2):599–603.

34. Thomson CA, Stopeck AT, Bea JW, et al. Changes in body weight and metabolic indexes in overweight breast cancer survivors enrolled in a randomized trial of low-fat vs. reduced carbohydrate diets. *Nutr Cancer.* 2010;62(8):1142–1152.

35. Giovannucci E, Harlan DM, Archer MC, et al. Diabetes and cancer: a consensus report. *Diabetes Care.* 2010;33:1674–1685.

36. Balter K, Moller E, Fondell E. The effect of dietary guidelines on cancer risk and mortality. *Curr Opin Oncol.,* 2012; 24(1):90–102.

37. George SM, Irwin ML, Smith AW, et al. Postdiagnosis diet quality, the combination of diet quality and recreational physical activity, and prognosis after early-stage breast cancer. *Cancer Causes Control.* 2011;22(4):589–598.

38. Chlebowski R, Blackburn G, Thomson C, et al. Dietary fat reduction and breast cancer outcome: Interim efficacy results from the Women's Intervention Nutrition Study. *J Natl Cancer Inst.* 2006;98(24):1767–1776.

39. Pierce J, Natarajan L, Caan B, et al. Influence of a diet very high in vegetables, fruit, and fiber and low in fat on prognosis following treatment for breast cancer: the Women's Healthy Eating and Living (WHEL) randomized trial. *JAMA.* 2007;298(3):289–298.

40. Brunner C, Davies NM, Martin RM, et al. Alcohol consumption and prostate cancer incidence and progression: a mendelian randomization study. *Int J Cancer.* 2017;140(1):75–85.
41. Nielsen SF, Nordestgaard BG, Bojesen SE. Associations between first and second primary cancers: a population-based study. *CMAJ.* 2012;184(1):E57–E69.
42. U.S. Department of Health and Human Services. *The Health Consequences of Smoking: 50 Years of Progress. A Report of the Surgeon General.* Atlanta, GA: U.S. Department of Health and Human Services, Centers for Disease Control and Prevention, National Center for Chronic Disease Prevention and Health Promotion, Office on Smoking and Health; 2014.
43. National Comprehensive Cancer Network. NCCN clinical practice guidelines in oncology: smoking cessation. https://www.nccn.org/professionals/physician_gls/pdf/smoking.pdf. Published 2015.

# Index

abdominal cramping, 106
acetyl cholinesterase inhibitor.
  *See* donepezil
ACSM. *See* American College of Sports
  Medicine
acupuncture
  for pain, 36
  for xerostomia, 25
acute toxicity
  breast
    breast pain, 81
    skin, 79–83
  esophagus
    acute esophagitis, 69–70, 73
    esophagitis, 101–105
    hiccups, 73
  female sexual dysfunction, 142
  head and neck cancer, 19–22
    alopecia, 34–35
    depression, 33–34
    dermatitis, 19, 23–24
    dysgeusia, 26
    fatigue, 31–33
    mucositis, 26–29
    nausea, 30–31
    oral infection, 29–30
    pain, 35–37
    xerostomia, 24–25
  liver/bile duct system
    liver enzyme increase, 107
    radiation-induced liver disease, 107
  lungs, radiation pneumonitis, 62, 65, 68–69
  pancreas, pancreatitis, 107–108
  skin, 168–169
  small bowel
    diarrhea, 108
    duodenitis, 108–109
  stomach
    abdominal cramping, 106
    anorexia, nausea, vomiting, 105–106
    gastritis, 106

alcohol intake, healthy lifestyle
  behavior, 311
alopecia, 34–35
  temporary, 187
alternative therapies, 144
American Cancer Society, 301–302
American College of Sports Medicine
  (ACSM), 306
American Society of Clinical Oncology
  (ASCO), 301–302, 306
amifostine, 218–219, 224–225
anejaculation, 150–151
angiotensin converting enzyme (ACE)
  inhibitors, 219
angiotensin II receptor blockers (ARBs),
  219
anorexia, 105–106
  definition of, 204
  patient assessment, 204
  time course, 204
  treatments for, 205, 206
antidepressant medications, 34
antinausea agents, 31
anxiety
  definition of, 199–200
  patient assessment, 200
  time course, 200
  treatments for, 200–201
APC. *See* argon plasma coagulation
ARBs. *See* angiotensin II receptor
  blockers
argon plasma coagulation (APC), 128–129
ASCO. *See* American Society of Clinical
  Oncology
avascular necrosis, 173–174
axillary deodorant use, 243

BBB. *See* blood-brain barrier
benzodiazepines, 21, 31–33, 89, 93, 105,
  198, 201
bevacizumab, 214–215
biliary stenosis, 113

biliary stricture, 113
bladder, pelvic organ toxicity
  acute cystitis, 133
  chronic cystitis, 133, 137–140
  incidence and prevention, 131–133
blood-brain barrier (BBB), 212
BMD. *See* bone mineral density
bone
  in children
    avascular necrosis, 173–174
    bone growth abnormalities, 179
    bone marrow, 174, 179
    bone mineral density, 179–180
  pelvic organ toxicity, 153–154
bone fracture, 170–171
bone growth abnormalities, 179
bone marrow
  in children, 174, 179
  pelvic organ toxicity, 153–154
bone mineral density (BMD), 179–180
bowel perforation, 112–113
brachial plexopathy, 89–90
brachial plexus, 46
brachytherapy, 119
brain. *See also* central nervous system
  site-specific effects, 8, 10
    brainstem, 9
    cochlea, 11–12
    hippocampus, 12–13
    hypothalamic-pituitary axis, 12
    optic structures, 9, 11
  whole-organ and non–site-specific effects
    cerebrovascular syndrome, 2–3
    radiation-induced cognitive decline, 3–4
    radiation-induced edema, 7–8
    radiation-induced white matter changes, 3–4
    radionecrosis, 7–8
    secondary malignancy, 7
    somnolence syndrome, 4
    stroke, 4, 7
brainstem, 9
  in children, 180
breast cancer, 286–287, 307
  acute toxicity
    breast pain, 81
    skin, 79–83
  late radiation toxicity
    brachial plexopathy, 89–90
    fibrosis/chest wall pain, 84–86
    heart, 90–91
    in lung, 91
    lymphedema, 86–88

    telangiectasias, 84
  overview of, 79
breast pain, 81
bronchial strictures, 74

CALGB. *See* Cancer and Leukemia Group B
Cancer and Leukemia Group B (CALGB), 87
Cancer of the Prostate Strategic Urologic Research Endeavor (CaPSURE), 148
cancer. *See* radiation-induced cancers
cancer survivors, 277, 295
cancer survivorship
  epidemiology of, 295
  follow-up care, 301–302
  health status and needs
    emotional effects, 300
    physical effects, 298–299
    social and financial effects, 300–301
  healthy lifestyle behaviors
    alcohol intake, 311
    diet/nutrition, 310–311
    overweight/obesity, 308–309
    physical activity, 306–308
    strategies to improve, 312
    tobacco use, 311–312
    weight management, 308–309
  special populations, 302–303
  transitions of, 295–298
cannabinoids, 205
CaPSURE. *See* Cancer of the Prostate Strategic Urologic Research Endeavor
cardiotoxicity, 90
cataracts, radiation-induced, 10
CCSS. *See* Childhood Cancer Survival Study
CDC. *See* Centers for Disease Control and Prevention
CDT. *See* complete decongestive therapy
Centers for Disease Control and Prevention (CDC), 251
central nervous system. *See also* brain
  cognitive impairment
    donepezil, 213
    memantine, 212–213
    methylphenidate, 213–214
    radiation necrosis, 214
      bevacizumab, 214–215
cerebrovascular syndrome, 2–3
cervical necrosis, alternative therapies, 144

cGMP. *See* cyclic guanosine monophosphate
chest wall pain, 84–86
Childhood Cancer Survival Study (CCSS), 290
children, radiation toxicity
  bone
    avascular necrosis, 173–174
    bone growth abnormalities, 179
    bone marrow, 174, 179
    bone mineral density, 179–180
  brainstem, 180
  central nervous system injury, 180
  cochlea, 180–181
  craniospinal axis, 181–182
  gastrointestinal tract, 182
  gonads (testes and ovaries), 182
  heart, 183
  hippocampus and temporal lobes, 183–184
  hypothalamic-pituitary axis, 184–185
  kidneys, 185
  lungs, 185–186
  posterior fossa syndrome, 186
  second malignancy, 186
  skin and hair follicles, 187
  thyroid, 187
  total body irradiation, 187–188
  vasculature, 188
  vision, 189
chronic toxicity, female sexual dysfunction, 142–144
cisplatin, 27, 43
cochlea, 11–12
  in children, 180–181
cognitive decline, radiation-induced, 3–4
cognitive impairment
  donepezil, 213
  memantine, 212–213
  methylphenidate, 212–213
colon cancer, 307–308
complete decongestive therapy (CDT), 37, 87, 88, 92, 152
conductive hearing loss, 44
corticosteroids
  anorexia, 205
  fatigue, 203
craniospinal axis, 181–182
curcumin, 244
cyclic guanosine monophosphate (cGMP), 238
cystitis
  acute, 133
  chronic, 133, 137–140

dental quality of life, 40
depression, 33–34
dermatitis, 19, 23–24
diarrhea, 108
diet/nutrition, healthy lifestyle behavior, 310–311
donepezil, 213
dose-volume constraints, 119
doxepin, 25, 28
dronabinol, 31, 198, 205
duodenitis, 108–109
dysgeusia, 26
dysphagia, 38–40
dysphonia, 45

edema, 169–170
  radiation-induced, 7–8
emotional effects, cancer survivorship, 300
erectile dysfunction, 146–150
  phosphodiesterase 5 inhibitors, 239
  preclinical data interventions, 239
  statins, 239–240
esophageal dysmotility, 74
esophageal fibrosis/stricture, 74–75
esophagitis, 101–105
  acute, 69–70, 73
esophagus
  acute toxicity
    acute esophagitis, 69–70, 73
    esophagitis, 101–105
    hiccups, 73
  late toxicity
    esophageal fibrosis/stricture, 74–75
    fistula, 109, 112
    stricture, 109
evidence-based interventions, acute skin toxicity, 155
exercise, 200
exocrine insufficiency, late toxicity, 113, 114
external lymphedema, 36–38
extremity, late toxicity
  bone fracture, 170–171
  edema, 169–170
  joint stiffness, 170

fatigue, 31–33
  definition of, 201
  nonpharmacologic treatments, 202
  patient assessment, 201–202
  pharmacologic treatments, 202–204
  time course, 202
FDA. *See* U.S. Food & Drug Administration

fecal incontinence, 129
female reproductive organs, pelvic toxicity
  early menopause, 144–146
  female sexual dysfunction, 140–144
  fertility, 144–146
female sexual dysfunction (FSD)
  acute toxicity, 142
  chronic toxicity, 142–144
  incidence and prevention, 141–142
  overview of, 140–141
fertility, pelvic toxicity
  female reproductive organs, 144–146
  male reproductive organs, 150–151
fibrosis, 36–38, 84–86
  radiation-induced
    pentoxifylline, 245–246
    vitamin E, 245–246
filgrastim, 251
financial effects, cancer survivorship, 300–301
fistula, 109, 112
5As for behavior change, 312
fluconazole, 29–30
FSD. *See* female sexual dysfunction

gastric outlet obstruction, 112
gastric ulceration, 112
gastritis, 106
gastrointestinal malignancies, 288
gastrointestinal mucositis, acute
  amifostine, 236
  immunosuppressive agents, 236
  miscellaneous interventions, 236
  probiotics, 230, 236
gastrointestinal tract, in children, 182
Gelclair®, 28
genitourinary malignancies, 288–289
GM-CSF. *See* granulocyte macrophage colony stimulating factor
gonads (testes and ovaries), 182
granulocyte macrophage colony stimulating factor (GM-CSF), 28, 225, 251, 256
gustatory stimulants, 25
gynecologic malignancies, 287–288

hair follicles, in children, 187
HBOT. *See* hyperbaric oxygen therapy
head and neck cancer
  acute toxicity, 35–37
    alopecia, 34–35
    depression, 33–34
    dermatitis, 19, 23–24
    dysgeusia, 26
    fatigue, 31–33
    mucositis, 26–29
    nausea, 30–31
    pain, 35–36
    xerostomia, 24–25
  anemia, 226
  oral mucositis
    amifostine, 224–225
    palifermin, 224
    pharmacologic and nonpharmacologic interventions, 225–226
    supportive measures, 225
  osteoradionecrosis and late tissue injury, 227–228
    hyperbaric oxygen, 228
    pentoxifylline, 228–229
    vitamin E, 228–229
  xerostomia
    miscellaneous interventions, 227
    pilocarpine, 226
    pilocarpine alternatives, 226–227
healthy lifestyle behaviors
  alcohol intake, 311
  diet/nutrition, 310–311
  importance of, 305–306
  overweight/obesity, 308–309
  physical activity, 306–308
  strategies to improve, 312
  tobacco use, 311–312
  weight management, 308–309
hearing loss, 43–44
heart
  in children, 183
  late toxicity, 90–91
hematologic malignancies, 281–286
herpes simplex virus (HSV), 30, 69
hiccups, 73
hippocampus, 12–13
hippocampus and temporal lobes, 183–184
HSV. *See* herpes simplex virus
hyperbaric oxygen, 42, 46, 228, 238
Hyperbaric Oxygen Radiation Tissue Injury Study (HORTIS) III, 138
hyperbaric oxygen therapy (HBOT), 130
hypothalamic-pituitary axis, 12
  in children, 184–185

ICRP. *See* International Commission on Radiological Protection
ICSI. *See* intracytoplasmic sperm injection
IG. *See* image guidance
image guidance (IG), 118–119
immunosuppressive agents, 236

IMRT. *See* intensity-modulated radiation therapy
intensity-modulated radiation therapy (IMRT), 118–119
International Commission on Radiological Protection (ICRP), 10
intracytoplasmic sperm injection (ICSI), 151
intravesical endoscopic procedures, 139

joint stiffness, 170

kidneys, in children, 185

laparoscopic ovarian transposition, 145
late toxicity
  esophagus
    esophageal fibrosis/stricture, 74–75
    fistula, 109, 112
    stricture, 109
  extremity
    bone fracture, 170–171
    edema, 169–170
    joint stiffness, 170
  head and neck cancer
    dental QOL, 40
    dysphagia, 38–40
    external lymphedema, 36–38
    fibrosis, 36–38
    hearing loss, 43–44
    osteoradionecrosis, 40–43
    peripheral neuropathy, 46–47
    psychosocial/economic effects, 47
    voice dysfunction, 45–46
  liver/bile duct system, biliary stricture, 113
  lung
    bronchial strictures, 74
    lung fibrosis, 73–74
  pancreas, chronic pancreatitis and exocrine insufficiency, 113, 114
  skin, 169
  small-bowel complications, 114
  stomach
    gastric outlet obstruction, 112
    ulceration, bleeding, and perforation, 112–113
left-sided breast cancers, 90
Lhermitte's syndrome, 45–46
Littman somnolence syndrome scale, 4
liver/bile duct system
  acute toxicity
    liver enzyme increase, 107
    radiation-induced liver disease, 107
  late toxicity, biliary stricture, 113
liver disease, radiation-induced, 107
liver enzyme increase, 107
lung
  bronchial strictures, 74
  in children, 185–186
  lung fibrosis, 73–74
lung fibrosis, 73–74
lymphatic system, pelvic organ toxicity, 152
lymphedema, 86–88, 152

male reproductive organs, pelvic toxicity
  anejaculation, 150–151
  erectile dysfunction, 146–150
  fertility, 150–151
manual lymphatic drainage, 88
megestrol (Megace), 205
memantine, 212–213
menopause, early/induced, 144–146
methylphenidate, 213–214
methylphenidate (Ritalin), 203
moisturizing lotions, 244–245
mucositis, 26–29

National Cancer Institute (NCI), 277
National Coalition of Cancer Survivorship, 295
National Comprehensive Cancer Network (NCCN), 301–302, 306
National Suicide Prevention Lifeline, 34
nausea, 30–31, 105–106
NCCN. *See* National Comprehensive Cancer Network
NCI. *See* National Cancer Institute
*N*-methyl-D-aspartate (NMDA) receptor antagonist, 211–213
NMSCs. *See* nonmelanomatous skin cancers
nonmelanomatous skin cancers (NMSCs), 167
nonnarcotic agents, 36
nutritional counseling, 205

olanzapine, 31
optic chiasm, 9–10
optic nerves, 9–10
optic neuropathy, radiation-induced, 9
optic structures, 9, 11
oral infection, 29–30
oral mucositis, radioprotection
  amifostine, 224–225
  palifermin, 224

oral mucositis, radioprotection (cont.)
    pharmacologic and nonpharmacologic interventions, 225–226
    supportive measures, 225
Oratect gel, 28
ORN. See osteoradionecrosis
osteoradionecrosis (ORN), 40–43
overweight/obesity, 308–309

pain
    assessment, 197
    definition of, 197
    head and neck cancer, 35–36
pain flare
    potential treatments for, 197–199
    time course of, 197
palifermin, 28, 224
pancreas/pancreatitis
    acute toxicity, 107–108
    chronic, 113, 114
    late toxicity, 113, 114
parasympathomimetic agents, 25
patient assessment
    anorexia, 204
    anxiety, 200
    fatigue, 201–202
patient-reported outcomes vs. physician-reported toxicity, 118
pediatric malignancies, 289–290
pegfilgrastim, 251
pelvic insufficiency fractures (PIF), 153
pelvic organ toxicity
    bladder
        acute cystitis, 133
        chronic cystitis, 133, 137–140
        incidence and prevention, 131–133
    bone, 152–153
    bone marrow, 153–154
    female reproductive organs
        early menopause, 144–146
        female sexual dysfunction, 140–144
        fertility, 144–146
    lymphatic system, 152
    male reproductive organs
        anejaculation, 150–151
        erectile dysfunction, 146–150
        fertility, 150–151
    radioprotection
        hyperbaric oxygen, 238
        miscellaneous interventions, 238
        pentoxifylline, 237
        statins, 237
        vitamin E, 237
    rectum
        acute proctitis, 119–120, 127
        chronic proctitis, 120, 128
        incidence and prevention, 120, 125–127
    skin, 154–156
PENTOCLO regimen, 43
pentoxifylline, 42, 228–229, 237, 245–246
pentsanpolysulfate (PPS), 129
peripheral neuropathy, 46–47
permanent alopecia, 187
PFS. See posterior fossa syndrome
phosphodiesterase 5 (PDE5) inhibitors, 239
physical activity, healthy lifestyle behavior, 306–308
physical effects, cancer survivorship, 298–299
PIF. See pelvic insufficiency fractures
pilocarpine, 226
pilocarpine alternatives, 226–227
posterior fossa syndrome (PFS), 186
PPS. See pentsanpolysulfate
PRET. See progressive resistance exercise training
probiotics, 230, 236
proctitis
    acute, 119–120, 129
    chronic, 120, 128
progressive resistance exercise training (PRET), 36
prostate cancer, 307
Prostate Cancer Outcomes and Satisfaction With Treatment Quality Assessment (PROSTQA) model, 148
proton therapy, 119
pseudoprogression, 8
psychosocial/economic effects, 47

radiation biology
    age and its role, 278–279
    delivery of radiation, 279–280
    radiation field size, 280–281
radiation dermatitis
    axillary deodorant use, 243
    curcumin, 244
    moisturizing lotions, 244–245
    skin washing, 243
    steroidal creams, 243–244
radiation-induced cancers
    breast cancer, 286–287
    gastrointestinal malignancies, 288
    genitourinary malignancies, 288–289

gynecologic malignancies, 287–288
hematologic malignancies, 281–286
pediatric malignancies, 289–290
radiation biology
  age and its role, 278–279
  delivery of radiation, 279–280
  radiation field size, 280–281
radiation myelopathy, 13
radiation necrosis, 7–8, 214
radiation pneumonitis, 62, 65, 68–69
Radiation Therapy Oncology Group (RTOG), 8, 24, 73, 212
radionecrosis, 7–8, 214
radioprotection
  acute gastrointestinal mucositis
    amifostine, 236
    immunosuppressive agents, 236
    miscellaneous interventions, 236
    probiotics, 230, 236
  central nervous system
    cognitive impairment, 212–214
    radiation necrosis, 214–215
  head and neck cancer
    anemia, 226
    oral mucositis, 224–226
    osteoradionecrosis and late tissue injury, 227–229
    xerostomia, 226–227
  pelvic organ
    hyperbaric oxygen, 238
    miscellaneous interventions, 238
    pentoxifylline, 237
    statins, 237
    vitamin E, 237
  peripheral neuropathy, 250
  radiation dermatitis
    axillary deodorant use, 243
    curcumin, 244
    moisturizing lotions, 244–245
    skin washing, 243
    steroidal creams, 243–244
  radiation-induced fibrosis
    pentoxifylline, 245–246
    vitamin E, 245–246
  thorax
    amifostine, 218–219
    angiotensin converting enzyme inhibitors, 219
    angiotensin II receptor blockers, 219
    other human studies, 219–220
    preclinical studies, 218
  total body irradiation
    endocrine effects, 253
    gastrointestinal radiation syndrome countermeasures, 252
    hematopoietic growth factors, 251
    mitigating agents, 253
    preventing agents, 252–253
    repurposed treatments, 252
rectal symptom treatment, radiation-induced, 121–124
rectum, pelvic organ toxicity
  acute proctitis, 119–120, 127
  chronic proctitis, 120, 128
  incidence and prevention, 120, 125–127
retinopathy, radiation-induced, 11
RT-induced thoracic toxicity, 71–72
RTOG. *See* Radiation Therapy Oncology Group

sargramostim, 251
SBRT. *See* stereotactic body radiation therapy
SCPs. *See* survivorship care plans
secondary malignancy, 7
  in children, 186
  of pelvis, 156
secondary malignant neoplasm (SMN), 277
sensorineural hearing loss (SNHL), 43–44
site-specific effects
  brain, 8–13
  spine, 13–14
skin
  acute toxicities in breast, 79–83
  acute toxicity, 168–169
  in children, 187
  late toxicity, 169
  pelvic organ toxicity, 154–156
SLP. *See* speech language pathologist
small bowel
  acute toxicity
    diarrhea, 108
    duodenitis, 108–109
  late toxicity, ulceration, obstruction, and fistula, 114
SMN. *See* secondary malignant neoplasm
SNHL. *See* sensorineural hearing loss
social effects, cancer survivorship, 300–301
somnolence syndrome, 4
speech language pathologist (SLP), 39
spine, 13–14
statins, 237, 239–240
stereotactic body radiation therapy (SBRT), 101
steroidal creams, 243–244

stomach
  acute toxicity
    abdominal cramping, 106
    anorexia, nausea, vomiting, 105–106
    gastritis, 106
  late toxicity
    gastric outlet obstruction, 112
    ulceration, bleeding, and perforation, 112–113
  stricture, 109
    biliary, 113
    esophageal, 74–75
stroke, 4, 7
stroke-like migraine attacks after radiation therapy (SMART) syndrome, 188
sucralfate, 28, 105, 126
Surveillance, Epidemiology, and End Results (SEER) database, 277
survivorship care plans (SCPs), 301
systemic effects
  anorexia, 204–206
  anxiety, 199–201
  fatigue, 201–204
  pain, 197–199

TBI. *See* total body irradiation
telangiectasias, 84
testicular cancer, 288–289
thorax
  acute toxicity
    acute esophagitis, 69–70, 73
    hiccups, 73
    lungs, radiation pneumonitis, 62, 65, 68–69
  for conventional fractionation, 62
  late toxicity
    bronchial strictures, 74
    esophageal fibrosis/stricture, 74–75
    lung fibrosis, 73–74
  pharmaceutical experimental agents, 66–67
  radioprotection
    amifostine, 218–219
    angiotensin converting enzyme inhibitors, 219
    angiotensin II receptor blockers, 219
    other human studies, 219–220
    preclinical studies, 218
  tumor types and RT fractionation, 60–61
thyroid, in children, 187
time course
  anorexia, 204
  anxiety, 200
  fatigue, 202
  pain flare, 197
tobacco use, healthy lifestyle behavior, 311–312
topical analgesic solutions, 28
topical short-acting pain control, 28
total body irradiation (TBI)
  in children, 187–188
  endocrine effects, 253
  gastrointestinal radiation syndrome countermeasures, 252
  hematopoietic growth factors, 251
  mitigating agents, 253
  preventing agents, 252–253
  repurposed treatments, 252

ulceration
  in small bowel, 114
  in stomach, 112–113
U.S. Food and Drug Administration (FDA), 34, 205

vaginal stenosis, 144–145
vasculature, in children, 188
viscous lidocaine, 20, 28
vision, in children, 189
vitamin E, 228–229, 237, 245–246
voice dysfunction, 45–46
vomiting, 105–106

WECARE. *See* Women's Environmental, Cancer, and Radiation Epidemiology
weight management, 308–309
WHEL. *See* Women's Healthy Eating and Living
WINS. *See* Women's Intervention Nutrition Study
Women's Environmental, Cancer, and Radiation Epidemiology (WECARE), 286
Women's Healthy Eating and Living (WHEL), 311
Women's Intervention Nutrition Study (WINS), 310
WR-274, inorganic thiophosphate, 218

xerostomia, 24–25, 226–227
  radioprotection
    miscellaneous interventions, 227
    pilocarpine, 226
    pilocarpine alternatives, 226–227